Conducting and Reading Research in Health and Human Performance

Third Edition

Ted A. Baumgartner
University of Georgia

Clinton H. Strong
Indiana University (Retired)

Larry D. Hensley
University of Northern Iowa

Boston   Burr Ridge, IL   Dubuque, IA   Madison, WI   New York   San Francisco   St. Louis
Bangkok   Bogotá   Caracas   Kuala Lumpur   Lisbon   London   Madrid   Mexico City
Milan   Montreal   New Delhi   Santiago   Seoul   Singapore   Sydney   Taipei   Toronto

McGraw-Hill Higher Education

*A Division of The **McGraw-Hill** Companies*

CONDUCTING AND READING RESEARCH IN HEALTH AND HUMAN PERFORMANCE
THIRD EDITION

Published by McGraw-Hill, a business unit of The McGraw-Hill Companies, Inc., 1221 Avenue of the Americas, New York, NY 10020. Copyright © 2002, 1998 by The McGraw-Hill Companies, Inc. All rights reserved. No part of this publication may be reproduced or distributed in any form or by any means, or stored in a database or retrieval system, without the prior written consent of The McGraw-Hill Companies, Inc., including, but not limited to, in any network or other electronic storage or transmission, or broadcast for distance learning.

Some ancillaries, including electronic and print components, may not be available to customers outside the United States.

This book is printed on acid-free paper.

3 4 5 6 7 8 9 0 QPF/QPF 0 9 8 7 6 5 4 3 2

ISBN 0–07–235388–0

Vice president and editor-in-chief: *Thalia Dorwick*
Executive editor: *Vicki Malinee*
Developmental editor: *Carlotta Seely*
Senior marketing manager: *Pamela S. Cooper*
Project manager: *Christine Walker*
Senior production supervisor: *Sandy Ludovissy*
Coordinator of freelance design: *David W. Hash*
Interior designer: *Kathleen Theis*
Cover image: © *David Bishop/PHOTOTAKE*
Supplement producer: *Sandra M. Schnee*
Media technology producer: *Judi David*
Compositor: *Electronic Publishing Services, TN*
Typeface: *10/12 Times Roman*
Printer: *Quebecor World Fairfield, PA*

Library of Congress Cataloging-in Publication Data

Baumgartner, Ted A.
    Conducting and reading research in health and human performance / Ted A.
Baumgartner, Clinton H. Strong, Larry D. Hensley. — 3rd ed.
    p.   cm.
    Includes bibliographical references and index.
    ISBN 0–07–235388–0
    1. Medicine—Research—Methodology. 2. Health—Research—Methodology.
I. Strong, Clinton H. II. Hensley, Larry D. (Larry Duncan), 1948–   . III. Title.

R850 .B365   2002
610'.7'2—dc21
    2001030403
    CIP

The Internet addresses listed in the text were accurate at the time of publication. The inclusion of a website does not indicate an endorsement by the authors or McGraw-Hill, and McGraw-Hill does not guarantee the accuracy of the information presented at these sites.

www.mhhe.com

Contents

PART ONE   THE RESEARCH PROCESS   2

PART TWO   TYPES OF RESEARCH   164

7   Experimental Research   166

PART THREE   DATA ANALYSIS   260

Preface

This book was developed based on the methods its authors have used to teach the master's-level introduction to research course for many years. It is assumed that students come to this course with varied backgrounds in areas related to health and human performance, such as dance, exercise science, health, kinesiology, physical education, recreation, and sports management. The two major objectives of our courses are to teach the student how to conduct their own research and how to read with understanding the research that others have done. The book is comprehensive yet practical and understandable. Many examples of the application of various research methods and techniques are presented in an attempt to increase the students' grasp of the research process.

Many students begin the introduction to research course with little research background, little interest in research, and considerable fear about their ability to succeed in the course. These students typically do not write a master's thesis. However, it is still important that they develop an appreciation for research and an understanding of how different types of research are conducted so they will become good consumers and readers of the research of others. The book is certainly written with this type of student in mind.

Other students begin the introduction to research course knowing they will write a master's thesis or complete a master's project. These students need to be aware of the many possible research approaches and the procedures that are basic to many types of research. This book will also serve the needs of this type of student.

Doctoral students and beginning researchers who want an overview of the research process should find this book helpful. However, the procedures and techniques specific to a certain type of research in a specialized area are generally not covered in this book.

In chapter 2 we suggest that a research project begins with the identification of a research topic and progresses through a series of steps until the research is conducted and a report describing the research project is written. The book's chapters are organized in this manner. The first six chapters are essential to cover. Portions of chapters 7 through 11 may be covered quickly if only certain types of research are of interest to the student. Likewise, some of the content in chapters 12 through 15 could be omitted depending on the particular interests and needs of the students.

The three chapters on experimental research, descriptive research, and qualitative research cover the common research approaches in Health and Human Performance. The two statistics chapters are inclusive but are presented with an orientation toward practical use and without emphasis on calculational ability. The computer programs accompanying the statistics chapters are presented with considerable explanation and use of examples. Even the emphasis on doing and understanding research is somewhat unique in this book.

New to This Edition

New Chapters

This edition has been expanded to include four new chapters. Chapter 4, Ethical Concerns in Research, focuses on ethics as a basic component of research. It highlights issues such as informed consent, privacy and confidentiality, research involving animals, and disclosure of research findings. Chapter 6, Reading and Evaluating Research Reports, explains the standard sections of a research report, with many examples provided. This chapter features a discussion of critiquing and evaluating published research material that is helpful to all levels of students. Chapter 10, Meta-analysis, presents an overview of this research process, discussing the steps in meta-analysis, featuring selected meta-analysis studies, and discussing criticisms of this approach to research. Chapter 11, Additional Research Approaches, summarizes the historical, epidemiological, single-participant, and creative activities approaches to research.

New or Expanded Topics

Chapter 1
- Research process and stages involved in the scientific method
- New material regarding various types of research questions
- New section on variables
- Expanded section on various types of research

Chapter 2
- Selecting the research problem
- Developing the research proposal
- Reviewing the literature
- Internet searching

Chapter 3
- Steps in the research process
- Discussion of hypotheses
- Data collection procedures

Chapter 4
- New chapter on ethics in research
- Historical events leading to the development of ethical standards
- Preparation of informed consent forms
- Role of Institutional Review Boards
- Ethics associated with disclosure of research findings

Chapter 5
- Random processes, including selection and assignment of research participants
- Steps in the sampling process

- Various sampling techniques
- Sample size determination, including Internet resources

Chapter 6
- New chapter on reading and critically evaluating research reports
- Typical sections of a published research report
- Examples of various sections of a research report
- Critiquing a research article

Chapter 7
- Updated material
- Additional practical hints

Chapter 8
- Updated material
- Improved format of examples

Chapter 9
- Qualitative research software
- Discussion of focus groups

Chapter 10
- New chapter on meta-analysis and basic procedures in meta-analysis
- Steps in meta-analysis
- Examples of meta-analysis

Chapter 11
- New chapter on alternative research approaches
- Overview of epidemiological research
- Overview of single-participant research

Chapter 12
- Use of SPSS version 10.0 computer program
- Directions for using SPPS
- Example printouts from SPPS

Chapter 13
- Use of SPSS version 10.0 computer program
- Directions for using SPPS
- Example printouts from SPPS
- Statistical design and sensitivity section
- Effect size section

Chapter 14
- New chapter on measurement issues in research
- Objectivity, reliability, and validity discussion
- Physical performance testing
- Use of SPSS version 10.0 computer program

Chapter 15

- Typical format of a published research report
- Preparation of a thesis or dissertation
- Updated examples of elements from theses and dissertations
- Recommended guidelines for preparing the research report

Appendixes

- Computer program for chapters 12 and 13 updated to SPSS version 10.0
- Update appendix material

Focus on the Internet

The Internet has revolutionized research study in many ways, offering access to the latest research information as it becomes available. This edition highlights the role of this powerful research tool by explaining the basics, such as search engines, and guiding the reader to specific research information sources on the Web. For both beginners and advanced students, this new focus makes research and research study easier, faster, and more wide-ranging.

PowerWeb

This book is packaged with *PowerWeb,* a new easy-to-use online resource from McGraw-Hill. This tool provides current articles, curriculum-based materials, weekly updates with assessments, informative and timely world news, related weblinks, research tools, student study tools, interactive tools, and much more!

Access to *PowerWeb* also gives you:

- study tips with self-quizzes
- links to related sites
- weekly updates
- current news
- a daily newsfeed of related topics
- web research guide

PowerWeb is a password-protected website. Ask your McGraw-Hill sales representative how you can create a student package with *PowerWeb*! Preview the site at www.dushkin.com/powerweb

Successful Features

This edition continues to include the following well-received and useful features:

- *Key Words*—The list of key words at the beginning of each chapter highlights the most important terms. When each key word is defined in the text, it appears in bold type for easy reference.

- *Objectives*—Each chapter begins with a list of objectives to focus the student's attention on the central issues addressed in the chapter.
- *Examples*—This book owes much of its strength to the integration of examples of research elements with the relevant text discussion.
- *Summaries*—The end-of-chapter summaries recap the content, reinforcing student learning and encouraging review.
- *Formative Evaluation of Objectives*—This list at the end of each chapter is an expanded discussion of the chapter objectives that guides the student in putting them into practice.

Acknowledgements

This book is the product of the influence of many people and occurrences. First, the professors who trained and educated the authors must be recognized. Second, the research experiences of the authors have been influential. Third, the experience of teaching the introduction to research course at both the undergraduate and graduate levels and the feedback from the students in the course is reflected in the book. Thanks must be expressed to people in the profession who reviewed this book and suggested improvements:

For the second edition:

Stan Bassin
California State University, Pomona

Mary L. Dawson
Western Michigan University, Kalamazoo

Mark Huntington
Manchester College

Mark Kelley
Southeastern Louisiana University

Beverly Mitchell
Kennesaw State College

For the third edition:

James M. DiNucci
Stephen F. Austin State University

Kurt A. Stahura
Arkansas State University

Donna J. Terbizan
North Dakota State University

Reuben L. Wright
Prairie View A&M University

In addition, thanks go to the editors at McGraw-Hill Higher Education, who improved the manuscript considerably.

Finally, the authors must thank their wives and families for allowing them to write the book. Adjustments and sacrifices were necessary by all in order for the book to be completed.

T.A.B.
C.H.S.
L.D.H.

Conducting and Reading Research in Health and Human Performance

Part One

The Research Process

Beginning graduate students in HHP frequently believe that research is foreign, abstract, and remote. They often feel totally incompetent, probably because they lack a basic understanding of the research process. A good course in research methods and statistics can lay the groundwork for attaining the high level of competency enjoyed by many of today's HHP professionals.

In Part I of this textbook, the foundation for the research process is described in six chapters. Chapter 1, "The Nature and Purpose of Research," details (1) the importance of research in the acquisition of knowledge by HHP professions, (2) how the scientific method of solving problems fits into the research process, (3) types of research, (4) the concept of variables, and (5) the significance of research in HHP. Chapter 2, "The Research Problem," discusses (1) how research problems are initiated, selected, and defined, (2) the importance of literature to the research process, and (3) the development of a research proposal. Chapter 3, "Selected Elements of the Research Process," covers (1) the concepts underlying various approaches to research, (2) the role of hypotheses in research, and (3) some of the more common approaches to research in HHP. Chapter 4, "Ethical Concerns in Research," describes (1) the history of research involving human subjects that led to the formation of ethical standards for the conduct of research, and (2) those standards and guidelines that are most applicable to research in HHP. Chapter 5, "Selection of Research Participants: Sampling Procedures," addresses (1) the importance of selecting participants appropriate for the research, (2) the concepts of population and sample, (3) various methods for selecting research participants, and (4) sample size. Chapter 6, "Reading and Evaluating Research Reports," discusses (1) the typical format for a research report, (2) evaluative criteria for the reading research reports, and (3) suggestions for becoming a wise consumer of the research literature.

1

The Nature and Purpose of Research

KEY WORDS

Applied research	Dependent variable	Imperfect induction	Research classifications
Basic research	Empiricism	Independent variable	Research question
Causal-comparative research	Experimental research	Induction	Scientific method
Correlational research	Extraneous variable	Perfect induction	Syllogism
Deductive reasoning	Historical research	Qualitative research	Theory
	Hypothesis	Quantitative research	Variable

OBJECTIVES

Members of the HHP professions have a wealth of information upon which they make decisions. Quite frequently, this information is passed down to us, as opposed to our discovering it through direct observation of our experiences. Many times we don't bother to examine the source of the information prior to using it. However, when members of a profession engage in various aspects of the research process, current information can be checked out—and new information acquired.

After reading chapter 1, you should be able to

1. Explain the relationship between research and a profession.
2. Know the various methods used in the past to obtain knowledge and how it is currently obtained.
3. Know the various types and classifications of research.
4. Distinguish between a hypothesis and a theory.
5. Explain the scientific method.
6. Recognize the different types of variables.

Each of us is a consumer of research on a daily basis. We cannot read the daily paper, watch television, explore the Internet, or even read signs along the highway without being exposed to the results of research. The choices we make and products we buy are frequently based upon the results of product research and the marketing of the results. For example, we choose one brand of toothpaste over another because it is more effective in preventing cavities, tastes better, or whitens our teeth better. The sunscreen we select is based on the fact that research has shown it to be effective in reducing the harmful effects of the sun's rays. Likewise, as professionals in HHP fields, our practices as a coach, a teacher, an exercise technician, or a health promotion specialist are greatly influenced by the results of research in our field. Research tells us, for example, that the use of straight-leg sit-ups poses problems for the lower back and therefore is not recommended as an exercise. A preponderance of research showing the beneficial effects of regular physical activity led to the publication of *Physical Activity and Health: A Report of the Surgeon General* (U. S. Department of Health and Human Services 1996). In effect, almost everything we do is influenced by research in one way or another. As professionals, many of you will also be producers of research, either as part of your formal educational experience or as an expectation of your employment. All of you will be consumers of research information in one way or another.

The Essence of a Profession: Knowledge

An essential quality that differentiates a profession from other vocations is the continuous pursuit and dissemination of new knowledge. The professions of HHP produce a variety of monthly, quarterly, and annual publications. The creation, reading, and interpretation of articles, books, theses, and dissertations are integral parts of the formal education and in-service education of the members of a profession. Moreover, the quality and quantity of such publications are an index of the vitality and soundness of a profession as a whole. The publications, and their use, also identify the professional stature of individual members. The information contained in the publications contributes greatly to the body of knowledge of a profession. A continuous flow of new facts and ideas must come from the laboratory and classroom, and this new information must be passed along. A profession's body of knowledge must grow and professional practices must adapt to new findings. If new knowledge suggests that an accepted practice is unsatisfactory, obsolete, or hazardous, then that practice must be modified or eliminated. The body of knowledge that characterizes a profession can be advanced, and must be for a profession to continue to contribute to the constituency it serves. The major vehicle by which a profession advances its knowledge base is the process of research.

Research is exciting and challenging, and it makes an essential contribution to the development of those who engage in it. Research accomplished by professionals in dance, exercise science, health, kinesiology, physical education, recreation, and sports management is exciting because the results frequently contribute to the pool of knowledge from which the fields of health and human performance can draw for purposes of application. It is challenging because the exploration of research ideas demands critical thinking and requires that judgment be exercised on both procedural and conceptual questions. Research contributes to the professional's development because the process builds a new set of skills that can be used to better comprehend the research literature and to recognize new questions that need to be researched.

Research: The Knowledge Pipeline

Research is a greatly misunderstood activity. For many people, the term conjures up the image of a person in a white laboratory coat, wearing black-framed glasses, and pouring the contents of one beaker into another. Others see a person sifting through volumes and volumes of numbers or statistics. And yet others may think of a person holding a clipboard and standing in a shopping mall, poised to interview an unsuspecting shopper. The perception is that this person, the researcher, is cold, shy, disinterested in people as individuals, interested in people only as subjects, and concerned primarily with test tubes, stopwatches, figures, and published articles. In effect, as soon as the word "research" is spoken, a barrier is raised as one's preconceived and misguided image of a researcher comes to mind.

Research is not like that. Nor is it a "mystical activity where the 'academic eggheads' go off to 'do their thing'" (Mobley 1980). In its simplest context, research is nothing more or less than finding answers to a question in a logical, orderly, and systematic fashion. Although there is not a single, universally accepted definition of research, the myriad of definitions that we see contain many similarities. Foremost, perhaps, is the fact that research is *systematic* in nature and focuses on a *question* of interest. Consider the following descriptions of research:

- The main goal of research is the gathering and interpreting of information to answer questions (Hyllegard, Mood, and Morrow 1996, 11).
- Research is a systematic attempt to provide answers to questions (Tuckman 1999, 4).
- Research may be defined as the systematic and objective analysis and recording of controlled observations that may lead to the development of generalizations, principles, or theories, resulting in prediction and possible control of events (Best and Kahn 1998, 18).
- Research is a systematic way of asking questions, a systematic method of inquiry (Drew, Hardman, and Hart 1996, 2).

As these examples illustrate, research is an organized, systematic attempt to find solutions to a problem or to answer a question; it searches for the truth in human feelings, values, behaviors, activities, processes, elements, and relationships. Virtually all definitions of research speak to its systematic nature and to the fact that it represents a process for acquiring information that may be used to posit answers to questions and to generally advance a body of knowledge. Professional practice in virtually every field, including HHP, involves many problems and questions that can be investigated through the research process. Answers to these research questions should be based on evidence that is as objective and free of bias as possible. Objectivity is a key element of research, which is why researchers employ the scientific method in their quest for knowledge and truth. In effect, research is the application of the scientific method to the study of a question. The scientific method offers researchers a structured means of finding the answers to research questions. Scientific solutions shape the body of knowledge for a profession, which, in turn, can be used to help synthesize, validate, or change the philosophy, theoretical relationships, and, ultimately, the practices of a profession.

The Search for Truth

Men and women have been searching for truth since the beginning of time. In doing so they have relied, in general, upon five sources of evidence: (1) custom and tradition, (2) authority, (3) personal experience, (4) deductive reasoning, and (5) scientific inquiry (Good 1972). The earliest search for truth was characterized by the first three sources, and each provided a modicum of truth. While there is something valuable, secure, serene, and peaceful about customs and traditions, many were found to be erroneous. The truth is, there is no Santa Claus or Easter Bunny. Reliance on an authority served people well in the past, but fell short as a complete source of truth. Many authorities have been wrong. There was a time when the word of a coach, a teacher, or even the president was considered unimpeachable, but we now are reluctant to accept the word of authorities merely because of the position they hold. There is also value in personal experience, but it, too, has limitations as a source of truth. First of all, one's experiences are limited. Moreover, one's response to a given situation is likely to be quite different from the response of another, depending upon previous experience, and personal values and beliefs. Brothers and sisters in a family grow up differently because they are affected differently and have different experiences in the same situation. Nevertheless, the use of personal experience is relatively high on the continuum of methods of acquiring knowledge. As humans have thought about problems over the ages, each of these sources of evidence has played an important role. The shortcomings of each source, however, dictated gross inadequacies in the search for truth. Thus arose the appeal to other sources for new knowledge, understanding, and insight.

Deductive reasoning (logic) was the first major contribution to the process of seeking truth systematically. In deductive reasoning, thinking proceeds from a general assumption to a specific application. Several pieces of rather general information, or facts, are woven together to produce a specific conclusion. Aristotle and other early philosophers ushered in the era of logic through statements referred to as a categorical **syllogism.** Here is such a statement:

All philosophers are mortal. Socrates is a philosopher. Therefore, Socrates is mortal (Sax 1979, 5).

Two ideas, or premises, form the basis for the conclusion. If the relationship between the two is true, then the conclusion is true. However, if either premise is false, the conclusion is also false. This represents the major weakness of deductive reasoning; that is, we have to accept the information contained in the premises as being true without really knowing that it is true.

All heavy cigarette smokers die from cancer. John smokes six packages of cigarettes a day. Therefore, John will die of cancer.

The ultimate truth or falsity of the conclusion concerning John's demise depends upon the truth of the first two statements. Do all heavy smokers die of cancer? Are six packs of cigarettes a day enough to cause John to develop cancer?

Sometimes rumors are true; other times, false. A teenager may observe that smoking marijuana is prevalent among his peers and conclude that such activity is okay for him. Peer pressure frequently leads to a deductive response. Phrases such as "It figures" or "That figures" also imply a conclusion based on deductive reasoning.

Deduction is valuable and is a part of almost every research project. Reasoning of this kind enables the researcher to organize the information already known to exist concerning the research problem of current interest, to theorize about the relationship of this information to the problem, and then deduce various hypotheses to be tested by the research. Despite the value of deductive reasoning in pointing up "new relationships as one goes from the general to specific, it is not sufficient as a source of new truth" (Ary, Jacobs, and Razaveih 1996).

The human thought process then turns to inductive reasoning in an attempt to get at the elusive truth. **Induction,** in which thinking proceeds from the specific to the general, is considered to be the basic principle of scientific inquiry. Conclusions about events are based on information generated through many individual and direct observations. In the inductive process, the researcher observes an individual or group of individuals from a larger population of similar individuals. Then, based upon these observations of the smaller group, inferences, conclusions, or generalizations are made back to the larger population. Hence, thinking moves forward from the specific to the general. Deduction moves backward from the general to the specific. Ary, Jacobs, and Razaveih (1996) have clearly illustrated the difference between deductive and inductive processes.

Deductive. Every mammal has lungs. All rabbits are mammals. Therefore, every rabbit has lungs.

Inductive. Every rabbit that has been observed has lungs. Therefore, every rabbit has lungs.

Induction, then, is based on seeking facts, which is a primary goal of science. There are two kinds of induction, **perfect** and **imperfect.** Perfect induction results in conclusions based on observations of selected characteristics of all members of a group or population. This is frequently not possible, especially when groups are large. Imperfect induction results in conclusions based on the observations of a small, specific number of members of a population. Most research is based on imperfect induction. The information obtained may not be absolutely perfect, or true, but is sufficient to make fairly reliable generalizations. It is generally conceded that Charles Darwin was responsible for integrating deduction and induction in his research on evolution in the nineteenth century. This integrated process became known as the scientific method.

The Scientific Method

The **scientific method** of solving problems and acquiring knowledge has been delineated in many different ways in the past. It is an approach, however, that is usually thought of as being accomplished in a series of logical stages that define a pathway for the acquisition of knowledge. Some authorities may specify four or five stages, others six, and some may even include seven stages in the scientific method. Although the number of stages may vary, authorities are in general agreement as to the overall process and the type and progression of activities undertaken. This is not to suggest, however, that the scientific method is governed by a strict adherence to a set of prescribed actions that must be followed faithfully during each stage in the process. Whereas the specific actions or steps undertaken within each stage may vary depending upon the participants, research approach taken, and techniques used, the general method for acquiring knowledge remains much the same and the logical progression from one stage to another reflects the systematic nature of the scientific method. A brief summary of the stages involved in the scientific method follows. In subsequent chapters, a more thorough discussion of each stage is presented.

1. **Identifying the Problem**

    The first, and arguably the most important, stage in the scientific method is the identification of the research problem. This is really an acknowledgment that a question needs to be answered and that at this time there is an insufficient knowledge base to answer the question. The research problem may arise from several sources. It may have a theoretical underpinning, it may derive from professional practice or personal experience, or it may simply be based on the curiosity of the researcher. While the choice of a suitable problem may be difficult, particularly for the beginning researcher, once identified and properly delineated, the research problem becomes the central focus of the research effort. Consequently, considerable thought and serious reflection should go into the identification of the research problem. One should also recognize that the research problem is inevitably broad in nature and must be narrowed or distilled into a potentially researchable question. This will lead to the specification of the problem statement that should provide direction for the research process.

2. **Formulating a Hypothesis**

   A **hypothesis** is a belief, hunch, or prediction of the eventual outcome of the research. It is a concrete, specific statement about the relationships between phenomena and is based upon deductive reasoning, following a thorough study of previous research related to the problem and considering the researcher's own past experience. Suppose a researcher wanted to study the effects of two different diets on selected health indices. Evidence from previous research suggests that a vegetarian diet provides a stronger and healthier person than does a nonvegetarian diet. If this theory holds true, what observable consequences could be expected? The deduced hypotheses, presented in a series of separate statements, would predict that the individuals on the vegetarian diet would show (a) lower cholesterol levels, (b) lower blood pressure, (c) greater energy, (d) a higher strength index, (e) less body fat, and so on, depending on the number of health indices observed. Not all studies have hypotheses, however. If a study is exploratory or simply descriptive in nature and not making comparisons between groups, no formal hypothesis is required. In such instances the researcher would carefully delineate the research questions that serve to provide focus for the study.

3. **Developing the Research Plan**

   In this stage, the strategy is developed for gathering and analyzing the information that is required to test the hypotheses or answer the research questions. Essentially, this becomes the "blueprint" or a "step-by-step plan" for conducting the research. The researcher will design a plan to test, measure, weigh, experiment, or observe the phenomena of interest in order to be able to answer the research questions. Typically, this plan consists of four parts: selection of a relevant research methodology, identification of the subjects or participants, description of the data-gathering procedures, and specification of the data analysis techniques. The choice of the research method is largely influenced by the questions being investigated. Certain types of questions require strategies that use quantitative methods, while others lend themselves to qualitative methods. Moreover, the research method selected then influences the specific details of the study, such as the participants, the instrumentation, and the actual procedures undertaken. In the diet study example, the researcher might select two groups of people and place one group on a vegetarian diet and the other on a nonvegetarian diet. The plan calls for each group to be tested on the selected health indices, then proceed with their respective diets for a preset period of time, and then be tested again on the health indices at the end of the experimental period. Lastly, the plan describes how the collected data will be analyzed in order to confirm or refute the stated hypotheses.

4. **Collecting and Analyzing the Data**

   At this point, the research plan is actually implemented and the data collected. Assuming that the research plan was carefully developed, this stage of the scientific method requires the investigator to systematically follow the pre-scribed procedures. This may include the management of an experimental treatment, or it may consist of actually testing or observing the participants, conducting an interview, or administering a questionnaire. Although it is critical to focus attention on the operational details of gathering the data, arguably the most important aspect of data collection is the preplanning—the development of a sound research plan. Once the data are collected, appropriate techniques are used to analyze the data. In quantitative studies, numerical data are typically analyzed statistically, first to simply describe the data and then, if appropriate, to determine if the evidence supports the hypotheses being tested. Inasmuch as qualitative studies generally result in non-numerical data, such as interview records or detailed descriptions of events, data analysis becomes inductive in nature, relying on coding and categorization processes.

5. **Interpreting Results and Forming Conclusions**

   While data analysis is an important step in the overall process, it is not an end in itself. At this point the researcher attempts to interpret the results of the data analysis and formulate meaningful conclusions. Does the evidence support or refute the hypotheses? Depending upon the nature of the research study and keeping in mind that not all studies have hypotheses, a decision to accept or reject each hypothesis is made. And most importantly, what does this mean? Conclusions should not be simply restatements of the results or findings of the study. Rather, conclusions attempt to provide an explanation of the results. It is important to recognize that the conclusions relate back to the question that prompted the study in the first place, yet inferences are typically made to situations beyond the specific study. Ultimately, researchers will report the details of their study to interested persons, describing the underlying basis for the study, the participants and procedures used, and the results and conclusions. In so doing, a researcher is thereby submitting his or her work for open and public review, a feature that distinguishes scientific inquiry from the other sources of knowledge.

The stages described above provide the framework of the scientific method. The research process, then, is the application of the scientific method to solve a problem or answer a question. It is important to note that the research process is cyclic in nature, whereby the first stage in the process begins with the identification of a problem or question. The process then proceeds through a number of other stages, ending with the researcher affirming or rejecting the research hypothesis and drawing conclusions that enable the question to be answered. In effect, the process begins and ends with a focus on the question of interest. Inevitably, however, the results of a single research study will give rise to other questions that warrant further investigation as the whole process starts anew and the body of knowledge continues to grow. Drew, Hardman, and Hart (1996) refer to this model as the closed-loop conceptualization of the research process. The cyclic nature of the research process is illustrated in figure 1.1.

FIGURE 1.1
Conceptualization of the
research cycle.

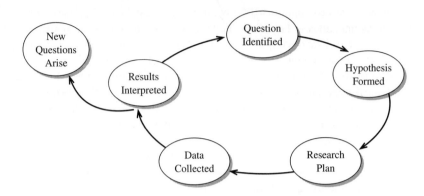

The essence of the scientific method is the objectivity and marked control it can provide the researcher. The structure and rigor imposed by the scientific method has served the natural sciences very well as investigations focus on physical and biological phenomena. But in the social sciences, including education and much of HHP, the strict application of the scientific method has proven to be more challenging. The use of human subjects diminishes our ability to administer some treatment conditions as well to control all factors that could affect an experiment.

For example, the use of performance-enhancing drugs in sports has received considerable attention in recent years. To truly determine the effect of these drugs, a sample of athletes should be drawn from the population, these individuals should be given drugs over a period of time, and then the effects on various body organs should be observed. Yet, performance-enhancing drugs may be harmful to the body. There are considerable moral, ethical, and legal reasons that would preclude studies designed in the manner described. Research participants have a right to expect researchers to prevent harm from coming to them and to pay attention to their safety and human dignity. Researchers cannot hope to know all the potential risks and hazards to the participants, but must inform them of all those that *are* known. There is much current evidence that indicates that performance-enhancing drugs are harmful. The use of drugs to see what happens to body organs five to ten years after they are ingested is a risk that should be avoided. Such a study would be difficult to justify from an ethical and moral standpoint. People cannot be treated in a harmful or dehumanizing way.

Also, many problems in HHP involve attitudes and personal opinions. While it is possible to determine the prevalence of one opinion or another, to fully explain the basis for such opinions is problematic because they are so subjective in nature and are influenced by many factors. A major limitation associated with research involving human subjects is the inability of the researcher to exercise the degree of control often required in scientific research. Not only are there moral and ethical issues that should be considered, but practicality also becomes a major factor when dealing with human behavior. Yet, the scientific method as previously described has provided the basic framework for research in the social and behavioral sciences and has led to the accumulation of a vast amount of knowledge. Despite the use of the scientific method, the social sciences have generally not attained the scientific stature of the natural sciences (Ary, Jacobs, and Razavieh 1996).

Since the social scientist is typically dealing with human subjects and their behaviors, problems of control, accuracy of measurement, and complexity of function are considerably greater than would be expected in the natural sciences. The major concern is that, whatever the problem, researchers try to be as scientific as possible in their attack. Control over the research situation will be more difficult in studies done in gymnasia, swimming pools, camps, and playing fields.

Types of Research Questions

The foundation of scientific inquiry and the first stage of the research process is the identification of the **research question.** While the research question will inevitably be refined and transformed into a specific statement of the problem that is amenable to investigation, it is especially useful for the beginning researcher to develop an understanding of what constitutes an appropriate research question. While chapter 2 provides a more detailed discussion of how to select and refine a research question, our focus now is toward a more global understanding of the nature of the research question. Obviously, there is a great variety of research questions that may be investigated. It is possible, however, to group research questions into three basic categories: descriptive, relationship, and difference (Drew, Hardman, and Hart 1996). Being able to identify the basic type of question being asked helps in understanding the very nature of the research, the preferred research design and methodology, and the appropriate methods for analyzing the data.

Descriptive questions, as the name suggests, seek simply to describe phenomena or characteristics of a particular group of subjects being studied. Such questions describe what is. Data are typically gathered by asking questions of a group of individuals, observing their behavior, or measuring (testing) their performance on specified tasks. Descriptive questions are often the basis for survey research as well as qualitative research. An example of a study centered around a descriptive question is illustrated by the School Health Policies and Programs Study (SHPPS) sponsored by the Centers for Disease Control and Prevention (CDC), a study which was designed to ascertain policy and program information of school health programs throughout the nation (Kann et al. 1995).

Difference questions seek to make comparisons between or within groups. They ask the question: Is there a difference? This type of question tends to be associated with experimental research, where at the simplest level a researcher is comparing an experimental group that has been exposed to some treatment to a control group that has not received the treatment. Similarly, comparisons that are made between pretest performance and posttest performance are also representative of research questions asking if there is a difference. Difference questions may also be the basis for nonexperimental research in which the researcher is interested in comparing one group to another on the basis of existing characteristics. For example, Faucette and colleagues (1995) used self-administered surveys to compare fourth grade boys' and girls' out-of-school physical activity levels and choices of activity.

Relationship questions investigate the degree to which two or more variables covary or are associated with each other. Rather than comparing groups, typically the researcher obtains measurements on two or more variables for a group of subjects and then computes some index of association, often a correlation coefficient. The intent of such questions is simply to determine the extent to which the variables are related, not to establish cause-and-effect. The work by Sallis and colleagues (1988) to investigate the relationship of cardiovascular fitness and physical activity to cardiovascular disease risk factors in children and adults provides a good illustration of a relationship question.

It is worth noting that most research studies, especially those that are ultimately published, usually contain multiple questions, including different types of questions. Whereas the definitive classification of a research question into one of these three types may be viewed as an academic exercise, comprehending the basic nature of the research question is an important part of understanding the research process.

In order to help the reader better understand the three types of research questions, the examples that follow have been adapted from published papers or theses and categorized according to the type of question being asked. It is noted that additional research questions may have been included in each study.

Descriptive

What are the attitudes of rural parents toward the inclusion of sexuality education in the school curriculum? (Welshimer and Harris 1994)

What is the perceived confidence of entry-level health educators related to specific responsibilities of health education professionals? (Balog and Scheidt 2000)

What is the extent of perceived ethnic/cultural violence among students in middle and high schools? (Hamdan and Martinez 2000)

What do physical education teachers think about the effect of block scheduling in secondary school physical education classes? (Bukowski and Stinson 2000)

What are the characteristics of highly successful high school football programs in the state of Iowa over the past 10 years? (Peters 1999)

Relationship

Is there an association between leisure-time physical activity and indicators of well-being and selected symptoms of medical conditions? (Brown, Mishra, Lee, and Bauman 2000)

What is the relationship between class size, lesson context, and students' engagement in physical activity during middle school physical education class? (McKenzie, Marshall, Sallis, and Conway 2000)

Is there an association between self-esteem and eating behaviors among collegiate female swimmers? (Fey 1998)

Is physical activity in childhood and adolescence a predictor of physical activity in young adulthood? (Telama, Yang, Laakso, and Viikari 1997)

What is the relationship between television viewing to physical fitness and obesity among adolescence boys and girls? (Tucker 1986)

Difference

Is there a difference in the participation in unhealthy behaviors between Mexican American adolescents who smoke and those who do not smoke? (Pesa 1998)

Does participation in Special Olympics affect the self-esteem of adults with mental retardation? (Major 1998)

Do expert and novice dancers use similar strategies to learn appropriately challenging routines in domain-relevant conditions? (Poon and Rodgers 2000)

What changes occur in the physical fitness of middle-aged adults with an intellectual disability over a period of 13 years and how does this compare to established standards of the nondisabled population? (Graham and Reid 2000)

Does psyching strategy have an effect on neuromuscular performance and motor unit activation of the biceps brachii and triceps brachii in well-trained individuals during a maximal isometric elbow flexion task? (Brody, Hatfield, Spalding, Frazer, and Caherty 2000)

Science, Research and Theory

The ultimate goal of science is the formation of theory based upon the synthesis and interpretation of facts and information. Through scientific research efforts, facts are discovered. As these facts grow, there is a need to organize and synthesize this information in order to make meaningful interpretations. Questions such as What do these facts mean? and What are the relationships among these facts? are asked. In an attempt to explain the phenomenon under study, theories must be postulated about the things inherent in the facts. Theories are formulated to bring order to the facts and to provide meaningful generalizations about the phenomenon being studied. The word "theory" is often misunderstood. Some believe that it is an esoteric term and that those who use it are "out in left field" or "in a world of their own." A **theory** is a belief or assumption about how things relate to each other. According to Best and Kahn (1998), "a theory establishes a cause-and-effect relationship between variables with the purpose of explaining and predicting phenomena" (p. 9).

Not only does theory summarize and organize existing knowledge, it also enables scientists to predict and, ultimately, control phenomena. Theories abound concerning the relationship between human behavior and the environment. Moreover, as these relationships are delineated and explained, predictions are offered as to what will happen if certain human behaviors are either changed or not changed, depending upon the circumstances. For instance, a growing body of scientific evidence clearly establishes the relationship between physical activity and one's health. The Surgeon General's Report (1996) concludes that people of all ages, both male and female, benefit from regular physical activity. The human body responds to physical activity in ways that have important positive effects on the musculoskeletal, cardiovascular, respiratory, and endocrine systems. These changes are consistent with a number of health benefits, including a reduced risk of premature death and reduced risks of coronary heart disease, hypertension, colon cancer, and diabetes mellitus (U. S. Department of Health and Human Services 1996).

Based on this evidence and our increasing ability to predict the consequences of specific health behaviors, various national organizations such as the American Heart Association (AHA) and the American College of Sports Medicine (ACSM), to name a few, have issued physical activity recommendations to the public. Theories can lead to civil laws to control various behaviors. Gun control laws, for example, have been offered because of certain theories about the relationship between guns and crime. Today, children with disabilities are mainstreamed by law into the regular classrooms in schools. This resulted from gathering sufficient facts through research that supported theory about the potential benefits—to both disabled and nondisabled children—of studying in the classroom together.

Theory is also a vehicle for obtaining new knowledge by providing hypotheses for additional research in a particular area. Frequently, scientists investigate theory under a different set of circumstances to determine if valid generalizations are possible. In effect, the theory is being tested. Theory, then, provides a framework for explaining phenomena and may serve as the basis for further research as well as practical application. In the quest for theory development, the veracity of the knowledge acquired is paramount. As a result, it is generally agreed that the scientific method represents the best means of acquiring knowledge.

Empiricism

As previously mentioned, the strict application of the scientific method to research investigations in the social and behavioral sciences has proved challenging. Moreover, research efforts in education and in HHP, in particular, have not always emphasized theory. **Empiricism** is acquiring information and facts through the observation of our world. In the past, professionals in these fields have demonstrated greater interest in empiricism, gathering facts in a particular area of interest through pragmatic observation. Consequently, theory development has occurred less than in the physical sciences. While inductive reasoning is the major medium for establishing generalizations and principles, empiricism is based on the idea that knowledge is obtained through experience and observation. It does not rely on theory or science. The empiricist focuses on "getting the facts," but has little interest in explaining the when, how, or why of the facts. Steroid and other performance-enhancing drug use by athletes is often the result of an empirical decision. These athletes may observe the apparent effect of steroid use in others without questioning its limitations. They do not seek the deeper questions with regard to rapid strength and muscular gains steroid use provides. They are interested only in the end result. They tend to overgeneralize! The scientist, however, digs deeper into all possible relationships associated with steroid use, seeking facts so as to theorize and explain such relationships.

While empiricism may yield a seemingly quick and practical solution to a problem, empiricism is not infallible. If we observe something occurring and base our conclusions on this single incident, then we run the risk of making erroneous conclusions, since an isolated incident may not represent true phenomena taking place. Moreover, the exclusive use of empiricism results does little to advance the body of knowledge within a field. The continued development of HHP as a field of study is dependent upon greater attention being given to theory development and the explanation of observed facts and relationships.

The Concept of Variables

The focus of the researcher's effort is always on the **variable.** A variable is a characteristic, trait, or attribute of a person or thing that can be classified or measured. Eye color, sex, and church preference are classifications. Skill, self-concept, strength, heart rate, and intelligence are variables that can be measured. The term *variable* indicates that a characteristic can have more than one value. There are two genders in the human race, male and female, and if both appear in a research project then gender becomes a variable. When a characteristic does not vary, it is referred to as a *constant*. In a study of the manual dexterity of second-year nursing students, the characteristic, second-year, is a constant; it does not vary among the student nurses.

Quantitative and Qualitative Variables

Variables can be *qualitative* or *categorical* if they are classified according to some characteristic, attribute, or property. People are categorized as to sex (male, female), eye color (blue, brown, green), church preference (Catholic, Protestant, Jewish), and political affiliation (Republican, Democrat, Independent). Qualitative variables are usually unmeasurable. Variables are called *quantitative* if they can be measured in a numerical sense. The heights of five starters on a basketball team may be 5'10", 6'2", 6'5", 6'8", and 7', respectively. Their ages range from 18 years, 6 months to 22 years, 3 months. There are two basic type of quantitative variables, *discrete* and *continuous*.

Discrete Variables. This type of variable is usually thought of as being a whole unit, one that cannot be fractionated or divided into smaller parts. Examples of discrete variables are football scores, and the number of correct answers on a test. Football scores are recorded in whole numbers (e.g., 3, 7, 10, 14) and cannot be divided into smaller parts like 7.5 or 11.75.

Continuous Variables. This type of variable can be divided into fractional amounts in large or small degrees. Strength and endurance scores, track and field times, height, weight, and girth measures are considered to be continuous variables. Time in a 100-meter dash is sometimes to the nearest tenth of a second, but in high-level competition it could be one one-hundredth of a second. The height of a person could be measured in feet and inches, in half-inches, or in quarter-inches, depending on the precision desired and the ability of the measuring instrument to measure height accurately.

Independent and Dependent Variables

In research, particularly experimental research, the terms **independent** and **dependent** variable are commonly used. Although sometimes confusing for beginning research students, recognizing the distinction between independent and dependent variables and being able to properly identify each in a research study is critically important in understanding the research process. The experimental approach involves observing what effect different amounts of one variable (independent) have on a second variable (dependent). The independent variable is referred to as the experimental treatment. It is the variable that is manipulated or purposively selected by the researcher in order to determine its effect on some observed phenomenon. The researcher controls what treatment will be selected and how much will be applied. The treatment, or independent, variable will not change during the research or as a result of the research. It is considered an antecedent or precursor to other variables. According to Ary, Jacobs, and Razavieh (1996), there are two types of independent variables, *active* and *attribute*. An active variable is one that is actually manipulated or selected by the researcher, such as method of training, form of reinforcement, or type of nutritional supplement. An attribute variable is one that cannot be actively manipulated or altered by the researcher since it represents a preexisting attribute or trait, such as gender, race, age, or grade level. Researchers are able to form comparison groups on the basis of such preexisting characteristics.

The dependent variable, on the other hand, is the one that is expected to change as a result of the treatment. It is the variable that is observed or measured in the research process. The dependent variable is not under the control of the researcher as it represents the response or outcome from the manipulation of the independent variable. It is the presumed consequence of the independent variable. Said another way, the independent variable is expected to *cause* some *effect* on the dependent variable. The changed, or affected, variable is referred to as dependent because its value depends upon the value of the independent variable (Tuckman 1999). In many instances, the independent variable forms or defines comparison groups in research; the dependent variable generates data.

Following are some examples of independent and dependent variables:

Problem 1: A study is designed to investigate the effects of different brands of toothpaste (e.g., Colgate and Crest) on the prevention of dental cavities.
Independent variable: brand of toothpaste
Dependent variable: number of cavities

Problem 2: A researcher wants to compare a dosage of 1200 mg versus 2400 mg of a popular over-the-counter pain reliever on delayed onset muscle soreness (DOMS) following an intense exercise bout.
Independent variable: dosage level
Dependent variable: some measure of muscle soreness

Problem 3: An investigator seeks to study the effects of different types of incentives on participation in a smoking cessation program.
Independent variable: type of incentive
Dependent variable: participation rates

Problem 4: A study is undertaken to compare male and female attitudes toward a television advertisement promoting physical activity.
Independent variable: gender
Dependent variable: attitudes toward advertisement

Some of the most common independent variables seen in HHP research are exercise, diet, medicines, drugs, motivation, programs, procedures, methods, techniques, gender, social class, attitude, and intelligence. Some of the most common dependent variables are performance, fitness, learning, health, knowledge, and behavior. It is also noted that variables may be used as an independent variable in one study and as a dependent variable in another study. Consider, for example, one experiment in which the investigator studies the effect of losing (independent) on motivation (dependent) among a group of athletes, while in another study the investigator studies the effect of motivation (independent) on physical performance (dependent). Motivation served as the dependent variable in one study and as the independent variable in the other. The purpose of the study determines whether a variable is considered independent or dependent.

While some research studies, as in the examples above, may have only one independent and one dependent variable, it is not uncommon for research studies to have more than one independent variable and/or more than one dependent variable. Consider the following examples:

Problem 5: A study is designed to investigate the effects of a new HIV (AIDS) education unit taught in a ninth-grade health class on students' attitude toward and knowledge about AIDS.
Independent variable: method of teaching AIDS (new versus traditional unit)
Dependent variable: attitude toward AIDS and score on a knowledge test

Problem 6: A researcher is interested in investigating the effects of a high-protein diet and two different modes of strength training on muscular strength development of college-age males.
Independent variable: type of diet and method of strength training
Dependent variable: muscular strength

Problem 7: An educational researcher seeks to determine the effects of block scheduling of classes on skill acquisition and attitude toward physical activity among junior high school students. Furthermore, the researcher is interested in determining if boys and girls respond to block scheduling differently.
Independent variable: type of scheduling (block versus traditional) and gender
Dependent variable: skill achievement and attitude toward physical activity

Extraneous Variables

While the independent variable is to serve as a stimulus to evoke a response from the dependent variable, there are usually other factors (variables) that could possibly cause the same response. In fact, it is quite likely that there are many possible variables that could have an effect on the dependent variable. To conclude that one type of physical fitness training is more effective than another, the researcher must be confident that other factors did not produce the same effect. Perhaps the most frequent and most serious mistake made by the beginning researcher is the failure to either control or account for the variables that could contribute error in an experiment.

These error-producing variables are generally referred to as **extraneous variables.** Although some authors may also describe error-producing variables as intervening variables, modifying variables, or confounding variables, we prefer to use the term extraneous variable to refer to any factor that is a source of unwanted or error variance. The task of the researcher is to eliminate or somehow control the potential influence of extraneous variables. Methods of controlling extraneous variables are discussed in some detail in chapter 3. The following examples illustrate the potential effect that extraneous variables could have on research findings.

A researcher studied the effect of motivation (independent) on the physical fitness test scores (dependent) of sixth-grade boys and girls. The two motivating conditions were team competition and level of aspiration (goal seeking). The subsequent finding that the group receiving level of aspiration was significantly better than the group receiving team competition was surprising because the literature contains much information proclaiming the superiority of team competition as a motivational vehicle. A detailed check into the composition of the groups participating under each condition revealed that they came from classes that were divided into high, average, and low academic achievement. The sixth graders who performed under the level of aspiration condition came from the high achievement category and possessed a mean intelligence quotient (IQ) of 132. The literature clearly indicates that, in general, the more intelligent an individual is, the easier it is to get that person "up," or motivated. So, IQ, a variable that was not included in the design of the study, served as an extraneous variable that slipped into the research situation, interacting with the dependent variable (fitness score) to make the condition (level of aspiration) look extremely potent and effective. The researcher presumed that IQ, while not a planned part of the study, was a substantive contributor to its results. This variable, like all extraneous variables, was not manipulated by the researcher.

There are many extraneous variables that can have a significant influence on the dependent variable and can invalidate research conclusions. Other such extraneous variables besides IQ, and depending on the specific type of experiment, are sex, socioeconomic level, teacher competence, personality, enthusiasm, physical health, emotional health, age, and the use of volunteers and intact groups as subjects. If a researcher conducted a study on the effect of three different methods of teaching outdoor education concepts on elementary students' appreciation and knowledge of the outdoors, with one recreation instructor assigned to each method, instructor personality could play an important role in the ultimate results of the study. Extraneous variables are difficult, if not impossible, to control. A good design of a study can help to play down the effect of such variables. In the teacher personality example above, the outdoor education teachers could be screened for personality characteristics; the one with the best personality would then be assigned to teach the outdoor education concepts under the three different methods. Teacher personality would be the same for all three groups of subjects and so, in this case, the teacher personality variable would be controlled, or neutralized. However, it is assumed here that the teacher is equally effective in teaching with each method.

Types of Research

While the underlying framework of research is founded upon the scientific method, there are various types of research that have differing purposes and approaches to the process. In order to bring some order to the numerous types of research, several systems, called **research classifications,** have been proposed. While experts in the field may differ in their classification criteria, virtually every research methods textbook provides some system for classifying research. It is also noted that the various research categories are not mutually exclusive, meaning that a given research study could be identified in several different classification systems. For instance, a study to determine the physiological characteristics of elite distance swimmers could be classified as applied research, quantitative research, or descriptive research, among others. Virtually every research study could be identified in multiple categories. The ability to classify research is not important in itself, but has value in making the research processes more understandable, particularly for the beginning researcher. Moreover, by developing knowledge of the various types of research, you will acquire an understanding and appreciation of the goals, methodologies, and activities that guide the research efforts. It is important to understand, however, that how a given research problem is attacked depends largely on the nature of the problem being investigated and the question being asked.

Basic and Applied Research

Generally, **basic research,** which is sometimes referred to as pure or fundamental research, is theoretical in nature: its primary purpose is the discovery of new knowledge and the development of theory. It is motivated by intellectual curiosity and interest in a specific problem area. Fundamental knowledge about such phenomena as the environment, space, human behavior, exercise, and the human gene makeup is sought. Broad generalizations and principles, such as the overload and cross-transference principles and laws of learning, frequently result from basic research. The results of this type of research may have no immediate practical application or utility since such an approach often leads to knowledge for knowledge's sake. It may take years before the results from basic research find some practical utility. The majority of this research is done in highly controlled experimental settings in which selected variables are formally manipulated by the researcher in order to test causal relationships. This type of research often involves animal subjects, as illustrated by the early work of psychologist B. F. Skinner on reinforcement using birds and rats. Some examples of what might be considered basic research studies include the following:

1. A study to determine the effect of lactic acid concentration on breast milk following different levels of exercise.

2. A study to determine the effect of various compounds on ventilation during normoxia and hypoxia.

3. A study to test the dynamic systems theory that infants learn motor skills through exploration and selection of adaptive responses.

Applied research, on the other hand, has as its central purpose the solution of an immediate practical problem, yet seeks to make inferences beyond the group or situation studied. Most research in HHP is applied research in which professionals in the field are confronted with real-world problems and are interested in solving them. A health educator may try out a new smoking-cessation technique or a leisure services professional may seek to utilize a new method of training recreation program supervisors. A new theory of motor skill acquisition may be tested by the physical education teacher. The idea is to improve products and processes and to test theoretical concepts. We are interested in improving our HHP practices and services. The results of this type of research are intended to be generalized and to extend to the target population and setting. An adapted physical education researcher who finds that a particular motor activity is successful in improving the social skills of a sample of individuals with mental retardation is likely to want to apply those results to all similar individuals with mental retardation. Seat belt studies and smoking and drug research are usually geared to producing results that will apply to the entire population. Some examples of what might be considered applied research studies include the following:

1. Application of the theory of self-efficacy to recreation supervisors' years of experience and number of employees supervised.
2. A study to determine if female children of divorce have more problems with trust and male children have more problems with intimacy when compared to children of a similar age from intact families.

Although sometimes presented as a distinct type of research, action research, in our view, represents a special form of applied research in which the interest is in local, not universal, applicability. This research is typically very pragmatic in nature, albeit objective, but the problem exists in a local setting. For instance, in an effort to increase the distance of his kicks, a football coach may experiment with having his punter utilize a new kicking technique. Although the coach's approach is scientific in nature, he is interested only in this local situation. Methods, techniques, and practices are tried out which may promise better results and provide the basis for improved decisions. Behavioral modification, intervention, and in-service training skills are frequently employed in action research studies. To be successful, the researcher must adhere to sound research procedures. The approach should be as scientific as possible given the less-controlled, local setting in which it takes place.

Quantitative and Qualitative Research

Another system of classifying research is based largely upon the approach taken to collect and analyze the data. It may be useful to think of these approaches to research as existing along a continuum or scale-continuing gradations. At one end of the continuum is quantitative research and at the opposite end is qualitative research. The terms quantitative and qualitative are conveniently used to differentiate one research approach from the other, but the terms themselves are generic in nature and refer to a family of research methods that fall under these broad categories. In fact, specific family members of each research approach fall at various points along the quantitative-qualitative continuum, suggesting that some methods more fully embrace the principles of quantitative or qualitative research than others.

Quantitative research uses an approach that is designed for the collection and analysis of numerical data that are usually obtained through direct testing, questionnaires, or a multitude of paper-and-pencil instruments. This approach to research, which is also referred to as the traditional or positivist approach, has been and continues to be the predominant method used in HHP. Quantitative approaches are commonly used to describe existing conditions or phenomena, investigate relationships between two or more variables, and explore cause-and-effect relationships between phenomena. The general procedures for carrying out the research activities, analyzing the resultant data, and deriving the conclusions have been widely accepted. Although the nature of the data collected serves as an easy and useful means of regarding quantitative research, a quantitative approach involves more than simply the use of numerical data. First of all, a quantitative approach is based on a paradigm adopted from the natural sciences that subscribes to the assumption that reality is relatively stable, uniform, measurable, and governed by rational laws that enable generalizations to be made. Moreover, a quantitative approach involves (1) clearly stated questions, (2) rationally conceived hypotheses, (3) fully developed research procedures, (4) controlling extraneous factors that might interfere with the data collected, (5) using relatively large samples of participants in order to provide meaningful data, and (6) employing data analysis techniques based upon statistical procedures (Gay and Airasian 2000; Drew, Hardman, and Hart 1996).

Although long used in anthropology and sociology, **qualitative research** methodologies are relatively new to HHP, gaining popularity only during the past 10 to 15 years. Although there is not complete agreement by qualitative researchers as to what qualitative research is, most would agree that qualitative research generally includes research methods that rely heavily upon extensive observations and in-depth interviews that result in non-numerical data. Furthermore, qualitative research is often conducted in natural settings and does not attempt to control the context or conditions surrounding the research setting, thus prompting the use of the term "naturalistic research" to describe this approach. Founded upon beliefs and assumptions different from those of quantitative research, qualitative research does not subscribe to the viewpoint that the world is stable and uniform and can be explained by laws that govern phenomena. Rather, qualitative research takes on a constructionist perspective, suggesting that meaning and reality is situational specific, thus allowing for many different meanings, none of which is necessarily more valid than another. Thus, there may not be an attempt to generalize the results of qualitative research since the context of the study is situational specific. In qualitative research, the researcher tends to not state hypotheses before the collection of data. Moreover, the research procedures are not fully articulated prior to conducting the study since the methods tend to evolve as the research proceeds. Analysis and interpretation of data collected using a qualitative research approach is mainly interpretative and descriptive in nature, resulting in a categorization of the data to identify trends and patterns. Statistical procedures are rarely used. Further discussion of qualitative research methods is presented in chapter 9.

Although some researchers perceive qualitative and quantitative approaches as oppositional and incompatible, a more prudent course is to consider them as complementary methods in the pursuit of truth and knowledge. Each has its advantages and disadvantages, and taken together, they allow us to know and understand different things about the world in which we live. In fact, we are seeing both approaches being utilized in the same studies. For instance, a study to investigate the nature of authentic assessment techniques in school physical education first administered a questionnaire to a randomly selected group of teachers (quantitative) and then followed up with a small number of detailed interviews and classroom observations (qualitative) in order to obtain a deeper understanding (Mintah 2000). The nature of the question or the problem to be investigated will usually determine the preferred research approach, whether it is quantitative, qualitative, or both.

Experimental Research and Nonexperimental Research

A major distinction is generally made between experimental and nonexperimental research. While the general purpose of research is to increase our understanding and the body of knowledge within a given field, there are substantial differences in the approach one may take in pursuit of this end. While the previous introduction to quantitative and qualitative research methodologies characterizes the nature of research activities using each respective approach, understanding the distinction between experimental and nonexperimental research adds yet another perspective to fully understanding the research process and the wealth of methodologies available. The following sections briefly discuss experimental research and the most prevalent forms of nonexperimental research in HHP.

Experimental Research.   In experimental research, the researcher explores the cause-and-effect relationship between variables by manipulating certain variables (referred to as independent variables) to determine their effect on another variable (referred to as the dependent variable). Furthermore, the researcher attempts to control all other factors that could possibly influence the dependent variable. Consider, for example, a situation in which a researcher is interested in investigating two different methods of training (free-weights and weight machines) on strength development. In this case, the method of training represents the independent variable and is being manipulated by the researcher. Ideally, the researcher would be able to randomly assign subjects to either a treatment group that utilizes free-weights or a treatment group that utilizes weight machines, have the subjects train for a specified length of time, and then determine if there were differences between the two groups in terms of strength development. [One could also add a control group to the study that did not perform any training.] In such a study the researcher would attempt to ensure that both groups trained for the same length of time, for the same duration, and at the same intensity. Moreover, the researcher would attempt to control other factors that could reasonably affect the outcome, factors like diet, physical activity, and even motivation, to name a few. The researcher would compare the two groups based on the subjects' strength scores (dependent variable) at the end of the training period. Assuming that there were no differences in strength when the study commenced, if the final strength scores were significantly higher for the group using free-weights, the researcher would be able to conclude with some confidence that training with free-weights was more effective than training using weight machines.

Experimental research is designed to answer the question "What if . . . ?" by systematically manipulating one or more variables and observing the consequences on another variable. The researcher is interested in the future. Experimental research methods are quantitative in nature, typically begin with clearly stated hypotheses to fit the research questions, and are commonly associated with a laboratory setting. It is the most formally structured of all the various types of research. According to Ary, Jacobs, and Razavieh (1996), in its simplest form, experimental research has three characteristics: (1) an independent variable that is manipulated by the researcher, (2) control of other relevant variables, and (3) observation of the effect of the manipulation of the independent variable on the dependent variable. A more thorough discussion of experimental research is presented in chapter 7.

Causal-Comparative Research. **Causal-comparative research** is similar to experimental research in that it seeks to investigate possible cause-and-effect relationships. However, in causal-comparative research the independent variable is not manipulated by the researcher, either because it cannot be manipulated or because it would be unethical to do so. With causal-comparative research, the independent variable is often referred to as an attribute or organismic variable because it is some attribute or characteristic that the subject already possesses due to the natural course of actions (e.g., gender, ethnicity, medical malady, family background, employment status). As a result, the subjects are already members of a particular class or group of individuals that possess the same attribute. The researcher then compares groups that differ on the attribute (independent variable) to determine if there are differences on some dependent variable of interest. Since the researcher has no control over the independent variable, which is either innate or has already occurred, this type of research is also called *ex post facto* (after the fact) research.

A good example of causal-comparative research is represented by many studies that have investigated the effect of smoking (independent variable) on lung cancer (dependent variable). Because of the potential harm to subjects, it would be unethical to assign some subjects to a group and force them to become heavy smokers and other subjects to a group that is forbidden to smoke; researchers would instead compare the incidence of lung cancer in a group of nonsmokers to a group of long-time smokers. Clearly, the researcher did not have control over the independent variable in this example, or in causal-comparative research in general. The group membership, either smoker or nonsmoker, was determined before the study commenced; the researcher merely selected subjects from each of the preexisting groups and compared them on the dependent variable—in this case, lung cancer. Because of the lack of control, especially the capability to manipulate the independent variable, the ability of the researcher to draw cause-and-effect conclusions is significantly limited compared to experimental research. This has been one of the arguments used by the tobacco industry in refuting the findings of most research pointing to a linkage between smoking and lung cancer, although a preponderance of the evidence today clearly shows such an association. Causal-comparative research generally functions to identify group differences and discover relationships among variables, but stops short of establishing causality. Although there are limitations associated with causal-comparative research, it nevertheless is frequently used in HHP research.

Descriptive Research.   **Descriptive research,** as the name suggests, attempts to gather information from groups of subjects in order to describe systematically, factually, and accurately specific characteristics of interest or conditions that presently exist. Quite simply, a descriptive study first determines and then describes the way things are. Nonexperimental in nature, a descriptive study is concerned with the present and describes *what is*. It typically precedes experimental research. There is no manipulation of an independent variable in descriptive research since there is no intent to explore a cause-and-effect relationship. Descriptive research utilizes a wide variety of methodologies to collect data—surveys, interviews, direct measurement, and observational techniques being the most prevalent. Frequently, descriptive research is interested in comparing relevant subgroups (for example, groups based on gender, age, grade level, socioeconomic status, or ethnicity) with the results being reported according to each subgroup as well as for the total sample. Although descriptive research is similar to qualitative research in some regards, there are important distinctions: (1) methodology for descriptive research is more structured and standardized; (2) variables of interest are predetermined in descriptive research; (3) descriptive research inevitably uses more subjects, often selected through randomization procedures; (4) data are analyzed predominately through the use of statistical procedures in descriptive research; and (5) there is typically less in-depth researcher interaction with the subjects in descriptive research.

Descriptive studies have been commonplace in HHP as well as in education and the social and behavioral sciences. Best and Kahn (1998) indicate that descriptive research is the predominant research method used in the behavioral sciences. Furthermore, many doctoral dissertations and master's theses involve descriptive research.

Descriptive research methodology is particularly suited to studies that seek to identify the attitudes or opinions of human subjects or to those that purport to detail behaviors that may naturally occur in the classroom, gymnasium, workplace, playing field, or home, for example. Since descriptive research commonly seeks to generalize the information collected from a sample (e.g., opinions, attitudes, abilities, behaviors) to a target population, researchers often employ randomization procedures in an attempt to obtain a sample that is representative of the population of interest.

Some of the best examples of descriptive research are represented by public opinion surveys in which the respondents are asked their opinion or attitude on a multitude of topics ranging from presidential preference, to physical activity and exercise, to abortion. The Centers for Disease Control and Prevention (CDC) regularly conduct a number of national probability studies aimed at describing health behaviors of Americans (e.g., Youth Risk Behavior Survey [YRBS], National Health Interview Survey [NHIS], and Behavioral Risk Factor Surveillance System [BRFSS]). In addition, a study to identify the physiological characteristics of elite women distance runners or a study to ascertain the leisure-time physical activity behaviors of adolescent males and females are good examples of descriptive research in HHP.

Correlational Research.   Nonexperimental in nature, **correlational research** is closely related to both descriptive and causal-comparative research. It is similar to descriptive research in that it describes currently existing phenomena; it is similar to causal-comparative research in that it explores relationships between or among variables. According to Gay and Airasian (2000), the purpose of correlational research is to either determine whether, and to what extent, a relationship exists between two or more variables or to use these relationships to make predictions. That is, it may be either relational or predictive in nature. If a relationship exists, the degree of relationship is usually expressed as some type of correlation coefficient. A good example of a relationship study in HHP would be an investigation to determine how self-esteem corresponds [relates] to physical fitness among adolescent females. Measures of self-esteem and physical fitness would be collected on a representative group of adolescent girls and the association between the variables measured as a correlation coefficient.

Contrasted to experimental research, there is no manipulation of variables in correlational research, therefore it is important to recognize that correlational studies never establish cause-and-effect relationships between variables, even in the presence of a high correlation. Therefore, even if we found a high correlation between self-esteem and physical fitness in the example above, this does not mean that self-esteem causes physical fitness or that physical fitness causes self-esteem. It simply means that adolescent girls who have high levels of self-esteem tend to have high levels of physical fitness and those who have lower self-esteem tend to have lower levels of physical fitness. Although similar to causal-comparative studies in the fact that causal relationships cannot be definitively established, correlational research methodology differs in that usually there is only a single group of subjects from which data on two or more variables are collected for each participant, while causal-comparative research methodology takes into consideration scores from two distinct groups of subjects (e.g., smokers and nonsmokers). It is noted, however, that the existence of a high correlation does permit more accurate predictions based on the relationship. For example, correlational research has established that there is a relationship between one's grades in high school and college grade-point average (GPA). As a result, we can now establish a prediction model [equation] whereby we can predict, with a certain degree of accuracy, a student's college GPA on the basis of the student's high school GPA. In fact, other variables, such as performance on the Scholastic Aptitude Test (SAT), could be added to the prediction model to improve the accuracy. As this example illustrates, often the results of prediction studies are used to facilitate decision-making or selection processes, as in the case of admission to college.

Historical Research. Authorities differ as to whether the activities undertaken in historical inquiry can be considered scientific or not (Best and Kahn 1998). Moreover, it is not easy to classify **historical research** into a particular category, although it seems obvious that it is nonexperimental. Most historical research can be regarded as qualitative and descriptive in nature, yet relationships can be explored and hypotheses tested in certain types of well-designed and well-executed historical studies. In the historical approach, the researcher endeavors to record and understand events of the past in order to provide a better understanding of the present and suggest possible directions for the future. For instance, a researcher might be interested in investigating the "evolution of football in Texas public schools." Such a study would likely based upon official records and reports of state education agencies, school officials, and local school boards, as well as newspaper and magazine articles, school yearbooks, and interviews with selected individuals who had some involvement with Texas school football programs in past years.

The historical approach is oriented toward the past as the researcher seeks to provide a new perspective on a question of current interest by conducting an intensive study of material that already exists. Yet, historical research differs from other forms of research because its subject matter, the past, is difficult to capture and the researcher cannot generate new data, but can only synthesize and interpret data that already exist. Moreover, locating all the relevant data and information concerning a particular question from many, widely scattered sources is typically a difficult and tedious process. Sources of data for historical research can generally be classified into two main categories, primary sources and secondary sources. Primary sources of data consist of original materials prepared by individuals who were participants or a direct eyewitness of an event under investigation. On the other hand, secondary sources of data are one step removed from the historical happenings of interest and consist of materials based upon secondhand accounts of events, accounts that are prepared by individuals who were not present or witness to the events. Historical research studies can be one of two types—descriptive or narrative, in which the researcher provides a recounting of "what happened," and analytical, in which the researcher attempts to explain "how" and/or "why" something happened (Thomas and Nelson 1996). In chapter 11 we provide a more extensive description of historical research methods.

The Significance of Research in HHP

The body of knowledge in each of the fields of health and human performance (HHP) is currently expanding at a rapid rate. Tremendous progress has been made because scholars in these fields have focused on all aspects of the human being—the physical, mental, and emotional. The whole person is studied in relation to movement, attitude, and lifestyle. The research has been both theoretical and practical and has reflected a sharp increase in quality, range, and depth.

Health education has produced a variety of conceptual and methodological approaches for dealing with problems in health promotion and disease prevention. Important attitudes, beliefs, intentions, and norms for people of all ages with regard to human sexuality, alcohol and drug use, smoking, family relationships, obesity, and nutrition have been identified. The thrust of health education research has been on promotion and prevention as opposed to researching ways to eliminate or treat existing health problems. Torabi, Seffrin, and Yarber, along with various colleagues, have done excellent studies with regard to these variables (Torabi, et al., six studies dealing with attitude, tobacco, alcohol, cancer, and HIV). In addition, Torabi has published several articles on the statistical evaluation of research studies in applied health science. Many epidemiological studies have recently produced an abundance of scientific knowledge concerning the relationship between exercise and longevity; controlling chronic illness; retarding the aging process; and the important roles of nutrition, sleep, exercise, and lifestyle in providing good health.

Physical education research continues to make essential contributions to the better understanding of the various physiological responses to exercise and stress through biochemical and histochemical studies. Research in motor learning and motor control has added a great deal to the understanding of the acquisition and retention of motor skills, motor response processing, and the varied roles of the nervous system in movement. Adapted physical education has produced significant information as a result of biomechanical and energy cost studies of the activity performance of disabled individuals. The area of measurement and evaluation has developed increasingly more reliable and valid measures of physical fitness, motor skill, and mental ability and has contributed excellent theoretical work concerning reliability and validity, measurement scales, probability and sampling theory, and statistical design. Biomechanics, sport psychology, sport sociology, sport history, and motor development have generated research data which have been indispensable to the understanding of how people behave as they interact with the environments of physical education, exercise, and sport.

Recreation and park administration has long provided exceptional services to people so they may improve the quality of their lives. Research has been a major tool for obtaining the knowledge that has led to better delivery of these services, such as physical and mental health, administrative behavior, leadership evaluation, facility design, outdoor recreation, and leisure counseling (Pelegrino 1979, 5). Studies relating life-span development to the effects of recreation on people, the cultural impact of increased leisure time on society, the improvement of playground surfaces and equipment, the impact of recreation on the environment, the effect of tourism on society, and the spiritual and moral aspects of recreation have led to better recreation programs, practices, and services.

Dance is a unique and dynamic field of study whose research is best characterized as a creative activity. Choreography, the act of forming and performing dances, is a method of research unique to dance. Movement notation research has provided, for movement, a complete and accurate language and vocabulary. Rhythm has been studied as a language which transmits ideas and meaning through the "signs, symbols, sounds, and motions of the human body" (Cooper and Andrews 1975, 61). The biomechanics of dance, physiological responses resulting from dance, and injuries peculiar to dance performers are other popular dance research topics.

The rapid progress in HHP research has resulted, at least in part, from improved instrumentation and the development of new methods, techniques, and procedures. These developments have led to better research designs, a more objective research approach, and more reliable and valid data. Better data have enabled HHP researchers to increase the quality of their generalizations.

The volume of research emerging from the fields of HHP has increased in the past five to ten years. The HHP professional journals are facing an increasing backlog of both basic and applied research articles waiting to be published, and not all of these studies are being done by professional researchers. The HHP practitioner has become more active in research, while the focus of the professional researcher appears to have become more fixed on research having utilitarian value. The so-called gap between the researcher and the practitioner appears to be narrowing. A stronger feeling of cooperation seems to be growing in both camps as it relates to both theoretical and applied problems. Theoretical applications can help solve practical kinds of problems, while basic research frequently needs the results from the applied research to round out its theoretical concepts.

In its simplest form, research is just another way of looking at the problems which permeate the fields of HHP. Research is for everyone, and everyone can and should engage in that process. Deep knowledge of statistics and research design is not necessary to carry out creditable research. All that is needed is someone who is interested and willing to undertake the activity and who has some background knowledge of the problem to be studied. Research should not be relegated to just a few "name" people in the profession, but rather it is the responsibility of many people. In the past, a few HHP "names" gave those fields good leadership and direction in research circles. This impetus was needed but resulted in research narrowly focused in just a few interest areas. Larger numbers of people engaging in research are needed to guarantee that the problems, questions, and interests of all fields of HHP are represented in research investigations. Research can help broaden the knowledge and improve the practices that have long been associated with HHP. It is, and should continue to be, an active and continuing ingredient of the scholarly efforts of those fields. It is a tool that HHP cannot do without. It is the lifeblood of a profession and must be pursued vigorously.

Summary

Research is the lifeblood of a profession because it produces information that adds to the profession's body of knowledge. The research process is a formal, systematic, and logical attack on a problem using the scientific method as the mode of inquiry. An organized endeavor to obtain facts about some subject and ultimately answers to a specific question, research attempts to discover truth. Properly conducted research requires a clear understanding of the functions research performs and the stages of the research process. We have seen that there are many different types of research as different problems require different approaches in seeking their solutions. Determining which type of research is appropriate for a given study is dependent upon the nature of the question being asked. The methodology should always follow the research question; it should never precede it. Health and human performance (HHP) scholars have produced a variety of conceptual and methodological approaches for dealing with all aspects of the human being (physical, mental, and emotional). Research productivity in the fields undergirding HHP has expanded at a rapid rate and reflects much quality, range, and depth.

Formative Evaluation of Objectives

Objective 1   Explain the relationship between research and a profession.

1. Select a piece of information that you have always assumed to be true (Examples: An aspirin a day prevents a stroke; there is only one sure way to make a free throw) and indicate how you would attack the study (research) of such information.

Objective 2   Know the various methods used in the way knowledge has been obtained in the past and how it is currently obtained.

1. Construct a categorical syllogism that makes sense and one that does not (also indicate why it doesn't make sense).

2. Select a problem in which you are interested and apply the scientific method to researching it.

Objective 3   Know the various types and classifications of research.

1. Provide examples for each of the following: pure or basic research, applied research, action research.
2. Provide a research problem example for each of the research classifications.

Objective 4   Distinguish between a hypothesis and a theory.

1. Explain the difference between a theory and a hypothesis.

2

The Research Problem

Assumptions
Computer search
Conceptual literature
Critical reading

Data collection plan
Definition of terms
Delimitations
Hypothesis

Internet
Limitations
Problem statement

Purpose statement
Related research literature
Working bibliography

OBJECTIVES

Beginners in the realm of research frequently have difficulty in selecting an appropriate problem. The inability of students to recognize the many problems that exist in a profession is the result of inexperience. They simply do not understand, through no fault of their own, the nature of research and problem-solving elements. The emphasis of this chapter is on the learning process of students faced with the necessity of selecting a researchable problem for the first time.

After reading chapter 2, you should be able to

1. Select a suitable research problem.
2. Know the various sources of research problems.
3. Understand the various steps of the research process.
4. Systematically review literature relevant to the selected problem.
5. Plan and develop an attack on the problem.

Steps in the Research Process

The research process operates in several stages: (1) identifying the problem, (2) formulating hypotheses, (3) developing the research plan, (4) collecting and analyzing the data, and (5) forming conclusions. Each stage is undergirded by certain necessary steps, and from each step definite results can be expected. Many of these steps combine mental activity, such as reflective thinking, and the physical activities of searching, evaluating, interpreting, and writing. In reality, there is no universally applicable order in which these steps are incorporated in a given research project. The order and importance of these steps will vary according to the type of research being conducted, the purpose for doing the study, and the whims of the researcher. In many instances, various steps will be combined or accomplished concurrently. For example, the steps of identifying the research question and definition of the problem for a research investigation involve, simultaneously, a literature search, an estimation of the success potential of the study, consideration of the way in which the research will be approached, and a statement of hypothesis. It is believed by the authors of this text that the following steps apply to most experimental and descriptive research projects. The content embodied in these steps is discussed in appropriate sections of the book. The steps are as follows:

1. **Identifying the research question or problem area:** Becoming aware of research problems, where to look for them, and how to select and define problems.

2. **Initial review of literature:** Reading sources that will provide an understanding of the basic body of knowledge surrounding the problem.

3. **Distilling the question to a specific research problem:** Judging the potential of the research and narrowing the research question to a specific researchable problem statement along with statements of why the problem is important and how it is delimited.

4. **Continued review of literature:** Becoming thoroughly knowledgeable in the problem area and obtaining ideas about methods, techniques, and instrumentation needed to attack the problem.

5. **Formulation of hypotheses:** Based upon the literature reviewed and the researcher's experience, establishing the expected outcomes of the research.

6. **Determining the basic research approach:** Depending upon the type of question being asked, determining the preferred research approach (e.g., experimental, nonexperimental, quantitative, qualitative) and basic plan of attack.

7. **Identifying the population and sample:** Determining the type of participants who will produce the needed data to answer the research question. Are the participants available? How many participants are needed? How will they be selected?

8. **Designing data collection plan:** Determining the techniques for experimental protocols, if required, as well as the methodological approach for gathering research data.

9. **Selecting or developing specific data collection instruments or procedures:** Considering the data collection plan as well as the availability and adequacy of available instruments; deciding what specific instrument(s) is (are) needed to procure the needed data.

10. **Choosing the method of data analysis:** Depending upon the nature of the variables and the types of data collected in the research, identifying what statistical procedure(s) will be applied.

11. **Implementing the research plan:** Conducting the research as planned.

12. **Preparing the research report:** Writing the report of the research in accordance with prescribed guidelines and disseminating the findings as appropriate.

Selecting the Problem

A researcher necessarily begins any study with a problem. The selection of a research problem, however, is often a major source of anxiety and frustration for graduate students. We have observed that students typically fall into one of three categories when it comes to selecting a research problem: (1) those who know precisely what they want to do and have a well-conceived problem, (2) those who have many interest areas and are having difficulty deciding exactly what they want to study, and finally, (3) those students who do not have any idea about a worthwhile research problem. While the source of research problems will vary according to the experience of the person contemplating an investigation, it is generally agreed that the process begins with an idea or question in the mind of the researcher. The initial question or problem area is typically broad in nature, lacking the specificity required of a researchable problem. The beginning researcher, most frequently graduate students with no previous research experience, oftentimes confuses a problem with a problem area. If asked, "What are you interested in studying?" they may reply, "Well, I am interested mostly in the area of sport psychology." Or, they may mention health promotion, outdoor education, corporate fitness, exercise science, or some other problem area, but are vague as to a specific, researchable problem. Each of these problem areas contains innumerable research problems. The challenge for the researcher is to narrow the initial question or problem area to a specific problem that is amenable to research.

In HHP there are many problem areas within which exist many potential research problems. Let's consider something as broad as "basketball" as an example of a problem area for someone who has teaching/coaching aspirations. Someone interested in basketball may have the *idea* that basketball officials can be classified as inferior, superior, or average, based on a measure of their personality characteristics, knowledge of the game, previous playing experience, and previous officiating experience. This *idea* might then be translated to a specific problem to be studied (Fratzke 1973). On the other hand, another basketball enthusiast may believe that there is a definite *need* to determine the physiological fitness of officials in relation to the demand placed on them during game situations. This *need* could then be translated into a researchable problem (Holland 1970). Gaunt, in 1979, saw a *need* to study basketball skills in an attempt to compile a battery of tests that might predict basketball playing ability. Henry, in 1974, studied the shooting accuracy of third graders when the basketball goal was less than ten feet high.

There are many reasons why people engage in research. Curiosity is as good a motivational factor as any. A recent graduate student was interested in the broad problem area of dietary disorders and illnesses, specifically, anorexia nervosa and bulimia. This student was curious about where the attitude began that led to the development of these disorders in teenagers and young adults. Is it possible that the dietary problems are rooted in childhood? Such curiosity led to an excellent study in which an attempt was made to determine and compare body figure perception and preferences among male and female preadolescent children, in grades 1 through 3 in Georgia and Indiana (Collins 1989). So, from a problem area, a definitive problem was identified.

Many methods for finding worthwhile research problems have been suggested to graduate students by their professors over the years. The following list represents some of the methods which have been helpful in the past:

1. Write out your philosophy of the field of HHP in which you are studying. Divide the field into its several parts and study them. When you come to something you would like to know, but do not know, write it down for your research "hope chest."

2. In reading, in discussions, at lectures, and at all times, write down at once any hunches or ideas that come to you. Many times reading or philosophizing will reveal gaps in your present field of knowledge. Write these down. Read the best studies in your interest area. Think about a problem, and note the questions which arise. Criticize and challenge statements made in current professional periodicals, in books and research studies, and in your own and allied fields. Hundreds of research problems exist in those sources.

3. Prepare a paper on some subject that interests you and extend it into unknown realms. When you meet an obstacle in your thinking, analyze it for the problem it suggests.

4. With what in your field are you dissatisfied? What problems does it suggest? Investigate these.

5. Analyze, challenge, and criticize the popular beliefs and practices in your field of interest. You will be appalled by their unquestioned acceptance. Again, note your hunches.

6. What procedures or practices in your field interest you? Observe the problems inherent in those procedures and practices that could be researched. What problems have you observed during your work experiences? Could these be the source of a research question?

7. Browse reference and bibliographical lists in books, journals, magazines, and theses. Just running down a list of titles frequently sparks a viable idea for a research problem. Examine the lists of master's and doctoral studies done at your institution. Then, move on to the lists from other institutions or research centers.

8. Talk to your professors or other professionals that work in your interest area. You will find that most professors have an abundance of ideas about potential research problems and are eager to share them with interested students.

Several of the suggestions listed above involve the utilization of hunches. Becoming sensitive to such ideas can become a valuable mental habit. Upon inspection, most of them will not be viable research problems or will already have been studied. Occasionally, though, a hunch will lead to an important research problem that, when solved, will make a major contribution.

Defining the Problem

Once the idea for a problem has been decided upon, the student should then begin a literature search in an attempt to obtain additional background information to assist in rounding out or fully defining the problem. Fox (1969) delineated two kinds of literature that should be consulted. **Conceptual literature** includes books and articles written by experts or authorities in a problem area. Through their writing they have passed on their ideas, opinions, and theories about what is good, bad, desirable, and undesirable in the problem area. Most of the time conceptual literature is not to be considered research literature as such, but the information disseminated frequently is based on research. An article by Mull (1991) in the *Journal of Health Education* provides a good example of conceptual literature that discusses the role of the health educator in the development of self-esteem in children. Mull gave full support to the idea that self-esteem is an important part of the makeup of healthy people and used previous research to support her argument. Several concepts are presented for health educators assisting children in the development of their self-esteem.

A second type of literature is **related research.** This category includes previous studies in the problem area. Similar or related studies are reviewed to determine what is already known about the main issues inherent in the problem. Using the self-esteem example, examining previous research in that problem area would uncover what earlier work has shown about that characteristic as it relates to children.

In reality, the literature should be consulted throughout the research project. However, the majority of the review should be accomplished before the final plans for conducting the research have been completed. The first plunge into the literature will provide the neophyte researcher with a broader and deeper understanding of what facts are already known in the problem area. If a decision is made to actually investigate the problem, further review of the literature will provide helpful information on methods, techniques, instrumentation, and procedures for conducting the study.

In making the final determination as to whether or not the problem should be studied, three primary criteria should be considered:

1. **Does the problem interest you?**
   Arguably the most important criteria is your interest in the problem. It may be a splendid problem, but you should pass it by if you are not genuinely interested

in it. You should realize that you will spend anywhere from approximately six months to well over a year working on the problem. People tend to do a better job with a problem that was their own idea or something they created. Faculty advisors are sometimes reluctant to "give" a research topic to a graduate student for this reason. Even when a faculty advisor suggests a research topic, you would be advised to carefully consider the topic to insure that it interests you before proceeding with the research.

2. **Is the problem worthwhile?**

   This criterion is often difficult to judge. Most individuals believe that the problem they are studying is important and worthwhile. Ultimately, a graduate student's thesis or dissertation committee will make a statement about the value of a problem when they approve the proposed research topic. The acceptance or rejection of a manuscript for publication in a professional journal is often based on how the reviewer or editor judges the worthiness of a research problem. Does the problem and its solution make a contribution to the body of knowledge within the field of study? Oftentimes the significance of a research problem can be established through either the theoretical or practical contribution that it will make to a field. Is the research problem timely? Is there a recognized demand for a solution to the problem? Until the last twenty years there was no great demand for the solution of the world's AIDS problem. When the disease reached epidemic proportions, however, suddenly AIDS research became timely. It is incumbent upon the researcher to answer these questions affirmatively and be able to justify and provide the rationale for these answers in the research proposal or report.

3. **Is the problem manageable?**

   A researcher may have a deep interest in a particular problem, but he or she must determine if the problem is actually researchable. Moreover, it is important to select a problem that is not too large. Oftentimes a graduate student identifies a worthwhile problem in which he or she has an interest, but is unable attack the problem in a meaningful fashion because the problem is too large and complex. Whereas it is important to contribute to building the road of knowledge within a particular area, this contribution may well take the form of a grain of sand as opposed to a large boulder. This is particularly true for beginning researchers as they acquire an understanding of the research process. Does the researcher have sufficient training and expertise in the problem area to conduct the study? If not, can the expertise be acquired? Is a research problem feasible from the standpoint of time, expense, resources, and availability of data? All research studies involve certain expenses, whether they are for the purchase of electrodes, printing of questionnaires, postage, laboratory costs, travel, or the design of equipment. Who will pay these expenses? Sometimes an excellent research problem is conceived and developed only to find that the participants needed to produce the relevant data are unavailable. No subjects, no data, no study! Historical studies often require an extended period of time and can also be expensive and involve extensive travel as one seeks to obtain original materials and sources of information. Is the problem one that you can attack without prejudice? If the answer to this question is no, then it is better to pass the problem on to someone else. All researchers, beginners and veterans alike, need to be objective. Bias can creep into a study through the way participants are selected, instrumentation is developed, and procedures conducted. While it is desirable to have a strong conviction, letting this conviction mediate one's research efforts to the point of introducing bias in a study is out of place.

Another helpful exercise in defining one's problem, especially for the beginner in research, is to prepare an outline of the problem. Such an outline is usually created after the first review of the literature has been completed. The outline task will enable the student to think through the research problem from beginning to end. The process involves determining what research questions need to be answered as a result of investigating the problem. The questions, in turn, imply what data need to be collected, what methods need to be employed to collect it, and what statistical techniques need to be used to analyze it. The following is an example of such an outline of the problem as prepared for a causal-comparative study.

Outline of the Problem

I. *Topic:* **Student Attrition at the College Level**

II. *Statement of the Problem.* **The problem was to determine the extent to which students in teacher education programs drop out of college, the reasons for their dropping out, and the relationship of various facts to loss of enrollment.**

III. *Results of Previous Studies*

IV. *Questions to be Answered*
   A. What is the extent of the attrition?
   B. What is the nature of the attrition? (That is, among various groups of students?)
   C. What are the causes of the attrition?
   D. What is the relationship of the cause of attrition to each type of attrition?
   E. Are there any factors that explain the causes of attrition?

V. *Collection of Data*
   A. What specific questions need to be answered?
      1. What is the extent of the attrition?

Outline of the Problem—*Continued*

(a) In each semester or year?

(b) Among students matriculated for each degree?

(c) Among majors in each of various areas?

2. What is the nature of the attrition among what groups?

(a) Students entering at different ages?

(b) Boys and girls?

(c) Students in the different types of high school programs offering different patterns of entrance units?

(d) Students at different scholarship levels?

(e) Students of different intelligence levels?

(f) Veterans and nonveterans?

(g) Students with deficiencies in college entrance requirements?

(h) Combinations of the above?

3. To what extent is attrition due to:

(a) Poor scholarship?

(b) Economic reasons?

(c) Personal (other than economic) reasons?

(d) Personality (emotional) difficulties?

4. What is the relationship of the causes of attrition to each of the categories under VA?

5. Are there any particular causes for attrition due to:

(a) Poor scholarship?

(b) Economic reasons?

(c) Other personal reasons?

(d) Personality difficulties?

(e) Other reasons?

B. What data need to be obtained? and

C. What methods should be employed to obtain these data?

1. Obtain the official college record for each student who was dropped or resigned during the last five years.

2. Select record cards of all students who entered in August of the years 1992–1996.

3. Prepare a code for the following:

(a) Reason for being dropped or resigning

Outline of the Problem—*Concluded*

    (b) Class

    (c) Level at which student left college (lower freshman, etc.)

    (d) Achievement record at time of separation

    (e) Age at entrance

    (f) Sex

    (g) Type of high school program completed

    (h) High school achievement

    (i) Degree for which matriculated

    (j) College major

    (k) Entrance deficiencies

    (l) Veteran or nonveteran

VI. *Statistical Treatment to Which Data Need to Be Subjected*

  A. Tabulation of number of cases of separation for each of the five class groups by:

    1. Class level at time of separation

    2. Degree for which matriculated

    3. Major

    4. Other traits listed under VA

  B. Computation of appropriate means, percents, and other measures needed for interpretation of data.

  C. Preparation of a table for each item or group of items listed in VA.

VII. *Interpretation of Data*

VIII. *Conclusions*

The outline process helps solidify thinking about the problem. Many important details are less apt to be forgotten if this task is carried out conscientiously.

Developing the Research Proposal

The final definition of the problem occurs when the graduate student develops a research proposal for the thesis or dissertation that is being planned. In most instances the proposal consists of three chapters: introduction, review of related literature, and procedures for collecting data. Those three chapters ultimately become the first three chapters of a thesis. It is in the first chapter that the final definition of the problem is noted. Before discussing the content in chapter 1 in detail, a few words about the title of the research project are appropriate.

Proposal Title

Quite frequently, the title of the research project is the last decision made by the researcher. All proposals will be titled, but the name given to the project at this time is considered only temporary. It may be changed several times before being finalized. The title is important in that it is the first thing the reader sees. Based on the title, the reader will continue reading or lose interest. A brief title, one that is streamlined, is currently preferred. This title is too long:

> An Analysis of the Specific Curriculum Content for the Preparation of Recreation Majors and the Relationship between the Details of the Curriculum and the Details of the Majors' On-the-Job Duties

Not only is this title overly long, it also includes some redundancy and is confusing. The title should be long enough to cover the subject of the research, but short enough to be interesting. Usually, twelve to fourteen words is sufficient. The beginning researcher should ask these questions when contemplating a project title:

1. Does the title precisely identify the area of the problem?
2. Is the title clear, concise, and adequately descriptive to permit indexing the study in its proper category?
3. Does the title indentify the key variables and provide some information about the scope of the study?
4. Are unnecessary words avoided, such as "an analysis of," "a comparison of," "a study of," "the effect of," and "the relationship between"? (*Note:* These words and other catchy, misleading, and vague phrases unnecessarily lengthen titles and do nothing to add substance. They are superfluous.)
5. Do nouns, as opposed to adjectives, serve as the key words in the title?
6. Are the most important words placed at the beginning of the title?

Following are some examples of appropriate titles:

1. Self-Consciousness and Physical Self-Efficacy in Relationship to Exercise Adherence (Visker 1986)
2. Group Cohesiveness and Team Success Among Women's Intercollegiate Basketball Teams (Cotter 1978)
3. Body Figure Perceptions and Preferences Among Preadolescent Children (Collins 1989)

4. Special Olympics Participation and Self-Esteem of Adults with Mental Retardation (Major 1998)

5. A Health Knowledge Test for Male College Freshmen in Saudi Arabia (Hashim 1988)

All of these titles meet the criteria for a streamlined, yet complete, title. Each accurately reflects the research problem.

Writing Chapter 1: Introduction

Chapter 1 of the proposal usually begins with a brief introduction. Customarily, the researcher includes a paragraph or two (perhaps more, depending on the nature of the problem) to help lead the reader into the problem. The researcher specifies the problem being investigated, provides the underlying rationale and establishes why it is important. How the researcher became interested in the problem is usually indicated. Some references to the literature should be made in the introduction, although it should not be so extensive to resemble a review of literature, which is more properly done in chapter 2. The literature cited in the introduction, coupled with the researcher's own thoughts, should be used to stimulate interest and to establish the underlying rationale for the study. Again, it is not necessary that this section be long. Following are two examples that illustrate the essence of introductory sections:

1. The three major points of emphasis in the field hockey drive according to most coaches and authors are (1) quickness, (2) power, and (3) accuracy. In particular game situations, a player may desire to sacrifice some accuracy to execute the drive as quickly as possible, or he/she may choose to sacrifice some power to achieve a more accurate pass. What differences, if any, exist in the mechanics of the field hockey drive under various conditions? It was the nature of this question that prompted this investigation (Hendrick 1981).

2. Obesity is prevalent in our society and its treatment is constantly being explored. All proper weight loss programs for the moderately obese include aerobic exercise as well as dietary restriction. Obese individuals are often told to exercise two or three times a day for short periods in order to burn more calories. The goal of exercise is to mobilize fats from adipose tissue stores for energy production. It is, however, not known if this is the most effective method of achieving weight loss. The optimal exercise prescription for the moderately obese has not been determined. This study, then, examined the duration of exercise in an attempt to determine the most effective exercise prescription for moderately obese women (Sun 1988).

Statement of the Problem. Immediately after the introductory comments, the **problem statement** should appear. This will always be a declarative statement that indicates what question or issue was addressed in the research project. The problem should be stated clearly, concisely, and definitively. All of the problem elements, including the variables to be studied, should be expressed in an orderly system of relationships. The statement results from the researcher's analysis of all of the facts and explanations that might possibly be related to the problem. Typically, the statement of the problem begins in a manner similar to one of the following:

1. "The problem of the study was to . . ."
2. "The study was concerned with . . ."
3. "The focus of the research was on the . . ."

Although it is sometimes seen, the phrase "The study investigated . . ." is not a good choice. Inanimate objects cannot take action; hence, a study cannot investigate.

Following are a few examples of problem statements that meet the criteria for clarity and conciseness:

1. The problem was to investigate the influence of cohesiveness on the team success of women's intercollegiate basketball teams (Cotter 1978).
2. The problem was to apply the Feldt (1975) and Kristof (1974) formulas to motor performance tests consisting of several trials in order to compare the resulting estimates of reliability with those obtained by currently recommended methods (Frye 1977).
3. The problem of the study was to determine if the psychological facts of self-consciousness and physical self-efficacy discriminate between female adults who adhere to exercise programs and female adults who do not adhere to exercise programs (Visker 1986).

Purpose of the Study.　　The **purpose statement** must indicate *why* the study was done. Again, brevity is stressed. The researcher spells out the reason(s) or objective(s) for doing the study and answers the question, "What potential impact will the results of the study have on the current body of knowledge?" The problem and purpose are often confused by research neophytes and veterans alike. Consider the following:

1. The problem tells *what* was done in the study (i.e., what was tested, determined, effected, compared, analyzed, evaluated, etc.).

   The purpose tells *why* the study was done. What good could possibly come out of the study? How will the findings be used or applied?

2. It is incorrect under the problem statement to say, "The purpose of the study was to . . ." It is also incorrect in a purpose statement to say that the purpose of the study was to test, to determine, to analyze, or to compare something. Such a statement is a problem statement. Just remember that the purpose tells why you want to test, determine, analyze, or compare.

This example illustrates the difference between the two statements:

Statement of the Problem. The problem of the study was to evaluate five options of coping with smoking in the workplace: (1) improvement of ventilation, (2) installation of air-cleaning devices, (3) segregation of smokers and nonsmokers, (4) smoking only in designated areas, and (5) a total smoking ban. Included in the study was an attempt to identify the effects of these options on the economical and productivity aspects while an acceptable indoor air quality was maintained. (Padilla 1986)

Purpose of the Study. The purpose of the study was to provide employers with guidelines to initiate or improve smoking policies in the workplace. (Padilla 1986)

Following is the purpose statement for the cohesiveness problem previously mentioned:

> If cohesiveness is a significant factor in predicting team success, coaches should devote greater time, effort, and personnel to the development and cultivation of group cohesion. If low cohesiveness is a better predictor of success, coaches may seek to increase success by generating conflict among players. Cohesiveness may not show any prediction ability for team success, in which case the time and energy of the coach would be better spent on other aspects of coaching. (Cotter 1978)

In the body perception and preference study discussed earlier, the reason or purpose for doing the study was given as follows:

> If concerns for thinness and weight loss are occurring among children of normal weight, health education intervention and prevention strategies must be addressed at earlier ages than has been believed previously. It was believed that the information provided in the study would assist in targeting the age at which health education for counteracting an unrealistic standard of attractiveness should begin. (Collins 1989)

Significance of the Study (Need for the Study). This section of chapter 1 follows the purpose statement, and its function is to elaborate on the purpose. Moreover, this section serves to further establish the underlying rationale for the study and to justify its need. One of the two section headings listed above should be selected. Which of the two is most appropriate will depend upon (1) the nature of the study, (2) the reasons the study was undertaken, and (3) the researcher's preference. Use the literature to help show why the study is needed, to explain why it is significant, or to justify its content. This is the place to present examples of how the problem has manifested itself in society. The development of this section will attempt to show that one or more of the following is true:

1. Knowledge gaps exist between the theoretical and practical aspects of the problem.

2. More and better knowledge is needed in the problem areas.

3. Present knowledge in the problem area needs validation.

4. Current practices concerning the problem need to be clarified.

5. A solution to the problem needs to be found.

The following example of a need for the study section appeared in a research proposal in which the problem was to determine the impact of rotation from day shift to periodic night shift work on nurses' performance and frequency of medication errors during the night shift sessions:

> Medical accident and error statistics continue to reflect significant numbers of accidental injury, fatalities, and inadequate care related to improper dosage and/or route of administration of medicines in medical care facilities (Smith 1990). Further evidence indicates that nurses rotating to night shift work from other shifts are likely to encounter biorhythm interference that adversely affects performance (Klein and Bruce 1989). Management knowledge of hazards has been recognized as a key element in the prevention of various industrial accidents (Accident Prevention Manual for Industrial Operation 1981). This includes work environments such as nursing. Medication error rates will continue to be a major problem in health care settings until proper countermeasures are identified and controls are instituted to reduce occurrence. Therefore, management action through knowledge is essential to correct the situation. The focus of this study was to provide an accurate assessment of the relationship between night shift rotation and medication errors which should lead to a more informed management. This information could provide new insight into shift workers' performance and contribute toward better decisions on shift rotation assignments in the future. (Welcher 1991)

Delimitations.   In research circles, **delimitations** refers to the scope of the study. It is in this section of chapter 1 that the researcher draws a line around the study and, in effect, "fences it in." This segment identifies what is included in the research. Delimitations spell out the population studied and include those things the researcher can control. It establishes the parameters on such characteristics of the study as (1) number and kinds of subjects, (2) number and kinds of variables, (3) tests, measures, or instruments utilized in the study, (4) special equipment, (5) type of training program, (6) the time and duration of the study (e.g., date, number of weeks, time of year), and (7) analytical procedures. These are the ingredients that the researcher uses to attack the problem. If an item does not appear in the list of delimitations, then it is of no concern in the research. A particular population is targeted on which selected variables will be studied. The variables will be measured by specific test instruments. A certain training program may be involved and the study will be conducted over a specified period of time. Following is an example of the delimitations that appeared in a proposal for studying an obesity problem (Sun 1988):

The study was delimited to:

1. Thirty moderately obese and previously sedentary women subjects, aged 25–55, who had been obese for at least five years and were free of any diagnosed metabolic or cardiovascular disease.

2. The subjects were randomly assigned to one of three groups as follows: Exercise Group One; Exercise Group Two; Control Group.

3. All subjects followed a daily diet of 500 calories less than their current weight maintenance diet using dietary exchanges. The diets were well balanced and nutritionally adequate with the contribution of nutrients as follows: 12–15 percent protein, 50–55 percent carbohydrate, and 30–35 percent fat. Three-day food diaries and 24-hour recalls were used for diet analyses.

4. Exercise groups walked at 50–60 percent of maximal heart rate reserve, four days per week for six months.

5. Exercise Group One walked 30 minutes twice a day and Exercise Group Two walked 60 minutes a day. The Control Group did not participate in any formal exercise program.

6. Three of the exercise sessions per week were under the supervision of the Indiana University Adult Fitness Program. The other exercise sessions were supervised by the investigator.

7. Percent body fat was determined by skinfold measurements, circumferences, and hydrostatic weighing. All measurements were performed by the investigator.

8. Pretraining and posttraining concentrations of plasma FFA, glycerol, and lipolytic hormones (epinephrine, norepinephrine, adrenocorticotropin, triiodothyronine, tetraiodothyronine, growth hormone, glucagon, and insulin) concentrations were obtained from blood samples taken at 0, 10, 20, 30, 40, 50, 60, and 90 minutes of exercise or rest.

9. The study was conducted for a period of six months between February and August, 1988.

The section on delimitations in the research proposal does not have to be excessively long, but it should specify those parameters of the research proposal that the researcher can control. Typically, a proposal would list 5 to 10 delimitations. Another example of delimitations taken from a study to ascertain the realtionship between self-esteem, eating behaviors, and eating attitudes among female collegiate swimmers is presented below:

1. Twenty-four female collegiate swimmers, ages 18 to 21.

2. A purposive sample consisting of members of the University of _____ women's simming team during Spring 1988.

3. The use of the Rosenburg Self-Esteem Scale (1965) to measure self-esteem.

4. The use of the Eating Attitudes Tests (EAT-26) of the National Eating Disorders Screening Program to measure the construct and concerns characteristic of an eating disorder.

5. Administration of the data collection instruments during a single testing session held during a team meeting of the swimming team immediately following completion of the collegiate swimming season.

Limitations. In research terminology **limitations** refer to weaknesses of the study. All studies have them because compromises frequently have to be made in order to conform to the realities of a situation. Limitations are those things the researcher could not control, but that may have influenced the results of the study. The reader of a research report should always know at the outset those conditions of the study that could reflect negatively on the work in some way. Only those things that might affect the acceptability of the research data should be presented. The researcher will, of course, try to eliminate extremely serious weaknesses before the study is commenced. Among the items that typically involve statements of limitation are the following:

1. The research approach, design, method(s), and techniques
2. Sampling problems
3. Uncontrolled variables
4. Faulty administration of tests or training programs
5. Generalizability of the data
6. Representativeness of subjects
7. Compromises to internal and external validity
8. Reliability and validity of the research instruments

It is important that all statements of limitation sound like, or imply, weakness. The statement, "The sample size was small," is not sufficient, because a small sample does not necessarily assume a weakness of the study. However, the statement, "The sample size of the study ($N = 30$) is small, necessitating caution in extrapolation of the data to a larger obese population," implies a possible weakness of the study. Whereas the number of limitations listed will vary depending upon the nature of the study, the research design, and the methodology utilized, it is generally recommended that the number of limitations be less than the number of delimitations presented. While it is important that the researcher recognize from the outset potential weaknesses of the study, an exceedingly long list of limitations raises serious questions about why so many facets of the research were not controlled, thus questioning the overall veracity of the research.

The limitations of the obesity study were presented as follows.

The study was limited by:

1. The sample size of this study is small ($N = 30$) necessitating caution in extrapolation of the data to a larger obese population.
2. Daily activities of the subjects other than the exercise program were not controlled.
3. Although subjects were requested to stay on a diet that was well balanced and restricted by 500 calories a day, occasional variance from this could not be controlled. In addition, due to the nature of the diet analyses performed, changes in caloric intake may not have been detected.
4. The investigator was unable to personally conduct all of the maximal graded exercise tests in pretraining and posttraining as well as the exercise sessions. To insure standardization in testing and training, she met with the staff of the Indiana University Adult Fitness Program in order to discuss the testing and training procedures.

5. Resting metabolic rate was not measured following the exercise sessions and lipolytic changes during this time could not be determined.

6. Since plasma FFA, glycerol, and lipolytic hormones can be affected by conditions other than exercise, it is possible that such conditions did exist.

7. Plasma FFA do not reflect FFA flux in adipose or skeletal muscle tissue and, therefore, conclusions concerning fat metabolism must be interpreted with caution. (Sun 1988)

Assumptions.   **Assumptions** are derived primarily from the literature. Assumptions then become the basis for the hypotheses, or predictions of eventual outcome, of the study. In other words, what does the literature tell the researcher that can be assumed to be true for purposes of planning the study? The information gleaned from the literature frequently serves as the basis for much of the development of the research project. The literature provides information about a particular behavior being investigated and the various conditions influencing that behavior, and sometimes contains factual evidence explaining the behavior. The researcher undertakes a study with certain assumptions about this information. Assumptions are also made about the way the instrumentation, procedures, methods, and techniques will contribute to the study. In a study that involved teaching the overhand throwing pattern to children, the following assumptions were made:

1. The maturational and environmental influences are unique to each child.

2. The throwing force of children increases with age due primarily to improved coordination.

3. A mature throwing pattern conforms to mechanically correct execution patterns.

4. Distributed practice is essential in the proper learning of motor skills.

5. Elementary school children have limited information and are able to handle only a few items at a time.

6. A child's information processing abilities improve with age, experience, and training. (Luedke 1980)

The researcher may also assume that certain things that could not be controlled or documented may have happened in the study. The following are examples of this type of assumption:

1. All subjects completed the questionnaire honestly and correctly.

2. The subjects complied with the researcher's request to perform maximally on all trials of the test.

3. The test instrument was a reliable and valid measure of self-esteem.

Hypotheses.   The following provides a second example of assumptions made by the author of a study designed to investigate the effects of participation in Special Olympics on the self-esteem of adults with mental retardation:

1. The test instrument, as modified, was appropriate for the target population and was a valid and reliable measure of self-esteem.

2. The subjects understood the directions as they were intended.

3. The subjects completed the self-esteem inventory to the best of their ability.

4. The subjects were a representative sample of adults with mental retardation who reside in the state of Iowa.

5. The interviewers were sufficiently trained and capable of utilizing the recommended survey administration procedures.

This section of chapter 1 permits the researcher to predict the outcome of the study in advance, and to present tentative explanations for the solution of the problem. The assumptions made by the researcher provide the launching pad for hypotheses. A simple research hypothesis can be written as a single sentence in which the researcher describes the expected outcome. Consider the following examples of simple research hypotheses:

Example: There is a positive relationship between the level of intrinsic motivation and performance on a test of cardio-respiratory function.

Example: There is a difference in the self-reported alcohol usage of male collegiate athletes compared to female collegiate athletes.

Normally, a statement of hypothesis will be declared for each research question posed, although some descriptive questions may not warrant hypotheses. It is important to note that because of space limitations in some professional journals, authors often do not explicitly present their research hypotheses in the published research reports, although such hypotheses may be implied in the paper and undoubtedly have been made by the researcher. On the other hand, graduate students preparing their research proposal or writing their dissertation or thesis are normally expected to explicitly state their research hypotheses in clear, unambiguous terms. Stating hypotheses helps to make a researcher's thought process about the research situation more concrete. If a prediction of a specific outcome is made, this forces more thorough consideration of which research techniques, methods, test instruments, and data-collecting procedures should be employed. It is extremely important that the hypotheses be testable. Hypotheses also help set up the way the data will be analyzed and how the final report will be organized and written. A more detailed discussion about hypotheses is presented in chapter 3. Following is an example of hypotheses presented in a therapeutic recreation study (Pate 1987) to determine the effect of sea kayak touring on the self-concept of patients with low-level spinal cord injuries (SCI):

1. Patients with a low level of SCI of at least one-year duration exhibit an increased self-concept after participation in a two-week sea kayak tour.

2. Increased self-concept changes are significantly greater for those patients participating in the sea kayak tour than patients participating in a two-week camping experience or a regular rehabilitation program.

3. Self-concept does not change for those patients participating in a two-week camping experience or in a regular rehabilitation program.

4. For those patients participating in the sea kayak tour, self-concept remains elevated for six months after completion of the tour.

Definition of Terms.   **Definition of terms** is a necessity since many terms and concepts have multiple meanings. The researcher should define terms as they will be interpreted and used throughout the study. Always define operational and behavioral terms and concepts, and check special terms in technical dictionaries or have them reviewed by experts in the field. An operational definition gives meaning to a concept or term by indicating what operation has to be accomplished so as to be able to measure the concept. In experimental studies a researcher will cause a particular result to occur by using a certain procedure or operation. An operational definition of personality might refer to the "scores on the Cattell 16 Personality Factor Inventory" or some other personality test selected by the researcher. Directly quoted or accurately paraphrased time-honored definitions, if they fit the research situation, are considered superior to definitions made up or "coined" by the researcher. Once defined, a term should be applied consistently throughout the study so as not to confuse the reader. It is customary to alphabetize the terms in a list of operational definitions. Following is an example of a partial list of terms defined in a study of women victims of sexual coercion (Ogletree 1991):

> For consistency of interpretation the following terms are defined:
>
> *Acquaintance Rape*. "A forced sexual intercourse that occurs either on a date or between individuals who are acquaintances or romantically involved" (Meyer 1984, 2). This term excludes incest, authority rapes, spousal rape, and rape of children under age 14. This phenomenon is also called "date rape."
>
> *Assertiveness*. "A response, direct and specific, to an aggressive act" (Bakker and Bakker-Rabdau 1973, 59).
>
> *Self-esteem*. "A positive or negative attitude toward a particular object, namely the self" (Rosenberg 1965).
>
> *Sexual Coercion*. "Sexual intercourse subsequent to the use of menacing verbal pressure or misuse of authority" (Koss et al. 1987, 163) or attempted rape or rape.

The Use of Literature in Research

As discussed earlier, the literature is a big help in providing the beginning researcher with an initial understanding of the facts in the problem area. The information gained from the preliminary excursion into the literature helps to round out the problem. As the problem planning continues, the literature search becomes increasingly more pointed and specific. Related research becomes critical. Studies related to the proposed study are sought out in terms of problem, variable, and population similarity. The researcher will attempt to find out just how far human inquiry into the problem has progressed. What is known and what is not known concerning the problem? Are there any gaps in the literature with respect to the relevant information surrounding the problem? These questions can be answered by a thorough literature search.

The researcher will also become knowledgeable about methodology and procedures for attacking the problem, as well as ideas on instrumentation and design. Conceptual and theoretical relationships among the essential variables will be found. A major outcome of the search is that the researcher will develop a theoretical basis for the study and justification for its conduct. It has often been said that the more sound and thorough knowledge of the previous research, the better will be the planning of subsequent study in the problem area. As noted by Bookwalter and Bookwalter (1959) almost fifty years ago, "Knowledge of the literature in the field and critical insight into the research in the student's major field of interest is considered evidence of high scholarship."

It is recommended that the literature be searched by looking at the most current literature first, then working backward in time. This will familiarize the researcher with the newer methods, techniques, procedures, instrumentation, and data analysis designs that have been developed in the problem area. Chances are better that mistakes made in previous studies will have been corrected, old theories revised, new ones postulated, and more sophisticated designs developed. Again, all background reading should be completed before final plans for conducting the study are made.

Searching the literature is hard and demanding work. It is absolutely essential that graduate students contemplating a research project for the first time build plenty of library time into their schedules. The literature search can be a frustrating and not particularly romantic task. However, it can be exciting to increase the knowledge base on the topic to be researched. One of the more frustrating occurrences for the beginner is to discover that the proposed study, or closely related study, has already been done. In this situation the researcher must weigh the merits of replicating the previous study or of revising the proposed study to attack a different part of the overall problem.

The Working Bibliography

Once the literature search has identified promising sources, the researcher creates a **working bibliography,** a listing of all sources that are pertinent to the problem. People differ in their methods for developing a bibliography. Some prefer to record the information on 3" x 5" or 4" x 6" index cards, others record the information on notepads or writing tablets, and others may elect to use a computerized reference database such as EndNote®. Whatever the method, it is important to accurately note all the bibliographic information for each source. Typically, this information includes the author's last name and initials; title of the journal article, book, report, or review; volume or issue number, year, and month of the journal; publisher of the book; date of publication; edition; page numbers of the article or book reference; library call number; and the Internet address (URL) of an on-line source.

Research Reading

After the working bibliography has been completed, the sources have to be located. The majority of sources will probably be found in professional journals, although books, monographs, dissertations, reports, and Internet sites may also provide relevant information. The task of locating the desired references is usually accomplished through the use of the card catalog in the library, which is divided into a subject list and an author list. Most college and university libraries have developed computerized catalogs that list information about books, magazines, journals, newspapers, and other regularly published periodicals and serials that these libraries hold. Locating information on the World Wide Web (WWW) usually requires the use of some form of Internet search utility, including subject directories, search engines, and metasearch engines. A more thorough discussion of using the Internet as a source of information is presented later in this chapter.

Once a source is located, the researcher studies it to evaluate its potential value to the proposed research. This is done by quickly reading the description of the source and by scanning the table of contents, index, and chapter summaries, or abstract if an article. Even though a title may seem to indicate that the content will be useful, frequently it is not. As the scanning process continues, the working bibliography will change. Some references will be thrown out because they hold no promise of being helpful, while new ones may well be discovered that will be of use. The research focus may even change as the study develops. This in turn, would render changes in the working bibliography. During this critical review of the literature, note taking is kept very brief, since the primary purpose is to judge the appropriateness of the various sources for the research problem.

When it has been determined which sources will be valuable to the proposed study, each one must be read in depth. Bookwalter and Bookwalter (1959) referred to this process as **critical reading** or gleaning. This means reading a large amount of material while at the same time thinking about, reflecting upon, and analyzing what is being said. While doing critical reading it is essential that the researcher take notes. This has been referred to as developing an annotated bibliography. Even today, with the widespread availability of computers and other electronic equipment, the use of index cards for note taking remains a time-honored method for abstracting the article or report. The first card for each source will contain all the relevant bibliographic information. Each additional card will contain source notes pertaining to the items that have a close relationship to the proposed research. Particular attention should be given to the problem, hypotheses, procedures, findings, and discussion or implications. Figure 2.1 is an example of a note card containing the type of information usually recorded. Computerized bibliographic applications such as EndNote® generally include a notes or abstract field within the database that may be used to record pertinent information from the article or report.

Notes should be taken only from the sources most pertinent to the current problem of interest. In transcribing notes from the source to the cards or electronic database, use extreme care to ensure accuracy. If any of the information will be

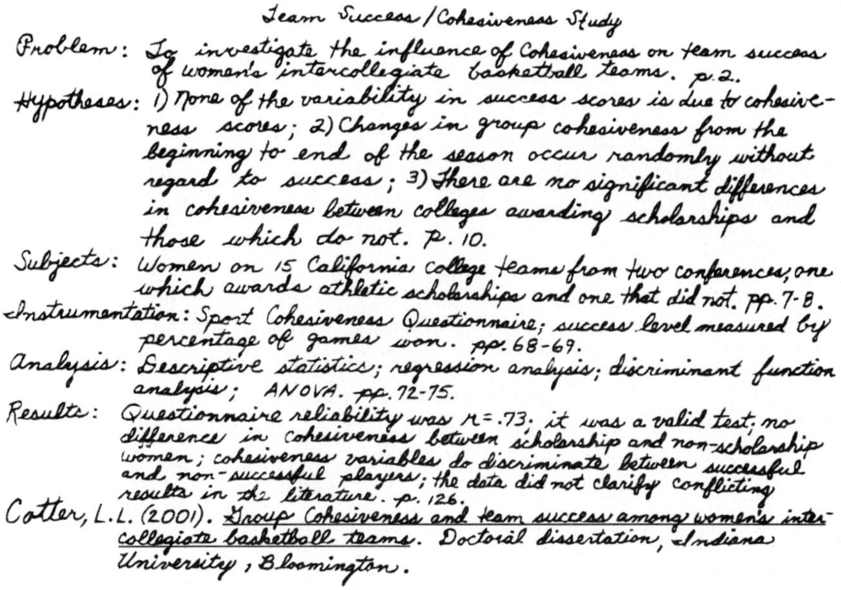

Team Success/Cohesiveness Study

Problem: To investigate the influence of cohesiveness on team success of women's intercollegiate basketball teams. p. 2.

Hypotheses: 1) None of the variability in success scores is due to cohesiveness scores; 2) Changes in group cohesiveness from the beginning to end of the season occur randomly without regard to success; 3) There are no significant differences in cohesiveness between colleges awarding scholarships and those which do not. P. 10.

Subjects: Women on 15 California college teams from two conferences; one which awards athletic scholarships and one that did not. pp. 7-8.

Instrumentation: Sport Cohesiveness Questionnaire; success level measured by percentage of games won. pp. 68-69.

Analysis: Descriptive statistics; regression analysis; discriminant function analysis; ANOVA. pp. 72-75.

Results: Questionnaire reliability was r = .73; it was a valid test; no difference in cohesiveness between scholarship and non-scholarship women; cohesiveness variables do discriminate between successful and non-successful players; the data did not clarify conflicting results in the literature. p. 126.

Cotter, L.L. (2001). Group cohesiveness and team success among women's intercollegiate basketball teams. Doctoral dissertation, Indiana University, Bloomington.

FIGURE 2.1
Sample research note card.

quoted directly when it appears in the research paper, use quotation marks to identify those items on the cards. Note page numbers accurately.

After the notes have been taken from all relevant and pertinent sources, they should be sorted and classified. The researcher should gain insight into agreements, differences, relationships, and trends as a result of this process. When two or more literary sources do not agree, both sides of the issue should be noted. Beginning researchers sometimes have the mistaken idea that they should seek out only those hypotheses, findings, and conclusions with which they agree.

While notes gathered from reading usually will be the most profitable, notes from speeches, lectures, class discussions, interviews, letters, and taped television programs can also represent related literature sources. The point is that no stone should be left unturned during the literature search. The annotated bibliography is an excellent mechanism for establishing control over a large amount of material. It is recognized that in this age of the copy machine and the highlighter pen, many graduate students will be tempted to duplicate book chapters and journal articles and highlight appropriate information. With the increasing popularity of the Internet, temptation exists to simply print out relevant information. This is a common way of "taking notes" today. Moreover, it is possible to use an article reproduction service such as UnCover (http://uncweb.carl.org) to obtain photocopies on a fee basis for articles not otherwise available. It is recommended, however, that photocopying be limited to only the key articles or reports, otherwise the expense becomes too great and the task of handling hundreds of sheets of paper becomes onerous.

Writing Chapter 2: Literature Review

After the literature has been thoroughly reviewed, the researcher will then organize the notes and transpose them into a chapter 2, which is usually called the "Review of Related Literature," "Related Literature," or "Literature." This section should be a well-organized chapter that consists of an insightful analysis and evaluation of each research source as it relates to the objectives of the current study. The literature review helps to justify the study. A careful analysis of related studies is important in verifying the worth of the study and in helping to establish the overall justification. Only those studies that have a significant relationship to the current problem should be included. It is also important to note that all references located will not be included in this chapter. Some will not be used at all or will be used in other chapters.

The review of literature should not merely present previous studies in chronological order, leaving it to the reader to assimilate the facts and to draw relationships between the cited research and the problem. Above all, the literature review should not be presented as a series of abstracts of various studies. Facts and theories should be presented and their relationships shown. Gaps in the existing knowledge in the problem area should surface.

Researchers vary in the way they organize the literature, but two methods are more common than others. In one, the sources are divided into literature related to the present study in content, and literature related in method. Discussion of the content literature will present relevant facts, theories, hypotheses, and background kinds of information. Method-related literature covers such items as design, techniques, instrumentation, and analysis.

A second method is to sort and classify the literature according to topics. For example, in the study "Two Speeds of Isokinetic Exercise as Related to the Vertical Jump Performance of Women" (Van Oteghen 1973) the literature reviewed was organized under the following topic headings:

1. Strength testing reliability of women

2. Nature of the vertical jump

3. Validity and reliability of vertical jump testing

4. Effects of weight training programs on vertical jump performance

5. Isokinetic training

6. Isokinetic training related to strength development

7. Summary

The introduction to chapter 2 should always contain an opening paragraph that relates the literature to the problem and explains how the chapter is organized. Following is an example from Collins's (1989) study:

The literature related to perception of bodily attractiveness in American culture is reported in this chapter. For organizational purposes, the literature is presented under the following topics: (1) Body Image and Self-Esteem, (2) Attractiveness in American Culture, (3) Influence of the Mass Media, (4) The Thin Standard of Bodily Attractiveness for Women, (5) Impact of the Thin Standard, (6) Body Dissatisfaction in Non-Clinical Populations, (7) Measurement of Body Image, and (8) Summary.

Chapter 2 is the only one in the proposal that may need a summary. It appears as the last section of the chapter and should be relatively brief. An attempt should be made to, in sum, indicate what the literature has told us. What is it that we know? Don't know? What gaps need to be filled? The summary should not be used to report or present any more specific references to the literature; this should already have been done in detail. Instead, the summary should be a series of statements that tie all of the previous reporting together. The following example (Hendrick 1981) illustrates the function of a summary.

> The majority of publications reviewed on the field hockey drive were considered conceptual. In addition, much of the information obtained from these sources was contradictory and inconclusive. Phrases like, the hands are to be placed 'close together,' the stick is to be held 'firm,' 'a strong forward foot,' and wrists should be 'cocked slightly,' but remain 'firm,' are just a few examples of the ambiguity that existed. How close is close? How firm is firm? Does 'cocked' mean flexed or extended? What is a 'strong foot'?

> Each author seemed to have his or her own viewpoint on the execution of the field hockey drive. There were no two descriptions that were completely alike. The two research studies available also led to inconclusive generalizations. There is definitely a large gap in the literature as to the components of the optimal field hockey drive. Cohen (1969) summed up the information well when she concluded that more research must be done in order to formulate any generalizations regarding the execution of the field hockey drive.

Sources of Literature

The first step in acquiring literature resource materials is to determine if they exist. It is necessary that students become familiar with the large range of references that are frequently housed in both public and academic libraries. Invariably, students will benefit from the assistance that can be provided by the reference librarians who are only too willing to help. These people are professionals who possess a sound knowledge of what sources are available and how to locate them.

Indexes.   Indexes provide a valuable resource for locating related literature. The *Education Index* includes comprehensive author and subject guides to educational literature from most significant American sources. The *Reader's Guide to Periodical Literature* leads to content in the mainstream popular magazines and journals. The *Physical Education Index* contains subject entries for nearly two hundred journals, including some foreign publications. Articles from journals representing almost all of the areas comprising HHP can be found in this index. The *Bibliographic Index of Health Education Periodicals (BIHEP)* is a comprehensive index to the professional literature through 1983 in the areas of Health Education, Health Business, Health Promotion, and the Social Aspects of Health. Other indexes frequently used by HHP researchers include the following:

Indices Medicus. Subject-author index of over two thousand biomedical journals.

Palmer's Index to the Times (London), 1790–1941. Indexes early period of the *Times*.

Engineering Index, 1884–date. Guide to engineering literature of the world.

U.S. Superintendent of Documents. United States government publications: Monthly Catalog 1895–date.

Book Review Digest, 1905–date. Excerpts from reviews of current books published in the United States.

Dramatic Index, 1909–1949. Index to articles on drama.

New York Times Index, 1912–date. Master key to news.

Industrial Arts Index, 1914–1957. A subject index to periodicals in the fields of business, finance, applied science, and technology.

Public Affairs Information Service (PAIS), 1915–date. A monthly index to books, current periodicals, government documents, and pamphlets pertaining to economics and public affairs.

Psychological Abstracts, 1927–date. A monthly bibliography listing new books and articles grouped by subjects, with a signed abstract of each item.

Applied Science and Technology Index, 1958–date. A cumulative subject index to periodicals in the fields of aeronautics, automation, chemistry, construction, electricity and electrical communications, engineering, geology and metallurgy, industrial and mechanical arts, machinery, physics, transportation, and related subjects.

Business Periodicals Index, 1958–date. A cumulative subject index to periodicals in the fields of accounting, advertising, banking and finance, general business, insurance, labor and management, marketing and purchasing, office management, public administration, taxations, specific businesses, industries, and trades.

Wall Street Journal Index, 1958–date. A monthly index with annual cumulation.

Biological and Agricultural Index, 1964–date. A cumulative subject index to periodicals in the fields of biology, agriculture, and related sciences. (Formerly the *Agricultural Index.*)

Social Sciences and Humanities Index, 1965–date. A quarterly guide to periodical literature in the social sciences and humanities. (Formerly the *International Index.*)

Current Index to Journals in Education. (CIJE) 1969–date. Monthly.

Dissertation Abstracts. University Microfilms, Inc. Monthly.

Research Quarterly Index. References in physical education, exercise, and sport. Yearly.

Reviews. Another excellent means by which to begin a literature search is to utilize the many reviews that are available. There are several in the areas of health and human performance (HHP) and others exist in the fields of education, psychology, physiology, and sociology. The following is a representative list of such reviews:

Exercise and Sport Reviews

Physical Fitness Digest

What Research Tells the Coach

Encyclopedia of Physical Education, Fitness and Sport

Science and Medicine of Exercise and Sport

Annual Review of Physiology

Annual Review of Psychology

Athletic Performance Review

Review of Educational Research

Encyclopedia of Educational Research

Annual Review of Public Health

Periodicals. As the fields of HHP have become specialized by several subdisciplines, the number of periodicals has increased dramatically. Added to those available in HHP are the many relevant journals from fields outside of HHP. It is not possible to mention all of them here, but the following list is representative of what is at the disposal of HHP researchers. The sources have been arranged by subject.

APPLIED HEALTH SCIENCE

Addictions

Alcohol Health and Research World
Bibliography on Smoking and Health
Bottom Line on Alcohol in Society
British Journal of Addictions
Changes
Prevention Pipeline

Smoking and Health Bulletin
Tobacco-free Young America Reporter

Diseases/Dying

Ca-A Cancer Journal for Clinicians
Journal of Cancer Education
Omega Journal of Death and Dying

Family Studies

American Journal of Family Therapy
Family Life Educator
Family Perspective
Family Process
Family Relations
Journal of Divorce
Journal of Family Issues
Journal of Family Violence
Journal of Marital and Family Therapy
Parenting Studies
Sage Family Studies Abstracts
Single Parent

Health Education

American Journal of Health Education
Health Education Quarterly
Health Education Research
Health Values
International Quarterly of Community Health Education

Human Sexuality

Current Research Updates in Human Sexuality
Journal of Sex Education and Therapy

Nutrition

American Journal of Clinical Nutrition
Annual Review of Nutrition
Clinical Nutrition
Food and Nutrition News
International Journal of Obesity
Journal of Nutrition
Journal of Nutrition Education
Journal of the American Dietetic Association
Nutrition Abstracts
Nutrition Action Newsletter

Nutrition & Cancer
Nutrition Reviews
Sports Nutrition News

Preventive Medicine

American Journal of Preventive Medicine
Behavioral Medicine
Indiana Medicine
Optimal Health
University of California, Berkeley Wellness Letter

Public Health

Accident Analysis and Prevention
Accident Facts
AIDS Education and Prevention
American Journal of Health Promotion
American Journal of Public Health
Canadian Center for Occupational Health and Safety
Canadian Journal of Public Health
Indiana State Board of Health Bulletin
Journal of American College Health
Journal of School Health
Public Health Reports

Youth and Adolescence

Adolescence
Adolescent Psychiatry
International Journal of Adolescence and Youth
Journal of Adolescent Health
Journal of Adolescent Research
Journal of Youth and Adolescence

Unclassified

American Health
Health

EXERCISE AND SPORT SCIENCES

Advances in Pediatric Sport Sciences
Canadian Journal of Sport Sciences
Exercise and Sport Sciences Review
Journal of Sport Sciences
Medicine and Science in Sports and Exercise
Research Quarterly for Exercise and Sport
Scandinavian Journal of Sport Sciences

SPORTS - Science
American Journal of Human Biology
Pediatric Exercise Science

PHYSICAL EDUCATION/KINESIOLOGY

Adapted Physical Education

Adapted Physical Activity Quarterly
Paleastra

Athletic Training

Athletic Training
NATA News
National Strength and Conditioning Association Journal

Biomechanics, Kinesiology, Physiology

Clinical Kinesiology
European Journal of Applied Physiology and Occupational Physiology
International Journal of Sport Biomechanics
Journal of Applied Physiology
Journal of Biomechanics
Journal of Motor Behavior
Journal of Sport and Exercise Physiology

Coaching/Referee

Coaching Clinic
Journal of Applied Research in Coaching & Athletics
Referee
Scholastic Coach
Spotlight on Youth Sports

Dance

American Journal of Dance Therapy
Dance Teacher Now
IDEA Today
Kinesiology and Medicine for Dance

History, Psychology, Philosophy, and Sociology of Sport

Arena Review
International Journal of Sport Psychology
International Journal of the History of Sport
Journal of Sport and Exercise Psychology
Journal of Sport and Social Issues
Journal of Sport Behavior

Journal of Sport History
Journal of Personality and Social Psychology
Journal of the Philosophy of Sport
North American Society for Sport History Newsletter
Personality and Individual Differences
Psychology and Sociology of Sport
Sociology of Sport Journal
Sport Psychologist

Individual Sports

International Gymnast
Journal of Swimming Research
Sports 'n Spokes
Swimming Technique
Swimming World and Junior Swimmer
Track and Field News

Physical Therapy/Rehabilitation

International Journal of Rehabilitation Research
Journal of Cardiopulmonary Rehabilitation
Journal of Orthopaedic & Sports Physical Therapy
Physical Therapy

Sport Medicine

American Journal of Sports Medicine
Annals of Sports Medicine
Archives of Physical Medicine and Rehabilitation
British Journal of Sports Medicine
Clinics in Sports Medicine
Electromyography & Clinical Neurophysiology
International Journal of Sports Cardiology
International Journal of Sports Medicine
Journal of Sports Medicine and Physical Fitness
Medicine & Science in Sports & Exercise
Physical Fitness/Sports Medicine (Index)
Physician and Sportsmedicine
Sports Medicine
Sports Medicine Digest
Yearbook of Sports Medicine

Sports Administration/Marketing

Athletic Administration
Athletic Business
Club Business International

College Athletic Management
Corporate Fitness
Employee Health and Fitness
Executive Edge
Fitness Management
Journal of Sport Management
Sports Careers
Team Marketing Report

Sports Law

Exercise Standards and Malpractice Reporter
Sports and the Courts

Teaching Physical Education

Great Activities Newspaper
Gym Dandies Series
Journal of Teaching in Physical Education
Physical Educator
Quest
Strategies

Unclassified

AAHPERD: Abstracts of Research Papers
Alliance Update
American Academy of Physical Education: Academy Papers
Athletic Performance Review
Completed Research in Health, Physical Education, Recreation and Dance
Computers in Human Behavior
Ergonomics
ERIC on CD-ROM
Futurist
Human Movement Science
International Journal of Physical Education
Journal of Aging and Physical Activity
Journal of Physical Education, Recreation & Dance
*Journal of the International Council for Health, Physical Education
    and Recreation*
Measurement in Physical Education and Exercise Science
Medline on CD-ROM
NCAA News
Olympic Message
Olympic Panorama
Physical Education Index

Sociology of Leisure Sports Abstracts
Soviet Sports Review
Sport Bulletin/International Union of Students
Sports, Parks and Recreation Law Reporter
Sportsearch (Index)
SPRE Annual on Education
The Kappan
Women's Sports and Fitness

RECREATIONAL SPORTS

National Intramural Recreational Sports Association
NIRSA Journal
NIRSA Proceedings
Rec Sports Report

RECREATION AND PARK ADMINISTRATION

Gerontology

Aging Research and Training News
Gerontologist
Journal of Aging and Health
Journal of Applied Gerontology
Journal of Gerontology
Research on Aging
Topics in Geriatric Rehabilitation

Leisure Studies

Journal of Leisurability
Journal of Leisure Research
Leisure Information Quarterly
Leisure Sciences
Leisure Studies
Loisir & Societe (Society and Leisure)
Newsletter, World Recreation and Leisure Association
Play and Culture
World Leisure and Recreation Association Journal

Outdoor/Environmental Education

Camping Magazine
Conservation Directory
Journal of Experiential Education
Journal of Outdoor Education

North American Environment
Outdoor Communicator
Outdoor Indiana
Restoration and Management Notes

Recreation and Parks

Design
Grist
Journal of Park and Recreation Administration
Marking Recreation Classes
Park Maintenance & Grounds Management
Park Practice Program Index
Parks and Recreation
Recreation and Park Education Curriculum Catalog
Recreation and Parks Law Reporter
Trends

Therapeutic Recreation

Programming Trends in Therapeutic Recreation
Therapeutic Recreation Journal

Travel and Tourism

Annals of Tourism Research
Cornell Hotel and Restaurant Administration Quarterly
Journal of Travel Research
Leisure, Recreation and Tourism Abstracts
Travel and Tourism Executive Report

Unclassified

Employee Services Management
Recreation Canada
Recreation Executive Report
Recreation Research Review
Recreation, Sports & Leisure

Computer Retrieval Systems.   The advent of the computer has added great speed to the process of searching the literature. Many reference sources are now available in the compact disk (CD-ROM) format, enabling complex searches to be performed that would be much more difficult, if not impossible, using paper resources. These reference sources include indexes to journals and other publications (sometimes accompanied by the full text of the cited article), abstracts, statistical reference materials, and compilations of useful data.

Learning to do a **computer search** for literature is a relatively simple matter. Select the key words, or descriptors, from the title or problem statement of the proposed research topic. These key words are entered into the computer, which uses them to search for related information from the databases upon which a particular system operates. The computer generates a printout with the titles of studies, reports, reviews, conference papers and proceedings, and other sources. Some systems include a brief abstract describing the content of each reference. These printouts may be available in a few hours; others may take up to a week to appear. There are many computer databases. Those that seem to be of the most value to HHP are the following:

Education Resources Information Center (ERIC). This very useful database contains thousands of materials from education and allied areas, including HHP, and houses information from the printed indexes, *Current Index to Journals in Education and Resources in Education,* from 1966 to the present.

Sport Discus. This is the primary research database for sport, physical fitness, sport science, and recreation. It is international in scope and covers such subjects as exercise physiology, leisure, biomechanics, coaching, sport psychology, and motor development.

Medline. This is an enlarged version of the printed *Index Medicus.* It contains references to journal articles in all areas of clinical and research medicine, including biomedical research, health administration, nursing, veterinary science, and others. It is of potential use for students and researchers in fields ranging from anatomy to zoology.

PsycLIT. This database provides users with information about articles in psychology-related journals. PsycLIT is a computerized version of *Psychological Abstracts.* It includes articles published from 1974 to the present.

Direct Access to Reference Information (DATRIX). This database focuses on the dissertation references at University Microfilms, Ann Arbor, Michigan, and is the computerized version of the printed *Dissertation Abstracts.*

Conducting a Computer Search.   Many computer reference sources are now available in most college and university libraries that subscribe to a variety of databases. The reference sources include indexes to journals and other publications, and may include the full text of the cited article, statistical reference materials, and compiled data. Most libraries utilize an on-line computerized information system that permits the researcher to gain immediate access to the needed literary citations.

Graduate students typically learn to do a computer search in one of two ways—through a seminar-type course sponsored by the institution or a HHP department, or with the help of a librarian highly skilled in using the various methods for retrieving information. In conducting the search, the following five steps must be performed:

1. **State the research problem precisely.** If the statement is too long and rather general, there will be too many descriptors. This will result in an unwieldy list of references, most of which will be irrelevant to the research problem. A brief

and specific statement like "physical fitness status related to improved self-esteem of elementary school students" is definitive and gives focus to the search. The descriptors (physical fitness, self-esteem, and elementary school students) will generate a limited number of references, yet provide the needed information.

2. **Determine what database(s) should be used.** In this step the researcher decides which database will provide the most information about articles pertinent to the research problem. One database, ERIC, may be sufficient; but, in some cases, two or more will need to be searched. In the physical fitness/self-esteem example, it may be necessary to use ERIC, Sport Discus, and PsycLIT to generate a helpful list of literature sources.

3. **Determine what descriptors will be used.** Select key words (descriptors) from the research problem statement. This tells the computer what direction the search should take. From the problem of fitness related to self-esteem, logical descriptors are physical fitness, self-esteem, and elementary school students. The computer will also want to know the year the search is to commence. If 1990 is selected, the resultant list of references will contain only those articles published from that year on. It is also necessary to indicate in what language the literature source should be written. This is usually English.

4. **Do the search.** The selected database software is inserted into the computer and the descriptors are entered. After a few minutes it is prudent to ask the computer to print out a small list of references to be sure the descriptors are providing helpful sources. If relevant sources are being obtained, the computer can then be asked to provide a printout containing all available references.

5. **Study the list of references.** The researcher obtains and reads, in detail, the articles that are determined to be the most pertinent to the research problem. Frequently, the bibliographic information in these articles provides other helpful sources and may prompt another computer investigation of the literature.

Searching the Internet. The **Internet** is a vast collection of interconnected computers throughout the world that provides access to a wealth of information. The resources available on the Internet are almost limitless. Today it is estimated that there are more than one billion web pages, accessible from computers located in libraries, classrooms, worksites, and even one's home. In fact, we are now seeing cellular phones and Personal Digital Assistants (PDAs) with Internet access capability, thus making it possible to connect to the Internet almost anywhere. The challenge, however, is to find quality information. Special care must be taken when obtaining information from the Internet, because anyone can put up a website and post information. Thus, just because you locate information on the Internet does not mean that it is accurate and credible. It is important to carefully read Internet sources and evaluate their content on the basis of intent, bias, reputation of the author or publisher, and verifiable accuracy.

The easiest way of locating information on the Internet is to use some form of search utility that is available on the Web, namely subject directories, search engines, and metasearch engines. *Subject directories* are essentially Internet "yellow pages" in which you are able to peruse Internet sources according to subject area. Subjects are organized and located within a hierarchy of topical categories. Yahoo! is an example of a large and perhaps the most popular subject directory. WWW Virtual Library is another example of a subject directory. The primary advantage of subject directories is that the content has been reviewed and organized by a team of editors who have knowledge of specific disciplines, thus enhancing the relevance and quality of the resources assembled for a given topic. Yet, despite their organizational integrity, subject directories index a relatively small number of web pages compared to the number of pages examined by Internet search engines. *Search engines* are websites that enable you to search Internet databases for specific information, based upon entry of a key word or words. The search itself is performed in an automated fashion using a "spider" or "robot" that moves from website to website, capturing information from each site it visits in an attempt to find relevant matches to the key word provided. Google, Excite, Alta Vista, HotBot, and Northern Light are examples of Internet search engines. Search engines index millions of web pages and provide a quick, convenient way to search the Internet, although the relevance of the results is often less than desirable. Furthermore, the various search engines do not obtain consistent results since their databases may differ, thus suggesting that it is wise for the researcher to use several search engines. A *metasearch engine* utilizes multiple search engines simultaneously to perform an Internet search of their databases. Within a short time, you get back results from several individual search engines, albeit only a portion of the results in any of the databases queried. Although no single metasearch engine includes all the search engines currently available, metasearch engines may be especially useful to researchers because of the inconsistent results obtained from each individual search engine. Dogpile, Copernic, Ixquick, and Metacrawler are examples of metasearch engines. Although the use of metasearch engines appears to hold much promise for the researcher, the user is somewhat limited in being able to specify search parameters, thus bringing to question the relevance of search results. In other words, the results obtained from a metasearch engine could easily yield large quantities of information, but only a relatively few sites are actually pertinent to the topic of interest.

Table 2.1 provides a listing of selected examples of each type of Internet search utility. Those interested in obtaining more information about Internet search capabilities, descriptions of the various directories, search engines, and metasearch engines, as well as strategies for successful Internet searching, may wish to consult the following websites:

- University of California, Berkeley Internet Resources (www.lib.berkeley.edu/TeachingLib/Guides/Internet)
- Search Engine Showdown (www.notess.com/search)
- Search Engine Watch (www.searchenginewatch.com)

TABLE 2.1 Internet Search Utilities	
SUBJECT DIRECTORIES	
Britannica Internet Guide	www.britannica.com
LookSmart	www.looksmart.com
Snap	www.nbci.com
WWW Virtual Library	www.vlib.com
Yahoo!	www.yahoo.com
SEARCH ENGINES	
Alta Vista	www.altavista.com
Excite	www.excite.com
Go/Infoseek	www.go.com
Google	www.google.com
HotBot	www.hotbot.lycos.com
Iwon	www.iwon.com
Lycos	www.lycos.com
Northern Light	www.northernlight.com
METASEARCH ENGINES	
Chubba	www.chubba.com
Copernic	www.copernic.com
Dogpile	www.dogpile.com
Ixquick	www.ixquick.com
MetaCrawler	www.metacrawler.com
WebFerret	www.ferretsoft.com/netferret

Writing Chapter 3: Procedures

The third chapter of a research proposal deals with the procedures for collecting data. Alternative titles for chapter 3 are "Procedures," "Methodology," "Experimental Procedures," and "Survey Procedures." All proposals must include a detailed and appropriate **data collection plan** for attacking the problem. Earlier in the proposal (primarily in chapter 1), the rationale for selecting certain methods, techniques, and procedures was presented as background information for the problem. However, a more detailed rationale is needed in chapter 3. The entire research proposal is like a contract between the student researcher and a faculty committee. If the research study is conducted as proposed, the committee cannot seriously complain about the procedures at the final defense meeting. Hence, the procedures section becomes extremely critical. The soundness of the study will depend on the appropriateness of the planned attack on the research problem. The reader will analyze this section closely and relate the methods, techniques, and procedures to the relative quality of the research data to be obtained.

The procedures chapter is considered to be the "cookbook" or "recipe" portion of the proposal or research report. Its presentation requires much attention to detail as the researcher illuminates the reader about where the data come from (sources), how the data were gathered (collection methods), and how the data were analyzed (treatment). This step-by-step set of instructions for conducting the investigation should be so detailed that if another researcher wanted to replicate the study, there would be no trouble in doing so. The reader should not have to make any assumptions about what or how something was done in the research situation.

The first paragraph of chapter 3 always includes a restatement of the problem (stated exactly as it was in chapter 1) and indicates how the chapter is organized. In general, most studies will include these items:

1. A discussion of the research participants and the sampling techniques used for obtaining them
2. A discussion of the tests, instruments, or measures that were used to collect the data
3. A discussion of the design of the study within which the data were collected
4. A discussion of the administrative procedures used to collect the data
5. A discussion on how the data were treated or analyzed

Depending upon the nature of the study, the advice of the faculty advisor, and the whims of the researcher, these five items are translated into a variety of section topics. Following are some of the topic headings typically found in this section:

1. Arrangements for Conducting the Study
2. Selection of Participants
3. Selection of the Test Instrument(s)
4. Development of the Test Instrument(s)
5. Instrumentation
6. Design of the Study
7. Training Program
8. Administration of Test
9. Procedures for Testing and Gathering Data
10. Data Collection Procedures
11. Preliminary Investigation

12. Pilot Study

13. Treatment of Data

14. Data Analysis Procedures

Format of the various topical headings selected will depend upon the style manual used at the various institutions. While some sections, Treatment of Data for example, do not have to be unduly long, they should clearly describe the procedures and methods that the researcher plans to follow in the conduct of the study. As stated earlier, chapter 3 constitutes a "recipe for conducting research" and should be written with enough detail and specificity that another researcher having similar expertise would be able to follow the procedures and conduct the study in the same manner in which it was originally done. The following questions can be used as a guide to providing the appropriate information in chapter 3:

1. Was the population clearly specified?

2. Is the design appropriate to the problem?

3. Were the sampling procedures clearly specified and the total sample adequate?

4. If a control group was involved, was it selected from the same population?

5. Were the various treatments (including control) assigned at random?

6. Were appropriate statistical treatment procedures selected and the level of significance selected in advance?

7. Were the reliability and validity of the data-gathering instruments and procedures established and reported?

8. Were the treatments and/or methods of the collection of data described so clearly and completely that an independent investigator could replicate the study?

9. Are the characteristics of the subjects clearly representative of the population?

10. Were extraneous sources of error either held constant or randomized among subjects of all groups?

See examples 2.1 through 2.5 for a demonstration of the various content areas of chapter 3 of a research report.

The problem of the study was to determine if an instructional emphasis on increasing the range of motion in the overhand throwing pattern of second and fourth graders results in improved throwing form and velocity. The conduct of the study included the following procedural steps: (1) arrangements for conducting the study, (2) selection of subjects, (3) development of instructional approaches, (4) selection of measurement tools, and (5) treatment of data.

EXAMPLE 2.1
An Opening Paragraph
(Luedke 1980)

All of the subjects were volunteers and were enrolled at Indiana University during the course of the investigation. The main criteria for participation included: (a) all subjects were males, (b) all subjects had previous high school competitive swimming experience with no collegiate experience (age-group swimming experience was considered to be an adequate substitute), (c) all subjects had a minimum of four years of competitive swimming background, (d) each subject had a personal best 50-yard time of 28.6 seconds or better, and (e) subjects had a minimum and maximum age of 18 and 22 years, respectively.

These criteria were selected to give the study an external validity factor that would allow the results to be generalized to a population of high school, or age-group swimmers. This population was selected because it has the largest number of participants relative to the total swimming population, and has the greatest potential for improvement. The number of years of competitive swimming experience, and the emphasis on minimum and maximum age added power to the analysis of the experimental data by reducing the intersubject variance in scores.

EXAMPLE 2.2
Selection of Subjects
(Wasilak 1988)

EXAMPLE 2.3
Selection of the Test
Instruments
(Umansky 1976)

Three measures were selected to assess perceptual-motor abilities of the subjects: the Perceptual Quotient score of the Frostig Developmental Test of Visual Perception (1966), and the developmental age scores from the Perceptual-Motor and Pre-Academic scales of the Assessment-Programming Guide for Infants and Preschoolers (Umansky 1973).

The Frostig DTVP is a five-part test that purportedly assesses five distinct perceptual functions: eye-hand coordination, figure-ground perception, form constancy, position in space, and spatial relationships. Standardized on a group of 2,116 children between three and nine years of age, the sample largely consisted of middle-class white children from southern California. The test yields raw scores from each subtest which are converted to scale scores, and then summed up to produce a Perceptual Quotient. Test-retest reliability for the Perceptual Quotient for first and second graders tested two weeks apart was .80, as reported by the authors of the test. Subtest scale score test-retest correlations were reported from .42 to .80 by the authors (Frostig 1964).

The Assessment-Programming Guide for Infants and Preschoolers (Umansky 1973) is an eclectic tool compiled by the investigator a number of years ago as a developmental evaluation instrument for young children. A list of sources upon which the Guide was based is presented in Appendix F. It is a criterion-referenced checklist composed of six developmental subscales. The Perceptual-Motor and Pre-Academic subscales were used for this investigation (Appendix B). The subscales consist of specific skills divided into appropriate age groups. A perceptual-motor age score and pre-academic age score were derived for the subscales.

The subjects were randomly assigned to either the Adventure Group or the Control Group. Both groups completed the pretest one day prior to the involvement of the Adventure Group in the Challenge Education Program. The Adventure Group participated in a six-hour sequentially based Challenge Education program conducted at Bradford Woods. The Control Group participated in the normal daily activities of the psychiatric hospital, which included various therapies, counseling sessions, and unstructured leisure time. One day following the Adventure Group's Challenge Education experience, both groups were administered the posttest.

Both the pretest and the posttest were administered by the investigator, in the company of a recreation therapist familiar to the subjects. The investigator also facilitates the Challenge Education experience for the Adventure Group. The Adventure Group was also accompanied by the same recreation therapist that assisted with the test administration. Additionally, a nurse accompanied the Adventure Group to monitor the health of the subjects, many of whom were under various forms of medication.

EXAMPLE 2.4
Design of the Study
(Miller 1990)

To test the hypothesis that there is no significant increase in vertical jump performance, a t-test for correlated samples, repeated measures design, was conducted utilizing pretraining and posttraining scores. The sum of a subject's three trials was used as his criterion score for a testing period. The null hypothesis was tested using a one-tailed test at the .05 level of significance.

The sum of the trials was also used as the criterion score for strength test measurements for testing the hypothesis of no significant increase in leg strength development. Again, pretraining performance was compared to posttraining performance by utilizing a t-test for correlated samples repeated measures design. The null hypothesis was tested using a one-tailed test and a .05 level of significance.

The difference between the pretraining and posttraining scores on each variable was determined for each subject. The relationship between muscle strength and vertical jump performance was tested by correlating the change in scores on the vertical jump with the change in scores on the cable-tensiometer using a Pearson product-moment r. The correlation coefficient which was obtained was tested for significance at the .05 level.

EXAMPLE 2.5
Treatment of Data
(Van Oteghen 1973)

Summary

The research problem is perceived, developed, and attacked in several steps as discussed in detail in this chapter. Crucial to the success of any research endeavor is a complete review of the related literature determined to be pertinent to the problem being investigated. This chapter has provided a compiled list of many sources of information useful to HHP research efforts. The usual procedures for conducting a research project have been delineated in some detail and have been illustrated using several examples extracted from successful graduate student research projects.

Formative Evaluation of Objectives

Objective 1   Select a suitable research problem.

    1. Select an area of HHP of major interest to you, and list five problems requiring investigation that have been published in the literature in the past year.

Objective 2   Know the various sources of research problems.

    1. Identify the more effective ways to find an appropriate research problem.

Objective 3   Understand the various steps of the research process.

    1. Select a research problem and:

        a) state the problem.
        b) indicate the purpose of the study.
        c) delimit the study.

Objective 4   Systematically review literature relevant to the selected problem.

    1. List the various sources of literature you would use in developing a background for the proposed problem in objective 3.

Objective 5   Plan and develop an attack on the problem.

    1. State the hypothesis for the problem, indicating how it will be tested, what data need to be obtained, and what data-gathering instruments or procedures will be employed.

3

Selected Elements of the Research Process

Controlling for variables
Data-collecting instruments
Directional hypothesis
Halo effect
Hypothesis

Internal consistency
  reliability
Measurement techniques
Nondirectional hypothesis
Null hypothesis

Objectivity
Observation techniques
Questioning techniques
Research approaches

Research hypothesis
Reliability
Stability reliability
Validity

OBJECTIVES

The process of developing a research project involves many interrelated elements. In the previous chapter various research procedures were discussed. The nature of problems, the importance of the problem, and the related literature were also addressed. Now it is important to consider the details of a research plan which include the research approach, methodological steps, instruments to be used, and how the instruments will be administered to capture the needed data obtained on the selected variables under study.

After reading chapter 3, you should be able to

1. Suggest one study that could be researched under each research approach.
2. Understand the role of hypotheses and hypothesis testing in the research process.
3. Know when it is appropriate to apply the different methods of collecting data.
4. Know the various techniques available for each data collection method.
5. State the criteria for selecting the appropriate research instrument.

Selecting the Research Approach

In chapter 1 we discussed various systems for classifying research and provided a description of the types of research that are most prevalent in HHP. As previously stated, the general purpose of research is to increase our understanding and the body of knowledge within a given field, yet there are substantial differences in the approach one may take in pursuit of this end. Regardless of the approach taken, however, all research involves elements of observation, description, and the analysis of what happens under certain circumstances (Best and Kahn 1998). Once a definitive problem has been identified and a thorough search of the literature has been accomplished, it is incumbent upon the researcher to decide on the best approach to take in systematically collecting the data, or information, needed to solve the research problem. According to Drew, Hardman, and Hart (1996), the approach selected will depend on several factors: the nature of the research problem, the setting in which the research is to be conducted, the disciplinary perspective of research, and the background of the researcher.

There is not a single way of conducting research. Many different approaches and procedures have been developed; the researcher must choose from these. We have found that the system proposed by Best and Kahn (1998) helps students, as well as veteran researchers, better understand the general approaches that may be taken in research. Best and Kahn suggest that practically all studies fall under one, or a combination, of the following **research approaches:**

- *Historical* – describes *what was* in order to discover generalizations that help to understand the past and the present
- *Descriptive* – uses quantitative methods to describe *what is* in order to gain an understanding of conditions that currently exist and the relationship between existing variables that are not manipulated
- *Qualitative* – uses nonquantitative methods for exploring existing phenomenon in order to describe *what is*
- *Experimental* – describes *what will be* when certain variables of interest are controlled or manipulated in order to seek causal relationships between variables

In general, the nature of the research problem will go a long way in determining what approach is best suited as the method of attack for obtaining the required knowledge. For example, if one wants to trace the evolution of worksite health promotion programs in the United States in order to better understand the basis for today's programs, an historical approach is needed. Research whose purpose is to investigate the effect of teaching method on sport skill development is seeking to establish a cause-and-effect relationship and thus would use an experimental approach. Such an approach would enable the researcher to deliberately manipulate the independent variable (teaching method in this example) while controlling all other variables and then observe the subsequent effect on the dependent variable (sport skill development). A descriptive approach utilizing survey methodology is called for when a researcher is interested in ascertaining the attitudes of citizens toward mandatory seat belt usage. Similarly, a correlational study in which an investigator seeks to determine the relationship between television-viewing behavior and physical fitness level of adolescent females utilizes a descriptive approach. In this situation there is no manipulation of the variables, only descriptions of the variables and their relationships as they naturally occur. A qualitative approach would best enable a researcher to investigate the role of community support for a local sports team. The researcher would likely study the community over an extended period of time and gather information through both interviews and personal observations. As the previous examples illustrate, the very nature of the research problem coupled with the intent of the researcher will generally reveal the preferred approach to be taken. Each of the four research approaches presented here is discussed more thoroughly in subsequent chapters in the textbook.

Hypotheses

Statements of **hypothesis** are important to almost all research projects. Most researchers proceed in their studies with the idea that a certain outcome will result. This idea is then stated as a "tentative explanation of the relationship between two or more variables" (Best and Kahn 1998). The predicted outcome is referred to as a **research hypothesis.** It has been hypothesized that extensive use of anabolic steroids by athletes leads to the deterioration of certain body parts and to disease. Many research studies have been done on the relationship between steroid use and serious illness, and the results have generally supported the hypothesis: There is a relationship.

In general, research hypotheses possess these characteristics:

1. They are based on theory or previous research findings.
2. They state a relationship between at least two variables.
3. They are simple and clear statements with no vague terms clouding the relationships.
4. They are testable; that is, the stated variables can be measured, and theoretical or previous research knowledge exists to permit a clear and testable hypothesis.
5. They have the capability of being refuted; the prediction can be evaluated in terms of "yes, it occurred" or "no, it did not occur."
6. They are related to available techniques of design, procedure, and statistical analysis.

Research hypotheses can be stated in a **directional** or a **nondirectional** manner. If, based on the research, the researcher believes that a particular relationship or difference exists between groups of subjects, he or she will state the hypothesis directionally, or in the direction of the expected result.

> **Example:**
>
> Children with a high IQ are more easily motivated than children with a low IQ.

The researcher is predicting that there is a difference between children in how easily they are motivated and that this difference favors or is in the direction of those with high IQs. A nondirectional hypothesis is stated when the researcher has no reason to believe that a difference or relationship exists in any direction.

> **Example:**
>
> There is a difference between the motivational level of children with a high IQ and those children with a low IQ.

In this case the researcher expects a difference but does not indicate the direction it will take. The topic of the directional versus the nondirectional hypothesis is related to a statistical analysis procedure that will be described in a later chapter.

The number of research hypotheses in a given study will depend upon the number of research questions being asked and the number of variables being investigated. The more variables, the greater the number of relationships; hence, the greater the number of hypotheses. This point is related to the scope of the study, which increases as the number of hypotheses increases. All research hypotheses are stated in the present tense and before collecting data on the variables.

The research hypothesis is not tested directly by the data. Rather, the research hypothesis is transformed into a **null (statistical) hypothesis,** symbolized by H_o, that is tested by the data. It states that there is no difference between the groups being studied. For example:

Research hypothesis. Students exposed to an experimental leisure activity program will show greater self-esteem than do students who have not been exposed to this program.

Null or statistical hypothesis. There is no difference in the self-esteem of students who have been exposed to an experimental leisure activity program and students who have not been exposed to the program.

The statistical procedures used for analyzing research data can test only hypotheses stated in the form of a null hypothesis. Moreover, hypotheses are neither proved nor disproved. Hypothesis testing involves determining the likelihood (probability) that the outcome observed is due to chance occurrence. If the data support the null hypothesis, it will be accepted (technically, we should say that we fail to reject the null hypothesis); if the data refute the null hypothesis, it will be rejected. Usually, the research and null hypotheses are stated in opposite terms. The research hypothesis is a positive statement of expected outcome, while the null hypothesis simply states that no difference or no relationship will be found.

> *Research hypothesis.* Children who perform on physical fitness tests under team competition obtain higher scores than children who perform on physical fitness tests under competition against someone of nearly equal ability.
>
> *Null or statistical hypothesis.* There is no difference in the test scores of children who perform on physical fitness tests under team competition and those children who perform on physical fitness tests under competition against someone of nearly equal ability.

If, on the basis of an appropriate statistical test, he or she fails to reject the null hypothesis, he or she concludes that there really is no difference between the two motivating conditions. If the data showed that team competition was the superior condition, the null hypothesis is rejected and the research hypothesis is accepted. Of course, the research hypothesis would also be rejected if, in fact, competition against someone of nearly equal ability was found to be associated with superior performance on the physical fitness test.

Sometimes the research hypothesis is stated the same way as the null hypothesis. A researcher may go into an investigation expecting no difference. In this case, whatever action is taken on the statistical hypothesis, as dictated by the data, will also be taken on the research hypothesis.

Stating hypotheses helps to make a researcher's thought process about the research situation more concrete. If a prediction of a specific outcome is made, this forces more thorough consideration of which research techniques, methods, test instruments, and data-collecting procedures should be employed. Hypotheses also help set up the way the data will be analyzed and how the final report will be organized and written.

Inasmuch as hypotheses are founded upon the research problem, they serve to guide the researcher in the selection of the approach and methods to be used to attack the problem. Hypotheses serve to focus the design of the study on the methods that are needed to collect the data that are required to test the null hypotheses. Once the research topic has been reduced to a specific and manageable problem and the type of approach needed to study it has been determined, the researcher then states the hypotheses or, more specifically, the predicted outcome(s) of the study. Any research project can include hypotheses. All experimental studies and those descriptive investigations in which comparisons are made will have hypotheses. Readers of those studies deserve to know what the researcher expected would be revealed by the experiment or the descriptive comparison. Hypotheses are also appropriate for causal-comparative research and correlational research. Simple descriptive and historical studies generally would not have hypotheses, although occasionally the researcher, by virtue of his or her experience or based on the literature, would want to make a prediction of the outcome and thus would include hypotheses. As a general rule, qualitative researchers do not state hypotheses *a priori,* but may formulate hypotheses based upon the results of their studies. A hypothesis is warranted whenever a reasonable expectation of outcome is anticipated. Usually the hypothesis will indicate an expected relationship between the variables (e.g., characteristics, traits, attributes) being investigated. The researcher may have several objectives for a research project, and a hypothesis should be stated for each one. The usual intent of a research study is to predict a series of outcomes based on the objectives of the research problem. Once the research data have been collected, the hypotheses are tested to determine their truth or falsity.

What happens if the research hypotheses are not supported by the results of the study? A frequent misconception is that the research was faulty and is of no value. Perfectly well-conducted research can reveal data that do not support what was expected. In such a situation, the researcher should review the assumptions that served as the basis for the hypotheses, the theoretical relationships involved, and the design of the study. On the other hand, the truth may be that the research hypotheses should have been rejected. There really may be no relationship between the groups.

Control of Variables

In chapter 1, we presented a detailed discussion of variables, including descriptions of various types of variables. It is critically important not only for the researcher but also for the consumer of the research literature to be able to identify the pertinent variables in a study. In designing a study, particularly an experimental study, the researcher should pay particular attention to controlling the influence of extraneous variables.

Many experiments in the fields of HHP are conducted outside of the laboratory, using human subjects, and many variables surround the research situation which could alter the results in some substantive way. It becomes imperative that the researcher maintain as much control over these variables as possible so as to prevent or reduce their effect. At the same time it must be recognized that not every variable that could make a difference can be controlled. Following are some of the procedures that are frequently used in an attempt to control extraneous variables:

Random Selection of Subjects.   When the laws of probability are permitted to operate in the selection of two or more experimental groups of subjects, systematic bias is removed and the effect of extraneous variables is minimized. It is assumed that the groups are equal and that if any difference does exist, it is due to probability or chance factors (Best and Kahn 1998).

Equating or Matching by Some Criterion.   The subjects are paired on some characteristic, such as age, sex, height, weight, ability, or the results of preliminary testing. After the pairing is completed, the members of each pair are assigned at random, one to the experimental group and the other to the control group. If a researcher wanted to use 15-, 16-, and 17-year-old boys and girls to study methods of developing flexibility, it might be desirable to match on age and gender so that the experimental and control groups would be comparable on those two variables at the beginning of the experiment. Each boy and girl in each age group would be randomly assigned to either the experimental or control group.

By matching subjects it is also possible to reduce the variation among them because of chance differences in initial ability. It is a relatively simple matter to match on one or two characteristics. As the number of traits to match increases, so does the difficulty in obtaining accurate pairs.

Excluding the Variable.   A researcher may simply choose to not include a particular trait in the study. The intent is to eliminate the possible effects of a variable by holding the variable constant, thereby removing it from the study. This is sometimes referred to as **controlling for the variable.** For instance, if a researcher suspects that gender might influence the outcome of a study designed to investigate the effect of extrinsic motivation on weight loss, the researcher could control for gender by limiting the participants to only females. In this case, gender has been held constant by excluding males from the study. Similarly, research participants could be selected from only one age group or grade level, thus removing age and grade as variables.

Data-Collecting Methods and Techniques

The research process includes three different methods of procuring information, or data. They are **observation, measurement,** and **questioning.** The researcher may watch subjects perform and record relevant data about them; he/she may test subjects or apply a device to subjects to measure certain qualities; or he/she may ask subjects questions to obtain information that cannot be obtained in any other way.

The relationship of each method of gathering information to the four research approaches described earlier in this chapter is illustrated in the following examples adapted from Fox (1969):

1. *Observation*
    a. This is accomplished retroactively in the historical approach by viewing museum artifacts, antiques, photographs, and printed material.
    b. In both the descriptive and qualitative approach, subjects can be watched in the research setting, although it is recognized that subjects' awareness of being observed could change their response and generate invalid data.
    c. Observations in the experimental approach represent only a small portion of some future reality.

2. *Measurement*

   a. With the descriptive and experimental approaches, the researcher can directly measure a large variety of variables (e.g., attitude, knowledge, physiological qualities, and personality traits).

   b. Direct measurement of cognitive and affective variables is not possible in the historical approach. The personality of a deceased famous person can be determined only by inference from other existing data. Physical remains (e.g., buildings, bridges, toys) can be measured directly.

3. *Questioning*

   a. In the historical approach, questioning has to be retroactive and must rely on the memory of those who were there at the time.

   b. The descriptive and experimental approaches permit questioning about past, present, and future activities.

A variety of techniques may be used to carry out each of these methods. Depending on the scope and objectives of the study, a research project may incorporate several methods and techniques.

Observation Techniques

Direct. Under the direct technique, subjects are cognizant of being observed and they usually know why they are being observed. *Example:* Subjects being observed exercising in different training programs using the biokinetics swim bench to determine front crawl stroke hand-speed patterns.

In many cases, it is important to the study that subjects be directly observed, but unaware they are being watched. *Example:* Any situation in which the researcher's presence might cause a change in the subjects that would inhibit them from reacting in a natural way. Elementary school subjects, knowing they were going to be observed performing a series of motor skill activities, might get nervous and feel intimidated, or become hyperactive in their behavior and not perform to their true ability. In this case, direct observation could be accomplished through the use of a one-way mirror so the youngsters would not know they were being watched.

Indirect. Indirect observation is a technique accomplished when a group of subjects are filmed or videotaped. *Example:* A group of physically disabled youngsters serve as subjects in a stress-challenge study. They are told that their performances will be videotaped first, and then they and the researchers will view the tapes to evaluate the various rope techniques, both good and bad. Observing the tape is indirect observation. The alternative to letting the subjects know they are being filmed is to use a hidden camera. In this situation, the term "bugging" could be applied. Whether or not the subjects know they are being taped, the direct observer is always the camera.

Participant.   In the technique of participant observation, the observer participates in the research situation. *Example:* The researcher is studying the attitude and behavior of teenage campers and participates in a two-week camp experience, engaging in all activities, attending meetings, and so forth. The subjects know that the researcher is an outside person who wants to learn as much as possible about teenage camper attitude and behavior. In certain instances it may be appropriate that the outside participant's motives be unknown to the subjects, as in the case of an undercover agent infiltrating an agency, association, or group to collect data on its activities.

Measurement Techniques

Almost anything can be measured, evaluated and assessed. Physical measures, cognitive measures, and affective measures are presented here. Although these three categories of measures by no means exhaust the possibilities, they are ones frequently applied in research.

Physical Measures.   The very nature of the activity inherent in the fields of HHP provides countless opportunities for physical measure. Physical education and the various areas of exercise science have produced a large variety of tests to measure physiological fitness, motor behavior and learning skills, sport skills, anthropometric attributes, and biomechanics variables. Following are a few examples of the thousands of research topics dealing with physical parameters.

1. Factor pattern differences in tests of physical fitness, motor ability, and skill in selected populations of men and women.
2. Static and dynamic strength tests for both sexes in various age groups.
3. Kinematic and kinetic factors involved in pole vaulting.
4. Task complexity effects on reaction times, movement time, and accuracy.
5. Sodium-calcium ratios and central body temperature in men during exercise and recovery.
6. Physiological responses to training.
7. Physical activity related to health promotion programs.
8. Distance, interval, and mixed methods of training for competitive swimming.

Cognitive Measures.   The HHP literature is profuse with tests developed to measure the acquisition of health, fitness, sport, and leisure knowledge. Typical examples include:

1. Oral and dental knowledge assessment of college students.
2. Health knowledge test for elementary school teachers.

3. A gymnastics apparatus knowledge test for college men in professional physical education.

4. Knowledge and practice of women physical education teachers regarding negligence.

5. Developing environmental knowledge and perceptivity in early childhood.

6. Cognitive learning related to motor performance in school orientation.

7. Leisure-time knowledge, activities, and interests of older Americans.

Affective Measures. Factors such as opinion, attitude, personality, motivation, interest, personal problems, mood, drive, and frustration are more difficult to capture quantitatively than are physical and cognitive variables. They are less objective and more unstable. Many change rapidly over time. The instruments developed to measure these variables have typically been paper-and-pencil self-report scales. If people are unwilling to provide information accurately and objectively, however, these measures may lack considerable validity. Nonetheless, there has been a considerable amount of research done on affective variables in the fields of HHP and better instruments have been developed to measure them. A few typical examples include the following:

1. Self-motivation and adherence to therapeutic exercise.

2. Leisure attitudes of selected populations.

3. Leisure-time activities and interests of aged residents.

4. Personality related to the sport of gymnastics.

5. Personality traits of highly skilled basketball and softball women athletes.

6. Attributes of nationally rated intercollegiate basketball officials.

7. Personality and attitude of selected traffic violators and nonviolators.

8. Adolescents' attitudes toward and beliefs about AIDS.

9. Self-concept related to lifestyle attitude and practice.

The measurement method utilizes more techniques than either of the other two methods.

Measurement Techniques in HHP. Following are descriptions of some of the techniques frequently used in HHP studies.

Inventory. With the use of this technique, the researcher tries to measure interests, attitudes, personality, personal problems, likes and dislikes, and motivation. Most inventories are self-report instruments on which subjects "take stock" of themselves. Questions are asked or statements are presented to which the research subjects are asked to respond. The total amount of information obtained represents a measure of the variable being studied. Following is an excerpt of ten statements from the Athletic

Motivation Inventory developed by Tutko, Lyon, and Ogilvie in 1969.[1] The original instrument contained some two hundred statements. "The purpose of the test is to provide information that can be personally beneficial to an athlete" (Tutko, Lyon, and Ogilvie 1969, 1).

I believe that the coach is not always right . . . . (A) sometimes (B) seldom (C) never
I seldom stay after practice to work out . . . . (A) true (B) somewhat true (C) false
I lose my temper during competition . . . . (A) sometimes (B) seldom (C) never
There is absolutely no excuse for being late
for practice . . . . (A) true (B) uncertain (C) false
There are usually one or two fellow athletes
with whom I can't get along . . . . (A) sometimes (B) seldom (C) never
When the team loses it is usually my fault . . . . (A) true (B) uncertain (C) false
I would like the responsibility of being a coach . . . . (A) very true (B) true (C) uncertain
I perform poorly after being harshly criticized . . . . (A) sometimes (B) seldom (C) never
Most athletes do not wear uniforms . . . . (A) true (B) seldom (C) never
When new athletes join the team or competition I . . . (A) try to show them up (B) hope they
compete well (C) try to help them

Sociometric Technique.   This technique attempts to describe social relationships among individuals in a group by having members of a group indicate individual preferences based on some social criterion. Though not applied on as large a scale in HHP as are some of the other measurement techniques, there appears to be a growing body of HHP research using sociometric analysis. The following question was used in a cohesiveness/cooperation study of a football team: "What member of the team would you select, regardless of the amount of playing time, as being the most inspirational leader on the team?" In a larger sense, it is well known that the sociometric technique is used when youngsters "choose up" sides for a playground or gymnasium game and when members of a team select a captain or most valuable player.

Projective Technique.   The use of this technique attempts to measure the internal feelings, values, attitudes, and needs of an individual (Best and Kahn 1998). A commonly used projective technique is based upon association, whereby participants are presented some type of ambiguous stimulus and then asked to project into the stimulus some psychological dimension, such as wants, fears, needs, and so forth. The Rorschach Inkblot Test is a good example of the projective technique. A spot of ink is dropped on a piece of paper, which is then folded. When the paper is unfolded, the subject is asked to indicate what the resultant inked figure looks like. Associations and perceptions can also be stimulated in subjects by having them view cartoons and pictures or having them listen to particular words. For example, word-association

---

1. From *Athletic Motivation Inventory,* by T. A. Tutko, L. P. Lyon, and B. C. Ogilvie, 1969, Institute for the Study of Athletic Motivation at California State University, San Jose. Reprinted with permission.

tests in which the tester says "I'll say a word and now you tell me the first thing that comes to mind" are among the most frequently used projective techniques based upon association.

Scaling Techniques.　Scales are devices used by researchers to attempt to quantify responses to various concepts and variables. A scale is actually an instrument with gradations or levels that is used to assign a numerical value to a subject's response to a concept, subject, or characteristic of interest. Scaling techniques measure the degree to which the subject values or exhibits the desired construct and are generally believed to obtain interval data. Scales can be used to obtain data on almost any topic, object, or subject. Attitudes, opinions, values, perceptions and even behaviors are frequently measured by some scaling device. Evaluation and assessment are often accomplished through the use of various scaling techniques. Several of the most popular types of scales are presented below.

Rating Scales. These scales can be numerical or verbal. Observers rate each item by selecting a verbal or numerical point on the scale that corresponds to their impression of the item. Table 3.1 represents a verbal rating scale administered to selected sport managers. The researcher's objective is to obtain data indicating how the importance of various administrative concepts relates to the successful operation of a sport management program.

Table 3.2 is another verbal scale that was used to determine the harmfulness of various controlled substances as perceived by undergraduate college students.

In both of these examples the subjects are presented a continuum of responses and will place an X in the preferred response column.

TABLE 3.1 Administrative Concept Scale

CONCEPTS	NO IMPORTANCE	MODERATE IMPORTANCE	GREATEST IMPORTANCE
Staff Discipline			
Communication			
Personnel Management			
Objectives and Goals			
Public Relations			
Computer Use			
Organizational Design			
Etc.			

Tables 3.3 and 3.4 are examples of numerical scales. Table 3.3 lists characteristics of an administrator that are to be rated on a scale of 1 to 10, with 1 indicating a low rating and 10 a high rating. Table 3.4 contains a scale to be used by graduate students who have completed a program in HHP.

Tables 3.1–3.4 are modified versions of the original instruments, edited here to conserve space. Because human beings do the rating, the rating scale technique is susceptible to the **halo effect.** A person may like or be favorably disposed to the person being rated, and so they may give that individual high ratings on all of the scale items. On the other hand, a dislike for the person being rated could

TABLE 3.2 Drug Evaluation Scale

DRUG	NOT HARMFUL	SLIGHTLY HARMFUL	VERY HARMFUL	DISASTROUS
Cocaine				
Crack				
Hashish				
Amphetamines				
Steroids				
Morphine				
Marijuana				
Etc.				

TABLE 3.3 Administrative Evaluation Scale

CHARACTERISTICS	RESPONSE
Honest and sincere	1 2 3 4 5 6 7 8 9 10
Treats faculty with respect	1 2 3 4 5 6 7 8 9 10
Motivates faculty in job performance	1 2 3 4 5 6 7 8 9 10
A good communicator; knowledgeable in all HHP programs	1 2 3 4 5 6 7 8 9 10
Empathic toward faculty concerns	1 2 3 4 5 6 7 8 9 10
Maintains equity in faculty salaries	1 2 3 4 5 6 7 8 9 10
Knowledgeable about research, etc.	1 2 3 4 5 6 7 8 9 10

TABLE 3.4 HHP Graduate Program Evaluation Scale

PROGRAM FACTORS	INADEQUATE; UNSATISFACTORY	ADEQUATE; SATISFACTORY	OUTSTANDING; EXCELLENT
My overall degree program	1 2 3	4 5 6	7 8 9
The courses in my major	1 2 3	4 5 6	7 8 9
The courses in my inside minor	1 2 3	4 5 6	7 8 9
The courses in my outside minor	1 2 3	4 5 6	7 8 9
Academic advisement in the School of HHP	1 2 3	4 5 6	7 8 9
Career counseling in the School of HHP	1 2 3	4 5 6	7 8 9
HHP facilities (in terms of my program)	1 2 3	4 5 6	7 8 9
Library resources for my area of interest	1 2 3	4 5 6	7 8 9
Academic competence of HHP faculty in my area	1 2 3	4 5 6	7 8 9
Teaching effectiveness of HHP faculty	1 2 3	4 5 6	7 8 9
Methods of evaluating student achievement in HHP	1 2 3	4 5 6	7 8 9
My experience as grad assistant	1 2 3	4 5 6	7 8 9
Etc.			

result in low ratings on all of the scale items. Since ratings are subject to considerable error, thus reducing their reliability and validity, instruments must be carefully designed and participants sufficiently instructed as to the appropriate use of rating scales.

Semantic Differential Scale. This is a technique that has been shown to be quite versatile and valid in measuring attitude and concepts. Research participants are asked to make judgments on a concept based on the use of bipolar adjectives. They will respond by placing an X in one of the spaces between each pair of adjectives. Table 3.5 contains an example of the semantic differential where the concept to be rated is "athlete." The responses made by the subjects are converted to numerical values and are treated statistically. For a more detailed discussion of this technique, students are referred to Best and Kahn (1998) and Alreck and Settle (1995).

Rank Order Scales. In this technique the research participants are asked to rank, usually in order of importance, a series of concepts or items. Table 3.6 presents an example of the rank order technique. The twelve qualities of conduct are to be ranked from 1 to 12, with 1 representing the most important quality and 12 representing the least important.

TABLE 3.5 Athlete								
Kind	___	___	___	___	___	___	___	Cruel
Bad	___	___	___	___	___	___	___	Good
Beautiful	___	___	___	___	___	___	___	Ugly
Slow	___	___	___	___	___	___	___	Fast
Strong	___	___	___	___	___	___	___	Weak
Masculine	___	___	___	___	___	___	___	Feminine
Soft	___	___	___	___	___	___	___	Hard
Active	___	___	___	___	___	___	___	Passive
Wise	___	___	___	___	___	___	___	Foolish
Unsociable	___	___	___	___	___	___	___	Sociable
Graceful	___	___	___	___	___	___	___	Awkward
Small	___	___	___	___	___	___	___	Large

TABLE 3.6 Qualities of Conduct Scale	
Ambitious (hard working, aspiring)	_____
Broad-minded (open-minded)	_____
Capable (competent, effective)	_____
Courageous (standing up for your beliefs)	_____
Helpful (working for the welfare of others)	_____
Honest (creditable, commendable)	_____
Imaginative (daring, creative)	_____
Logical (rational, consistent)	_____
Obedient (dutiful, respectful)	_____
Responsible (dependable, reliable)	_____
Loving (affectionate, tender)	_____
Independent (self-reliant, self-sufficient)	_____

Paired-Comparison Scale. Several pairs of concepts are presented in this technique. The research subjects are asked to indicate which item of each pair is the most important by underlining or circling it. Table 3.7 is a paired-comparison example containing several pairs of value preferences. The subjects are to select which value of each pair is the most important or most preferred.

Likert Scale. This is a five-point scale designed to measure a particular attitude, belief, or judgment about something. The continuum of response runs from strongly agree (SA), agree (A), undecided (U), disagree (D), to strongly disagree (SD). The subjects responding to a Likert-type attitude scale are asked to circle the letter of the point on the scale that represents their opinion, belief, or judgment. An example of the Likert technique appears in table 3.8.

If the Likert intervals (SA to SD) are presumed to be equal thus resulting in interval data, a scoring system can be applied to allow the responses to be treated statistically. If the Likert intervals are not presumed to be equal but rather ordinal in nature, a sum of the scores is not legitimate and the scale may

TABLE 3.7 Value Preferences Scale

VALUES

A prosperous life (wealth)
An exciting life (stimulating, active)

Salvation (saved, eternal life)
Human equality

Human freedoms
A world at peace

Family well-being
Social recognition

National unity
Inner harmony

Etc.

TABLE 3.8 Team Cohesiveness

I feel that being on this team gave me a chance to make friends.	SA A U D SD
Most of my teammates believe in things I do not.	SA A U D SD
The coach always tried to do the right thing for the team.	SA A U D SD
I didn't like the members of this team very much.	SA A U D SD
The coach of the team didn't really know basketball; she just got stuck with the job.	SA A U D SD
Most of my teammates were out for their own glory and cared little about the team.	SA A U D SD
I believe playing on this team was boring.	SA A U D SD
The other players on the team were willing to help me if I needed it.	SA A U D SD
I feel that I have some really good friends among my teammates.	SA A U D SD
I cared less what the coach or other players said; I believe in making my own decisions.	SA A U D SD

have to be analyzed item by item. Whether the items all measure the same or different concepts influences, to some degree, whether the sum of the item scores is correct. A discussion of this issue is beyond the scope of this book.

Questioning Techniques

Structured Questionnaire.   Also called the *closed-ended questionnaire,* this instrument includes questions that can be answered with yes-no or true-false responses, or by selecting an answer from a list of suggested (multiple-choice) responses. The short, quick response format takes less time and effort from the sub-jects and tends to be fairly objective. The analysis of the data from this type of instru-ment is relatively simple.

The following examples from an instrument used in a breast cancer study, illustrate the structured type of item:

How would you classify your knowledge of breast cancer, in particular the various methods of detection?

_____   quite knowledgeable

_____   some knowledge

_____   very little knowledge

How have you learned about breast cancer? Check any appropriate answer.

_____   media (newspaper, TV, radio, etc.)

_____   literature from cancer societies

_____   physician

_____   health course

_____   experience (yourself or family member)

Unstructured Questionnaire.   Also called the *open-ended* or *essay question-naire,* this technique provides an either-or or multiple-response opportunity. Subjects answer freely in their own words. While this format tends to produce answers of greater depth, it takes considerable time on the part of the subject. It requires a highly motivated person to wade through several open-ended questions. This type of questionnaire is frequently used in exploratory situations, those in which the researcher is trying to gain information that may or may not exist in any particular manner, shape, or form. The unstructured item is not always easily tabulated, ana-lyzed, and interpreted. The following examples from a study of applicants for an Assistant Athletic Director/Athlete Advisor position illustrate the open-ended item:

How would you motivate a student-athlete who has demonstrated excellent athletic ability, but is very apathetic toward academic responsibilities?

A coach has an athlete who appears marginally ineligible. He asks your assistance in getting this athlete eligible. What would be your response to the coach, the athlete, and any faculty involved?

Checklist.   A relatively simple instrument, the checklist is basically a very highly structured questionnaire. Usually, a long "laundry list" of items is presented and the subject is asked to check those that apply. Sometimes a yes or no response is necessary. A "things to do today" list or a "things to do to get ready for vacation" list are examples of the typical checklist. The example shown in Box 3.1 appeared in a park and recreation interest survey.

Structured Interview.   In large measure, the structured interview technique is an oral questionnaire. The researcher poses the questions, along with the expected answers, much the same as the structured questionnaire. The questions are asked in order and no repetition is permitted. Questions other than those listed are not permitted. The questions and expected answers are written down in what is called an *interview guide.* Distinct advantages of this technique are that (1) less bias prevails because whatever is in the guide is asked without alteration, and (2) the interviewer may not

BOX 3.1

		Your Leisure Interest			
Do Now	**Would Like to Do**		**Do Now**	**Would Like to Do**	
_____	_____	Little League baseball	_____	_____	Football
_____	_____	Slow-pitch softball	_____	_____	Square dancing
_____	_____	Community Center activities	_____	_____	Tennis
_____	_____	Attending sporting events (outdoors)	_____	_____	Swimming
_____	_____	Attending sporting events (indoors)	_____	_____	Boating
_____	_____	Fishing	_____	_____	Hiking
_____	_____	Family camping	_____	_____	Golf
_____	_____	Picnicking	_____	_____	Playground
_____	_____	Shuffleboard	_____	_____	Ice skating
_____	_____	Basketball	_____	_____	Horseshoes
		List below any others	_____	_____	Rifle range
_____	_____	_____			
_____	_____	_____			
_____	_____	_____			

need to know a lot about the research dynamics being studied. Public opinion pollsters frequently use this technique by employing high school or college students as interviewers. They are screened for good interpersonal skills (essential to this technique) and then are sent out to do the interviewing without a lot of information concerning the variables and dynamics involved.

Unstructured Interview.   This technique utilizes no set format of questions and expected answers. The open-ended question format applies in that the person being interviewed is supposed to answer in his or her own words and provide all relevant information in as long or brief a period of time as is necessary. The interviewer may have a guide with possible questions, but is not tied to it. Usually the interviewer will know the areas of the research dynamics being studied and will select questions from each one. There usually is no set order for the questions and they can be repeated to ensure complete understanding on the part of the interviewee. No question implies a particular response. One major advantage of this technique is that follow-up or clarifying questions can be asked to preclude misconceptions on the part of both the interviewer and interviewee. Good interpersonal skills on the part of the interviewers are important, but perhaps even more so is the amount of knowledge they have concerning the research dynamics to which the questions are tied. Limited knowledge about the research topic provides a dull, boring, and weak data collection interview. The more informed interviewers are, the better decisions or judgments they will make as the interview process unfolds.

Focus Group Interview.   A relatively new technique to HHP, focus group interviews have become a popular qualitative research technique for gathering information, particularly for research in education, health, and recreation. The results of focus group interviews have made significant contributions to product-marketing research as well as program evaluations. Greenbaum (1998) indicates that there are three major types of focus groups: full groups, minigroups, and telephone groups. Full focus groups, the most common of the three, typically involve eight to twelve individuals who discuss a particular topic or issue under the guidance of a group facilitator or moderator. The moderator poses questions to the group, leads the group discussion to insure that it stays on track, and attempts to stimulate discussion from all participants. Often, focus group interviews are video or audio recorded in order to minimize the need for the moderator to record the views expressed. Alternatively, a research assistant could be utilized to record pertinent information during the conduct of the focus group. It is noted that focus groups are qualitative in nature and do not represent scientifically drawn samples, thus there are substantial limitations in being able to generalize the results to larger populations. Further discussion of focus group interviews is presented in chapter 9.

Delphi Technique.   This technique is unique in the questioning method employed and is used to get consensus from a defined group of individuals on a specific issue. Individuals respond to the questions to produce the collective input of the group.

Then each one reviews his or her position based upon group trends and revises that position as warranted. Ultimately, a group consensus is obtained. The Delphi technique has not been extensively used in HHP, but has wide application potential for topics in those fields. In brief, the Delphi technique is accomplished through the following procedures (Rubinson and Neutens 1997):

1. Identify group members whose consensus opinions are sought.
2. Use initial questionnaire to solicit concerns, goals, and problems for which consensus is sought (e.g., knowledge competencies needed for a particular field of study, such as adapted physical education teachers, health educators, outdoor educators, and exercise specialists).
3. Arrange initial results in a second questionnaire. Each member ranks these items in terms of importance.
4. Present a third questionnaire containing an initial trend toward consensus on each item along with each member's initial response. Again each item is rated.
5. Administer a fourth questionnaire. It contains the data obtained from the third questionnaire and each member's most recent ranking. A consensus trend appears as the items are ranked for the third and final time.
6. Present the data from the fourth questionnaire, representing the final group consensus.

Criteria for Selecting Methods and Techniques

The selection of the data-gathering method(s) and technique(s) is always based on the type of data needed to solve the research problem, and many underlying factors must be considered. The researcher will examine the needs of the research in terms of (1) the demands on the subjects, (2) the cost in terms of energy, money, and time that will be required, and (3) personal ability to handle the selected methods and techniques, including data analysis procedures. The process usually follows this sequence: Problem → Data → Approach → Method(s) → Technique(s). The problem of the research implies a certain kind of data obtained by the selected research approach. The approach will incorporate one or more methods that will be carried out by one or more techniques. Once a technique has been determined, the instrument needed to collect the data must be determined.

Data-Collecting Instruments

A **data-collecting instrument** is any paper-and-pencil test or measure, mechanical or electronic equipment measure, or physical performance test used to collect information (data) on the variable under study. The choice of the instrument to be used in the data collection process involves deciding whether it will be one that has already been developed and will be used as it is, one that already exists but will be revised, or one that will be new and needs to be developed. This decision will be based on the needs of the research and what instruments are available.

Whenever data are to be collected, the researcher must keep in mind that, at a minimum, there are three characteristics or attributes data must have to be worth using in a research study: (1) objectivity, (2) reliability, and (3) validity. **Objectivity,** sometimes called *rater reliability,* exists if the same or similar scores would occur no matter who collected the scores. In other words, the data are not unique to the person who collects them. Objectivity of the data are estimated by having two or more people independently score the performance of each individual in a group as he/she performs. Then the scores of the two or more persons are compared as to agreement. An example for physical performance data is each of two people independently scoring each person in a group as to the number of sit-ups correctly executed as he/she takes a sit-up test. For paper-and-pencil test data each of two people would independently score the test. If there is good agreement, objectivity is demonstrated. An intraclass correlation coefficient is calculated to determine the degree of agreement. The maximum value of the coefficient is 1.0 and a value of at least .70 and maybe .80 would be required to indicate acceptable objectivity. (More on objectivity, including the calculation of an intraclass correlation coefficient, can be found in Baumgartner and Jackson [1999].) Once the objectivity of the data from a test or measuring procedure has been demonstrated, it is not necessary to estimate objectivity each time the test or measuring procedure is used. If the scores from a test or measuring procedure are found to be sufficiently objective, then reliability of the data is estimated.

Reliability is declared for the data to the extent that a test or measuring procedure yields the same or basically the same score for a person on two or more occasions. This could mean administering the test or measuring procedure two or more times within a day, called **internal consistency reliability.** This is commonly done with non-fatiguing physical performance tests and measures. An example is administering three trials, one after another, of a sit-and-reach test to measure flexibility. For knowledge tests or any paper-and-pencil test where a total score is obtained, internal consistency reliability is calculated as an indicator of consistency of performance across test items. If the test or measuring procedure is administered once on each of two or more days, **stability reliability** can be determined. An example is administering a one-minute sit-up test on one day and then administering the test again three days later.

Reliability for physical performance measures is estimated by calculating an intraclass correlation coefficient. Reliability for paper-and-pencil tests is commonly estimated by calculating the Cronbach alpha coefficient or a Kuder-Richardson coefficient. The maximum reliability no matter the technique used is 1.0 and usually a value of at least .70 is required to demonstrate acceptable reliability. Once the reliability of the data from a test or measuring procedure has been demonstrated it is not necessary to establish reliability each time the test or measuring procedure is used. However, reliability can be influenced by factors such as the gender, or age of the group tested, so be sure any previously reported reliability coefficients apply to the group used in your research. (More on reliability and the calculation of reliability coefficients can be found in measurement books like Baumgartner and Jackson [1999].) If the scores from a test or measuring procedure are found to be sufficiently reliable, then the data has the potential to be valid.

Validity is declared for the data from a test or measuring procedure if the data really are measures of what they purport to measure. For example, if you administered a paper-and-pencil test that was supposed to measure fitness knowledge and it really did measure fitness knowledge because the more fitness knowledge a person had the higher the person scored on the test, the test would be declared valid. Validity is not all or none; there are degrees of validity. Thus, to the extent that things other than fitness knowledge influenced scores on the test, the test would not be perfectly valid. Validity can be estimated using a variety of techniques too numerous to discuss here. Consult any measurement book for information on estimating validity. The important thing for a researcher to remember is that before data are collected make sure the test or data collection procedure will yield valid data. As a consumer of research, when reading a research report, check that the tests or measuring procedures are known and/or documented to yield valid data.

Selecting the Instrument

Selecting a research instrument for any project is usually the result of a thorough search of the literature. The researcher who wants to study the effect of improved physical fitness on the self-concept of adolescents will probably find that several tests measuring self-concept are available. Once it is determined that such an instrument exists, the next step is to assess its acceptability. We have just finished a discussion of certain characteristics of data. Some of these same criteria apply to the selection of the data instrument as well. Whether the instrument is *reliable* (measures consistently each time the test is used), whether it is *objective* (free of tester bias), and whether it is *valid* (measures what it is suppose to measure) are important characteristics in this part of the process also. In this case, an acceptable instrument would be shown to, in fact, measure self-concept the same way on repeated applications of the test. Quite frequently an instrument will be selected on the basis of its reliability and validity as reported by the researchers who have used it in earlier studies. If measures of reliability and validity are not provided, various statistical techniques can be applied to quantitatively determine the reliability and validity of the instrument. Measurement books such as Baumgartner and Jackson (1999) discuss these techniques. Sometimes, researchers must make their own determination of the reliability and validity of the instrument they plan to use. Part of determining validity is analyzing whether or not the instrument is *appropriate*. Can the subjects meet the demands of the instrument, or is it too hard or too easy for the ability of the subjects? The vocabulary of an instrument may be appropriate for one age group and not for another. The same can be true for certain physical performance tests. If the instrument is not appropriate, it will not produce valid data. Without reliability and validity the data are of no use in answering the research question.

In selecting an instrument, a researcher will also consider other criteria. How easy the test is to administer, how much it costs in time and money, and how easy it is to score are other factors the researcher must consider. Ideally, the researcher selects the most reliable and valid instrument. In reality, however, if that test is difficult, time consuming, costly, and very demanding of the subjects, the researcher may instead select a test that is a little less reliable and valid, but is less difficult to handle, has a shorter administrative time span, is less costly, and is less demanding of the subjects.

Revising the Instrument

Quite often a researcher locates an instrument that is not quite acceptable for the intended research situation, in which case the instrument must be revised. Permission should be obtained before revising a paper-and-pencil instrument originally developed by someone else. Permission is sometimes needed to revise a physical performance instrument. When a standardized instrument is used or revised, permission from the instrument's publisher is required.

Changes in an original instrument may take many forms, but are usually done to better fit a particular group of subjects. Self-concept has been studied with different age groups, sexes, and races, and various kinds of disabled populations. Obviously, one instrument designed to measure self-concept cannot be used with all subject groups. The same can be said concerning the study of countless numbers of variables of a research interest. Collins, in her 1989 study of body figure perceptions and preferences among male and female preadolescent children, used a pictorial instrument modified from the original instrument developed in 1983 that used adult male and female subjects (Stunkard, Sorenson, and Schulsinger 1983). Basically, the major change was that Collins revised the Stunkard adult figure drawings to reflect the figures of children. She also used seven figures for each gender, while Stunkard used nine figures. Revising an instrument may change its reliability and validity, and new measures must be determined for the revised instrument if changes are major enough. Note: Reliability and validity of an instrument are often specific to the age and gender of the subjects.

Instrument Development

It is difficult and time-consuming to develop an instrument and this procedure is avoided by both veteran and beginning researchers whenever possible. The task is undertaken only when it becomes obvious that no paper-and-pencil, electronic or mechanical, or physical performance test or instrument exists to generate the needed research data.

The starting point for instrument development is, once again, the literature. All of the dynamics in the prospective research problem must be thoroughly understood, and what instruments are available to use as models must be known before the instrument development begins. Suppose a researcher is interested in determining the motivation of high school students for participating or not participating in athletics. The dynamics involved in this phenomenon are many and are comprised of intellectual, sociological, psychological, and physiological components. A complete review of the literature must include related research and conceptual articles reflecting each of those components and what instruments others have used. The knowledge accrued from such a review will provide the basis for determining the content of the instrument. That is, what type of questions and/or statements will contribute most in the attempt to measure the motivation students have, or do not have, for athletic involvement during high school?

The usual next step is to select the questions or statements and produce a tentative instrument. In writing these research items, the researcher is careful to see that each item will provide a reasonable estimate of each relevant component of the athletic motivation problem. If, for example, one of the components related to athletic participation is the student's perception of whether or not athletic participation will enhance the chances of being successful in life, then the researcher's task is to develop questions or statements that will provide an estimate of this component. If the students perceive that athletic participation will enhance their self-concept and status among their peers, the instrument should contain items that will provide a measurable estimate of these components.

Once the tentative instrument has been developed, it is then submitted to a jury of experts or committee of authorities. The researcher invites selected individuals, who are considered to have expertise in the problem area, to review the content of the instrument. These can be people who have taught, researched, or written in the problem area. The task of the jury members is to review the research questions or statements and revise them as needed. Which items should be rewritten? Should any of the items be deleted? Should items be added? Which items are most significant to the essence of the problem? Which are relatively insignificant? Needless to say, the work of the jury suggests careful attention to the elimination of instrument flaws. Submitting the proposed instrument to a jury of experts is an excellent way to increase the content validity of the measured tool.

Based on the reaction of the jury, the researcher revises the instrument. In most instances the instrument is submitted to the jury only once, but it may be necessary to repeat the procedure two or more times.

The next step in the instrument development process is the pilot study or preliminary investigation. The intended instrument is administered to subjects selected from the same population of subjects who will make up the actual research sample, but who are *not* sample subjects. The pilot study serves as a trial run of the instrument to see if it is in further need of revision. The objectives of a pilot study are (1) to determine whether or not the subjects understand the content items in the instrument, (2) to determine whether the instrument will provide the needed data, (3) to familiarize the researcher and any assistants with instrument administration procedures, (4) to obtain a set of data for trying out the proposed data treatment techniques, and (5) to first determine the reliability and then the validity of the instrument.

The researcher will further revise the instrument if the pilot shows change to be necessary. A pilot study may not always be needed, but is a valuable research tool. The knowledge that the instrument is sufficient and will yield reliable and valid data, that the planned instrument administration procedure is appropriate, and that the planned attack on the research problem is the proper approach are the typical payoffs for conducting a pilot study. The actual research study may not be completely without problems, but the prospects of severe trouble occurring are diminished by having performed a test run. With a successful pilot study, the researcher can claim a finalized instrument.

This discussion of instrument development happens to be for a paper-and-pencil instrument. However, the same basic steps occur in the process of developing any instrument. These steps are: (1) survey the literature, (2) develop a tentative instrument, (3) reflect upon and revise the instrument, (4) obtain opinions of experts concerning the instrument, (5) revise the instrument, (6) conduct a pilot study, (7) revise the instrument, and (8) use the instrument.

Summary

The research problem can be attacked using a variety of approaches: historical, descriptive (quantitative), qualitative, or experimental. The nature of the research problem coupled with the intent of the researcher will generally point to a preferred research approach. Formulating hypotheses will provide direction to the research approach and guide the researcher in designing data collection methods and techniques that will elicit the information needed to complete the study. Since extraneous variables could likely influence the results of a study in an unknown or undesired way, the researcher must attempt to control or minimize their effect. Three methods of controlling extraneous variables are discussed. Data-collecting methods and techniques are determined based upon the selected research approach, and the research instrumentation relates to the techniques necessary to produce the needed data. Several examples have been provided to aid the student in applying these concepts.

Formative Evaluation of Objectives

Objective 1 Suggest one study that could be researched under each research approach.

1. Write out a statement of the problem for the following:
   a) a descriptive study.
   b) a historical study.
   c) an experimental study.
   d) a qualitative study.

Objective 2   Understand the role of hypotheses and hypothesis testing in the research process.

1. Using the problem statement developed above for an experimental study, write out the null hypothesis as well as a tentative research hypothesis.

Objective 3   Know when it is appropriate to apply the different methods of collecting data.

1. Name a topic that could be an appropriate study for

   a) observation.
   b) measurement.
   c) questioning.

Objective 4   Know the various techniques available for each data collection method.

1. What technique would be most useful in studying the health knowledge of junior high school students?

Objective 5   State the criteria for selecting the appropriate research instrument.

1. What are the three most important characteristics one should look for in selecting a research instrument?

Ethical Concerns in Research

4

KEY WORDS

Authorship	Confidentiality	Institutional Review	Plagiarism
45 C. F. R. 46	Ethics	Board (IRB)	Privacy
Belmont Report	Helsinki Declaration	Justice	Respect for persons
Beneficence	Human subjects protection	Nazi experimentation	Scientific misconduct
Common Rule	Informed consent	Nuremberg Code	Situational ethics
			Tuskegee Syphilis Study

OBJECTIVES

The public acceptance of the scientific method as a source of knowledge is founded, at least in part, on the integrity associated with the process. While it is impossible to legislate ethics, the scientific community has sought to develop ethical standards that provide direction for conducting research. The effectiveness of such standards is ultimately dependent upon the adherence and practices of individual researchers. Since most research in HHP involves the use of human subjects in one way or another, it is important for researchers to consider the ethical principles and regulations that guide their research activities.

After reading chapter 4, you should be able to

1. Discuss various instances of ethical misconduct in research involving humans.
2. Identify ethical codes and federal regulations that serve to guide research in the United States.
3. Understand the importance of informed consent in research involving human subjects.
4. Understand the role and function of Institutional Review Boards in approving research activities.
5. Explain ethical considerations involved in the disclosure of research results.

The Basis of Ethics in Research

As researchers work to contribute to the knowledge of a profession, they engage in a variety of activities that are critical to making the scientific method an effective and credible source of information in the search for truth. While the scientific method, with its orderly, systematic nature and built-in series of checks, has evolved to become highly respected as a source of knowledge, the integrity of this very system is founded upon the professional conduct of the researcher. Dishonest, fraudulent, or unethical researchers can circumvent the scientific method. While the quest for knowledge is important to a profession, and the application of such knowledge is important to professional practices and to society as a whole, we must also concern ourselves with the ethics of the researcher and the rights and well-being of the research participants.

History has taught us that without moral principles, protective measures, and a system of ethical standards that oblige researchers to follow certain rules, scientific misconduct and dishonesty will occur. It is noted, however, that the mere existence of ethical standards does not guarantee ethical behavior by researchers. Ultimately, it is the responsibility of individual researchers to conduct themselves in a way that promotes integrity and honesty throughout the scientific method. The following examples illustrate scientific inquiry gone askew.

Nazi Germany Experimentation During World War II

Perhaps the most grievous examples of unethical behavior in research were the "medical experiments" of Nazi scientists during World War II (**Nazi experimentation**). The charges brought against twenty-three German physicians in the Nuremberg War Crime Trials (the "Doctors' Trial") for their "medical experiments" upon prisoners, concentration camp inmates, and other living human subjects without the consent of these people shocked the world and exposed the dark side of humanity. The trials documented charges that, in the course of these "medical experiments," the doctors subjected thousands of people to cruelties, tortures, and other inhuman acts. Most of the people were murdered. Experiments included, but were not limited to the following:

> *Freezing Experiments.* These experiments were designed to determine how long it would take to lower the temperature of the human body to the point of death and also to determine how best to re-warm a frozen victim. Prisoners were outfitted in aviator uniforms or stripped naked and either placed in an icy tank of water or strapped to a stretcher and placed outside in freezing temperatures. Methods for re-warming a frozen body included placing the victim under extremely hot sunlamps, immersing the victim in a hot bath and slowly increasing the temperature, or internal irrigation whereby hot water was forced into the stomach, bladder, and intestines. The investigators claimed that they hoped to determine the most effective means of treating persons who had been frozen.

Malaria Experiments. Prisoners and concentration camp inmates were purposively exposed to mosquitoes that were known to carry the malaria virus, or were given direct injections of the virus, in order to investigate the effect of various antimalarial compounds. After having contracted malaria, the subjects were treated with various drugs to test their relative efficacy. Testimony revealed that victims not dying of malaria often suffered substantial and debilitating side effects from the various compounds being tested. The alleged intent of these experiments was to determine effective immunization and treatment for malaria.

High-Altitude Experiments. Supposedly to investigate the limits of human endurance and existence at extremely high altitudes, Nazi physicians placed concentration camp inmates in a low-pressure chamber capable of reproducing atmospheric conditions and pressures prevailing at extremely high altitudes. As the simulated altitude was progressively increased, victims experienced excruciating pain, spasmodic convulsions, grave injury, and, frequently, death—due to an enormous amount of air embolism that developed in the brain, coronary vessels, and other internal organs.

The international outrage over the atrocities revealed at the Nuremberg War Crime Trials led to the development of the **Nuremberg Code,** a set of basic principles to govern the ethical conduct of research involving human subjects. Although the code focused on biomedical experiments, since its publication in 1947 it has been widely recognized as the starting point for systematic protection of human subjects in all areas of research.

Tuskegee Syphilis Study

Even as the Nuremberg War Crime Trials were being conducted, the United States Public Health Service supported a research project that constituted an example of unethical behavior, and blatant misconduct—in the name of science. In 1932, the United States Public Health Service initiated a study in Macon County, Alabama, to investigate the long-term effects of untreated syphilis. At the time, Macon County was poor, semi-illiterate, and reportedly had the highest syphilis rate in the country, 36 percent, compared to less than 1 percent for the nation as a whole. While funding to support a treatment program was "not available," researchers believed that the high rate of syphilis in Macon County warranted further investigation. Moreover, there was speculation among some medical personnel that African Americans responded differently to the disease than did other racial groups. So the decision was made to conduct a prospective study and follow the long-term effects, all the way until death, of untreated syphilis among African Americans living in Macon County. It is also noted that at the time the study commenced, no cure for syphilis was available.

Various inducements, such as free physical examinations, free treatment for minor health problems, food, transportation to and from the clinic, and a burial stipend of $50, were used to recruit 399 males with syphilis and another 200-plus controls without syphilis to be a part of the study. (The burial stipend was needed in order to obtain permission to perform autopsies upon the death of the research participants.) Recruitment was easy. Most of the study participants had little money and almost no access to medical care. In some instances, this represented the first opportunity ever to receive a medical examination. The participants, however, were never told the real nature of the study and were not afforded the opportunity to provide informed consent. In fact, many were never told they had syphilis and others thought they were being treated for "bad blood," a term that presumably was a synonym for syphilis. In reality, however, they were either not treated or provided only aspirin and an iron supplement to relieve some of the symptoms.

The periodic examinations for monitoring the course of the disease continued year after year. Moreover, treatment for syphilis was withheld, even after the discovery and widespread use of penicillin to treat syphilis in the 1940s. In order to preserve the integrity of the "experiment" and prevent treatment of those infected individuals by other doctors, the Public Health Service solicited and obtained agreements from local health departments as well as from the U.S. Army (for those individuals who were drafted) to not treat those participants in the study who were detected to have syphilis. The study continued for forty years. In 1972, an article in the *Washington Star* by Jean Heller exposed the story about the **Tuskegee Syphilis Study** and led to its termination. Following a series of congressional hearings on the matter, in 1974 the government agreed to an out-of-court settlement of approximately $10 million, paying each living participant $37,500 and the heirs of each deceased participant $15,000 altogether. In 1997, President Bill Clinton, speaking on behalf of the U. S. government, formally apologized for the syphilis study.

History contains other examples of experiments in which researchers have perpetrated unthinkable acts on unsuspecting research participants. The human radiation experiments conducted in the United States from the end of World War II to the mid-1970s represents one such example. Those interested in reading more about instances of scientific misconduct may wish to consult sources such as *Human Experimentation: When Research Is Evil* (McCuen 1998).

Regulation of Research and Protection of Research Participants

Ethics is concerned with human behavior from a perspective of right or wrong. According to Drowatzky (1996), "ethical statements are developed to prescribe behavior as directives that tell us what we ought to do in the situations we encounter." Ethical statements essentially define our values in terms of acceptable behaviors, telling us what we ought to do. It is important to note that ethics applies to our daily life, just as it does to research activities. But ethics may vary from one person to another, from one group to another, and from one culture to another. How, then, can we define normative ethics that apply to all individuals in all situations? Proponents of **situational ethics** argue that no general rules can be applied to all situations, that each action is unique and must be evaluated on its own merits, or lack thereof. In other words, "it depends." Others, however, believe that fundamental ethical principles can be formulated and that behavioral norms constitute the basis for such an ethical system (Drowatzky 1996).

The philosophical debate not withstanding, governments and organizations have generally embraced a normative approach to ethics. While it is recognized that no ethical standards or codes will totally prevent scientific misconduct, it is also recognized that without ethical standards to serve as guiding principles for appropriate behaviors, responsible conduct in research may be jeopardized and scientific knowledge devalued. Developed in 1947, the Nuremberg Code (see Box 4.1) represents the first attempt to develop ethical standards for the conduct of research involving human subjects and has become the prototype for other ethical guidelines developed since.

The World Medical Association (WMA) subsequently codified ethical guidelines for medical research involving human subjects in its *Declaration of Helsinki:*

BOX 4.1
The Nuremberg Code

(*Trials of War Criminals before the Nuremberg Military Tribunals under Control Council* Law No. 10, 1949.)

The Nuremberg Code

1. The voluntary consent of the human subject is absolutely essential.

   This means that the person involved should have legal capacity to give consent; should be so situated as to be able to exercise free power of choice, without the intervention of any element of force, fraud, deceit, duress, over-reaching, or other ulterior form of constraint or coercion; and should have sufficient knowledge and comprehension of the elements of the subject matter involved, as to enable him to make an understanding and enlightened decision. This latter element requires that, before the acceptance of an affirmative decision by the experimental subject, there should be made known to him the nature, duration, and purpose of the experiment; the method and means by which it is to be conducted; all inconveniences and hazards reasonably to be expected; and the effects upon his health or person, which may possibly come from his participation in the experiment.

   The duty and responsibility for ascertaining the quality of the consent rests upon each individual who initiates, directs or engages in the experiment. It is a personal duty and responsibility which may not be delegated to another with impunity.

2. The experiment should be such as to yield fruitful results for the good of society, unprocurable by other methods or means of study, and not random and unnecessary in nature.

BOX 4.1
Concluded

3. The experiment should be so designed and based on the results of animal experimentation and a knowledge of the natural history of the disease or other problem under study, that the anticipated results will justify the performance of the experiment.

4. The experiment should be so conducted as to avoid all unnecessary physical and mental suffering and injury.

5. No experiment should be conducted, where there is an *a priori* reason to believe that death or disabling injury will occur; except, perhaps, in those experiments where the experimental physicians also serve as subjects.

6. The degree of risk to be taken should never exceed that determined by the humanitarian importance of the problem to be solved by the experiment.

7. Proper preparations should be made and adequate facilities provided to protect the experimental subject against even remote possibilities of injury, disability, or death.

8. The experiment should be conducted only by scientifically qualified persons. The highest degree of skill and care should be required through all stages of the experiment of those who conduct or engage in the experiment.

9. During the course of the experiment, the human subject should be at liberty to bring the experiment to an end, if he has reached the physical or mental state, where continuation of the experiment seemed to him to be impossible.

10. During the course of the experiment, the scientist in charge must be prepared to terminate the experiment at any stage, if he has probable cause to believe, in the exercise of the good faith, superior skill and careful judgement required of him, that a continuation of the experiment is likely to result in injury, disability, or death to the experimental subject.

Recommendations Guiding Medical Doctors in Biomedical Research Involving Human Subjects (1964). The **Helsinki Declaration**, as it has come to be known, has since been revised slightly and reaffirmed by the World Medical Assembly of the WMA in 1975, 1983, 1989, 1996, and again in 2000. Readers should consult the website of the WMA for a complete description of the international code of medical ethics: (www.wma.net/e/policy/17-c e.html).

A variety of regulations protecting human subjects have been established in the United States. The **scientific misconduct** associated with the Tuskegee Syphilis Study, government-sponsored human radiation experiments between 1944 and 1974, and other incidents of nonconsensual experiments on human subjects led Congress in 1974 to pass the National Research Act, establishing the National Commission for the Protection of Human Subjects of Biomedical and Behavioral Research. The commission was charged with formulating ethical principles and guidelines for conducting research activities with human subjects. The resultant **Belmont Report** (1979) serves as a fundamental document for current federal regulations for the protection of human subjects in biomedical and behavioral research in the United States. Three basic ethical principles were set forth in the report:

1. **Respect for persons.** Proclaiming respect for individuals as autonomous agents capable of self-determination, and special protection to persons of diminished autonomy.

2. **Beneficence.** Obligating researchers to protect persons from harm, and to maximize possible benefits and minimize possible harms.

3. **Justice.** Requiring that the benefits and burdens of the research be fairly distributed, thus impacting upon the selection of research subjects.

The complete Belmont Report is available on the Web at the following address: http://ohrp.osophs.dhhs.gov/humansubjects/guidance/belmont.htm

In response to the commission's recommendations, the Department of Health, Education, and Welfare (now the Department of Health and Human Services, DHHS) and the Food and Drug Administration (FDA) enacted in 1981 major revisions to their existing policies concerning research involving human subjects. These basic government regulations have since been revised, most recently in 1991, and currently serve as the federal rules and regulations that govern research involving human subjects in the United States. The DHHS regulations, those most applicable to HHP researchers, were codified in federal law as Title 45, Part 46 of the Code of Federal Regulations **(45 C.F.R. 46)** June 18, 1991. These regulations are sometimes called the "**Common Rule.**" Subpart A constitutes the Federal Policy for the Protection of Human Subjects. The policies established therein are applicable (with certain exceptions specified) to all research activities involving human subjects conducted, supported, or otherwise regulated by any Federal Department or Agency (45 C.F.R. 46, 1991). Moreover, the code requires that all research protocols involving human subjects be reviewed by an **Institutional Review Board** (IRB) to assure compliance with the requirements set forth in this policy. For further information you may wish to consult with your local Institutional Review Board or read the entire federal code at the following website: http://ohrp.osophs.dhhs.gov/humansubjects/guidance/45cfr46.htm.

In 2000, the DHHS established the Office of Human Research Protections (OHRP) to assume responsibility for the development, coordination, and monitoring of policies relative to the protection of human subjects in research. This office maintains oversight of compliance polices and provides educational guidance materials on **human subjects protection.** The OHRP website provides a wealth of information concerning ethical standards and the protection of human subjects: http://ohrp.osophs.dhhs.gov.

In addition to the ethical standards and regulations promulgated by the federal government, many professional associations have developed ethical codes of conduct to guide the research activities of their members. The American Psychological Association (APA), for instance, issued its first code of ethics in 1953 and has subsequently revised the code several times since, the most recent being in 1992 (American Psychological Association 1992). Other associations publishing ethical standards or research guidelines that may be of interest to HHP researchers include, among others: American College of Sports Medicine (ACSM) (1999), American Educational Research Association (AERA) (1992), American Sociological Association (ASA), and the American School Health Association (ASHA). Whereas the ethical standards of professional associations typically relate to all practices pertinent to its members, some standards relate specifically to research practices. The following websites provide online access to the code of ethics for the respective associations:

> American Psychological Association (APA)
> www.apa.org/ethics/code.htm
>
> American Educational Research Association (AERA)
> www.aera.net/about/policy/ethics.htm
>
> American Sociological Association (ASA)
> www.asanet.org/members/ecointro.html

Informed Consent

The first provision of the Nuremberg Code and arguably the most important pillar underlying ethical standards governing research involving human participants states that "the voluntary consent of the human subject is absolutely essential." Inherent to this principle are four important elements: (1) subjects are made fully aware of the nature and purpose of the research project, (2) consent is voluntarily given, (3) the person involved has the legal capacity to give consent, and (4) the responsibility for obtaining consent rests with the researcher. Thus, **informed consent** is often seen as the key aspect of obtaining approval for conducting research involving human participants. An example of a written consent form used at the University of Northern Iowa appears in Example 4. 1.

In the United States, the Department of Health and Human Services articulates the requirements for informed consent in 45 C.F.R. Subpart A, Section 46.116 (1991). As set forth in these regulations, the basic elements of informed consent should include:

> **(1)** a statement that the study involves research, an explanation of the purposes of the research and the expected duration of the subject's participation, a description of the procedures to be followed, and identification of any procedures which are experimental;

(2) a description of any reasonably foreseeable risks or discomforts to the subject;

(3) a description of any benefits to the subject or to others which may reasonably be expected from the research;

(4) a disclosure of appropriate alternative procedures or courses of treatment, if any, that might be advantageous to the subject;

(5) a statement describing the extent, if any, to which confidentiality of records identifying the subject will be maintained;

(6) for research involving more than minimal risk, an explanation as to whether any compensation is available, and whether any medical treatments are available, if injury occurs and, if so, what these consist of, or where further information may be obtained;

Project Title: Validation of Accelerometers During Health-fitness Activities

Project Director(s): Kevin J. Finn, Ph.D., Forrest A. Dolgener, Ph.D.   Phone No. (319) 273-xxxx

Please read (listen to) the following information:

1. **The purpose of the project is to validate two accelerometers comparing the sensor counts to a measure of energy expenditure (oxygen consumption) while performing various physical activities used to promote health and wellness.**

2. **If you consent to participate, you will be involved in one or both of the two phases of the project. The first phase involves performing a treadmill protocol and cycling in a laboratory. This first phase should take one hour of your time.**

   A. Report to the Human Performance Laboratory on an assigned day. Upon signing an informed consent, you will have an accelerometer attached at the waist, hip, wrist, and ankle. In addition, a Polar (Polar CIC Inc) chest belt transmitter will be positioned on the middle torso with an elastic strap. Finally you will be fitted with a mouthpiece attached to a directional valve headgear to collect all expired air. The expired air will be analyzed for oxygen consumption using standard gas exchange methodology by the Sensor Medics 2900 system.

   B. The treadmill protocol will consist of four 5-min stages walking on a level grade at 2.0 and 4.0 miles per hour, walking 2.0 miles per hour at 5% grade, and running at 6.0 miles per hour. One minute of quiet sitting will separate each of the four exercise stages.

EXAMPLE 4.1
Sample Informed Consent Form
(Courtesy University of Northern Iowa.)

EXAMPLE 4.1
Concluded

C. The cycling will be performed at a workload equivalent to 75W completing two 5-min stages at pedal rate 50 and 80 revolutions per minute.

3. **There are no risks above the normal daily risks associated with physical activity. You will not be asked to exert yourself at intensity above your regular level of physical activity.**

4. **There are no direct benefits from participating in the study. Feedback will be provided to the study subjects regarding the heart rate and oxygen consumption measurements that may contribute to a greater knowledge of the relationship of these measures with various physical activities.**

5. **Your responses are strictly confidential. When the data are presented in the written report, you will not be linked to the data by your name, title, or any other identifying item. A subject number will be assigned to you and only that number will be used on data forms. All data forms will be filed in a locked cabinet in the investigator's office.**

6. **Participation in this project is voluntary. You have the right to withdraw at any time without penalty (affecting your grade). If you have any questions about your rights or feel uncomfortable in any way, you may contact Kevin J. Finn, Ph.D. at the number listed above or the Office of the Human Subjects Coordinator in the Graduate College, University of Northern Iowa, (319) 273-xxxx.**

7. **There is no compensation for participation for this study. Study subjects in the course "Physiology of Exercise" will be given ten points of extra credit for completion of the required tasks.**

I am fully aware of the nature and extent of my participation in this project as stated above and the possible risks arising from it. I hereby agree to participate in the first phase of this project. I acknowledge that I have received a copy of this consent statement.

_____

(Signature of subject or responsible agent)   Date

_____

(Printed name of subject)

_____

(Name of Investigator)

(7) an explanation of whom to contact for answers to pertinent questions about the research and research subjects' rights, and whom to contact in the event of a research-related injury to the subject; and

(8) a statement that participation is voluntary, refusal to participate will involve no penalty or loss of benefits to which the subject is otherwise entitled, and the subject may discontinue participation at any time without penalty or loss of benefits to which the subject is otherwise entitled.

Furthermore, when appropriate, one or more of the following elements of information shall also be provided to each subject:

(1) a statement that the particular treatment or procedure may involve risks to the subject (or to the embryo or fetus, if the subject is or may become pregnant) which are currently unforeseeable;

(2) anticipated circumstances under which the subject's participation may be terminated by the investigator without regard to the subject's consent;

(3) any additional costs to the subject that may result from participation in the research;

(4) the consequences of a subject's decision to withdraw from the research, and procedures for orderly termination of participation by the subject;

(5) A statement that significant new findings developed during the course of the research which may relate to the subject's willingness to continue participation will be provided to the subject; and

(6) the approximate number of subjects involved in the study.

In addition, for research involving vulnerable groups such as children, prisoners, or pregnant women, federal guidelines prescribe additional protections. Since a considerable amount of HHP research involves the use of children, it is important to note that regulations require written parental consent before the minor child can participate in a research project. Researchers using children as research participants are encouraged to review the federal regulations for the protection of human subjects, 45 C.F.R. Subpart D (http://ohrp.osophs.dhhs.gov/humansubjects/guidance/45cfr46.htm) as well as local IRB policy concerning the acquisition of informed consent.

Although the federal requirements concerning informed consent are relatively straightforward, questions often arise about how much information the participant needs to know before consent can be given. Researchers often cite the Hawthorne effect or placebo effect in pointing out that participants in experimental studies may act differently if they are fully informed of the study, thus necessitating the use of deception in the research design. This deception might take the form of misleading the subject or withholding information about the true nature of the study. Furthermore, Dooley (1990) points out that some qualitative studies involving participant observation may not be possible if full disclosure is made *a priori.* As a result of legitimate dilemmas such as these, IRBs have been given the right to waive requirements for informed consent if (and only if) it is clear that (1) the goals of the research cannot be accomplished if full disclosure is made; (2) the undisclosed risks are minimal; and (3) when appropriate, participants will be debriefed and provided the research results (Belmont Report 1979). Nevertheless, there is continuing debate among scholars regarding the appropriateness of deceptive procedures in research methodology.

Prospective participants in a research study must be able to comprehend the information they are provided with respect to the study. The presentation of information should be adapted to the participant's capacity to understand it and researchers should strive to write informed consent forms that are understandable to the prospective research participants. This involves avoiding the use of technical jargon as much as possible and writing at the reading level of the desired participants. Cardinal, Martin, and Sachs (1996) recommend that if the researcher is uncertain of the reading level of the target audience, informed consent forms should be written at or below the eighth-grade reading level. For further information on this topic, see Cardinal (2000), Ogloff and Otto (1991), and LoVerde, Prochazka, and Byyny (1989).

Inasmuch as informed consent is the cornerstone of ethical principles regarding the participation of human subjects in research, professional associations such as the American Psychological Association (APA) and the American Education Research Association (AERA), among others, as well as leading journals in the HHP field, such as *Medicine and Science in Sports and Exercise* and *Research Quarterly for Exercise and Sport,* have developed policy statements regarding informed consent and the use of human subjects. Moreover, authors of research-based manuscripts in these and other professional journals are typically required to include some statement about the acquisition of informed consent from research participants.

For further information about informed consent, researchers are advised to consult materials published by the Office for Protection from Research Risks (OPRR) of the Department of Health and Human Services as well as their local IRB. The OPRR website contains considerable policy information about the protection of human subjects, in addition to useful guidelines designed to assist the researcher.

Informed Consent Checklist:
http://ohrp.osophs.dhhs.gov/humansubjects/assurance/consentckls.htm

Human Subjects Regulations Decision Charts:
http://ohrp.osophs.dhhs.gov/humansubjects/guidance/decisioncharts.htm

Privacy and Confidentiality

One of the major ethical concerns associated with conducting research involving human participants pertains to the issues of privacy and confidentiality. Yet, there is considerable debate over the precise definitions of these two terms. Some experts argue that the terms can be used interchangeably, while others argue that they are completely distinct. While further debate about the definitions of privacy and confidentiality is beyond the scope of this book, it does seem clear that the terms are closely related. The definitions that follow are consistent with federal guidelines concerning research involving human subjects. **Privacy** refers to the capacity of individuals to control when and under what conditions others will have access to their behaviors, beliefs, and values (Monette, Sullivan, and DeJong 1990). That is, it is simply the control we have over information about ourselves. In his book, *Privacy and Freedom*, Westin (1967) defines privacy as "the claim of individuals, groups, or institutions to determine for themselves when, how and to what extent information about them is communicated to others." **Confidentiality** refers to the ability to link information or data to a person's identity. The expectation is that information that an individual has disclosed will not be divulged to others without permission. Confidentiality, then, pertains to how the personal information that is disclosed may be used.

Virtually any research endeavor in which the investigator seeks to obtain information about human subjects brings forward the issues of privacy and confidentiality. Normally, these issues are addressed through informed consent, in which the prospective research participant, by indicating his or her consent to participate in the study, is providing authorization for the researcher to have access to certain specified personal information. Privacy issues do arise, however, in situations in which information is obtained without the consent of the subjects, for example, when a researcher seeks to obtain information from student records, patient records, or client files. It is noted that the Buckley Amendment to the General Education Provisions Act (20 USC 1232) requires parental permission for access to records of, or identifiable information about, children in public schools. The use of covert observation or participant observation (see chapter 9), however, presents even more serious concerns regarding privacy. While it is not possible to specify precisely the methods a researcher might take to reduce problems associated with privacy in such cases, it is incumbent upon the researcher to take all reasonable and appropriate action to honor a person's right to privacy. Researchers would be well advised to consult with their local IRB in situations where privacy may be an issue.

Additionally, the informed consent form should indicate how the researcher will go about protecting the confidentiality of the participants. In most cases, the researcher is interested in group data and will aggregate individual scores or information. Confidentiality is a major factor in determining whether certain types of research projects involving education tests, surveys, interviews, or the observation of public behavior may be exempt from the human subjects review process (45 C.F.R. 46).

According to federal policy (45 C.F.R. 46), researchers are responsible for insuring confidentiality of personal information obtained from human subjects unless express permission to the contrary is granted by the research participant. Procedures that the researcher might take to insure the confidentiality of his or her subjects include:

- Obtain anonymous information (best example being survey research in which responses are obtained with no identifying names or numbers).
- Code data in such a manner that identifying information is eliminated.
- Substitute surrogate names or information that could identify subjects.
- Do not release or report individual data.
- Limit access to data that could reveal a subject's identity. (For example, only the principal investigator would have access to the data).
- Report the data only in aggregate form.
- Use computerized methods for encrypting and storing data.

Where research involves collecting data about sensitive issues (such as illegal behaviors, alcohol or drug use, or sexual behaviors), it is essential that researchers are able to provide assurances of confidentiality to the participants. In fact, in certain instances researchers are able to obtain a "certificate of confidentiality" that protects the identities of research participants or research data even against subpoena by law enforcement agencies. In general, the more sensitive the data being collected, the more attentive the researcher needs to be in protecting confidentiality.

Research Involving Animals

Although the general nature of HHP research precludes the frequent use of animals in research endeavors, it is not uncommon to see in some professional journals in our field the results of learning studies or biomedical studies utilizing animals. Animal research has long been a part of biomedical research and has produced significant benefits for humans. Questions have arisen, however, about the way animals are selected and treated as research subjects.

Governmental agencies and professional associations have issued ethical guidelines and regulations for the utilization and care of animals in testing and research. While various guidelines for the proper care and use of animals in research have existed for many years, the *U.S. Government Principles for the Utilization and Care of Vertebrate Animals Used in Testing, Research, and Training* (Interagency Research Animal Committee 1985) is a primary directive in the United States. In general, the guidelines relate to the transportation, care, and use of vertebrate animals in ways that are judged to be scientifically, technically, and humanely appropriate.

Similar regulations are included in the *Guide for the Care and Use of Laboratory Animals* (now in its seventh edition) published by the Department of Health and Human Services, and the *Public Health Service (PHS) Policy on Humane Care and Use of Laboratory Animals* (Public Health Service 1996). The current version of the *Guide for the Care and Use of Laboratory Animals* is available at the following website: http://oacu.od.nih.gov/regs/guide/guidex.htm. Moreover, the Animal Welfare Act of 1985 established assurance procedures to monitor compliance with federal regulations for conducting research using animals. The American College of Sports Medicine (ACSM) has promulgated a policy statement on research with experimental animals, while the American Psychological Association (APA) has developed standards for ethical conduct in the care and use of animals in research and teaching (www.apa.org/science/anguide.html). For further information, readers contemplating research involving animals are advised to consult the sources named above as well as their local IRB.

Institutional Review Boards

Institutional Review Boards (IRBs) have been established by federal mandate to assure compliance with governmental regulations pertaining to research involving human subjects as well as animals. The "Common Rule" (45 C.F.R. 46) requires that all research protocols involving human subjects be reviewed by an IRB to assure compliance with the requirements set forth in this policy. IRBs have the authority to approve, require modifications in, or disapprove the research. In addition, local IRBs have the authority to grant waivers or alter certain requirements as specified in federal guidelines. Although regulations specify the general requirements for IRB membership, function, and operation, IRBs vary slightly from institution to institution. Therefore, it is important that a researcher review IRB guidelines pertinent to his or her institution.

For research involving human subjects, the "Common Rule" specifies that the following criteria must be met in order to obtain IRB approval for the research:

1. Risks to subjects are minimized.
2. Risks to subjects are reasonable in relation to anticipated benefits, if any, to subjects, and the importance of the knowledge that may be expected to result.
3. Selection of subjects is equitable in relation to the purposes of the research and its setting. Special attention is given to vulnerable groups such as children, prisoners, pregnant women, mentally disabled persons, or those economically or educationally disadvantaged.

4. Informed consent will be sought from each prospective subject or the subject's legally authorized representative.
5. Informed consent will be appropriately documented as required by federal statute.
6. When appropriate, the research plan makes adequate provision for monitoring the data collected to ensure the safety of subjects.
7. When appropriate, there are adequate provisions to protect the privacy of subjects and to maintain the confidentiality of data.

In addition, if the research involves vulnerable subjects, additional safeguards shall be included in the research plan to protect the rights and welfare of these subjects.

IRB approval is required before any aspect of the research that involves human subjects may commence. Institutions develop procedures that all researchers, from graduate students to full professors, must follow to obtain IRB approval. Typically, this includes completion of a standardized form and/or checklist that describes the proposed research and identifies the subjects, types of data to be collected, methods to be used, inherent risks and anticipated benefits, and procedures to assure confidentiality. Example 4.2 provides an example of such a checklist that is used at Indiana University. If appropriate, an Informed Consent Statement and, in some cases, copies of research instruments (e.g., questionnaires, inventories, interview schedules) may also be required by the local IRB.

Guidelines set forth in the code of federal regulations (45 C.F.R. 46) establish three categories of review, depending upon the amount of risk present to the research participants: exempt from review, expedited review, and full review. Please note that "exempt from review" does not mean that the researcher can simply ignore IRB guidelines and not submit required forms; it means that the proposed research is exempt from the full review process established by the IRB. Many institutions actually extend their requirement for IRB review beyond that specified by federal regulations, another reason to become familiar with local IRB policies. Expedited review pertains to research in which there is no more than minimal risk to the participants and the IRB review of the proposed research is conducted by the chair of the IRB or a designated member or members of the committee. Full IRB review is required in instances in which the proposed research project involves more than minimal risk to the participants (see Example 4.2).

Disclosure of Research Findings

The culmination of a research project generally results in the disclosure of the results in one form or another. Usual methods of disclosure include publication in a professional journal in one's field, presentation at a professional conference, report to a sponsoring organization, a news release, and, for student researchers, completion of

EXAMPLE 4.2
Sample Checklist
Required for Review by
Institutional Review Board

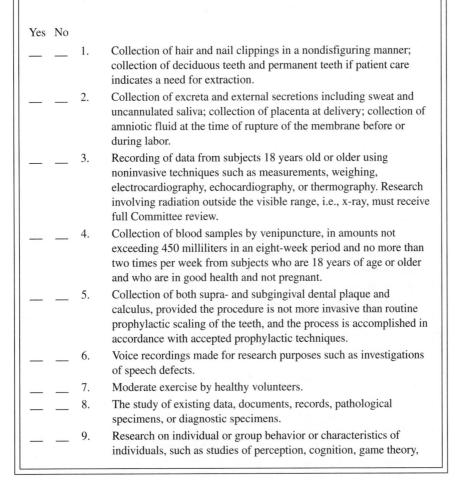

Protection of Human Subjects Form

DIRECTIONS: This form is to be completed and submitted to the Committee when the investigator plans a research project which, in the investigator's judgment, requires expedited or full Committee review. Items 1–13 are the categories which may qualify for expedited review. *If "yes" is the response to any of items 14–17, the study does not qualify for expedited review (full Committee review will be required).*

STUDIES INVOLVING MINORS AND ECONOMICALLY OR EDUCATIONALLY DISADVANTAGED PERSONS <u>MAY</u>, IN THE DISCRETION OF THE CHAIR, REQUIRE FULL COMMITTEE REVIEW.

STUDIES INVOLVING PREGNANT WOMEN, FETUSES, ABORTUSES, PRISONERS, OR PERSONS WITH MENTAL DISABILITIES <u>WILL</u> REQUIRE <u>FULL COMMITTEE REVIEW</u>.

Yes No

___ ___ 1. Collection of hair and nail clippings in a nondisfiguring manner; collection of deciduous teeth and permanent teeth if patient care indicates a need for extraction.

___ ___ 2. Collection of excreta and external secretions including sweat and uncannulated saliva; collection of placenta at delivery; collection of amniotic fluid at the time of rupture of the membrane before or during labor.

___ ___ 3. Recording of data from subjects 18 years old or older using noninvasive techniques such as measurements, weighing, electrocardiography, echocardiography, or thermography. Research involving radiation outside the visible range, i.e., x-ray, must receive full Committee review.

___ ___ 4. Collection of blood samples by venipuncture, in amounts not exceeding 450 milliliters in an eight-week period and no more than two times per week from subjects who are 18 years of age or older and who are in good health and not pregnant.

___ ___ 5. Collection of both supra- and subgingival dental plaque and calculus, provided the procedure is not more invasive than routine prophylactic scaling of the teeth, and the process is accomplished in accordance with accepted prophylactic techniques.

___ ___ 6. Voice recordings made for research purposes such as investigations of speech defects.

___ ___ 7. Moderate exercise by healthy volunteers.

___ ___ 8. The study of existing data, documents, records, pathological specimens, or diagnostic specimens.

___ ___ 9. Research on individual or group behavior or characteristics of individuals, such as studies of perception, cognition, game theory,

EXAMPLE 4.2
Concluded

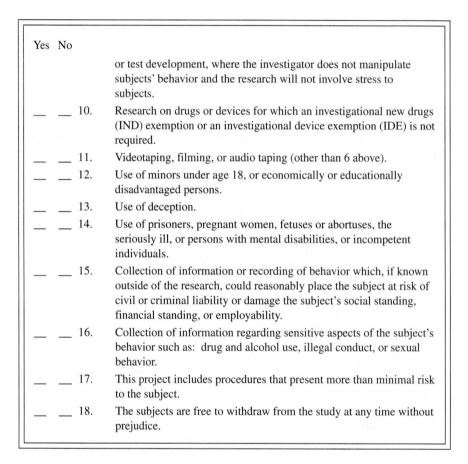

Yes No

			or test development, where the investigator does not manipulate subjects' behavior and the research will not involve stress to subjects.
__	__	10.	Research on drugs or devices for which an investigational new drugs (IND) exemption or an investigational device exemption (IDE) is not required.
__	__	11.	Videotaping, filming, or audio taping (other than 6 above).
__	__	12.	Use of minors under age 18, or economically or educationally disadvantaged persons.
__	__	13.	Use of deception.
__	__	14.	Use of prisoners, pregnant women, fetuses or abortuses, the seriously ill, or persons with mental disabilities, or incompetent individuals.
__	__	15.	Collection of information or recording of behavior which, if known outside of the research, could reasonably place the subject at risk of civil or criminal liability or damage the subject's social standing, financial standing, or employability.
__	__	16.	Collection of information regarding sensitive aspects of the subject's behavior such as: drug and alcohol use, illegal conduct, or sexual behavior.
__	__	17.	This project includes procedures that present more than minimal risk to the subject.
__	__	18.	The subjects are free to withdraw from the study at any time without prejudice.

a thesis or dissertation. Chapter 15 provides additional information on disseminating the results of a research study. It is through the disclosure of research findings that the scientific method furthers our knowledge, thus affecting professional practices and personal choices. In order for research to be viewed as a credible source of knowledge, the honest and accurate disclosure of research findings is essential. According to Monette, Sullivan, and DeJong (1990), the preeminent ethical obligation of the researcher [in terms of reporting the results of research] is to not disclose inaccurate, deceptive, or fraudulent results. So doing would undermine the very nature of the scientific process.

Scientific misconduct has been defined by the U. S. Public Health Service (1989) in the following statement:

"Misconduct" or "Misconduct in Science" means fabrication, falsification, plagiarism, or other practices that seriously deviate from those that are commonly accepted within the scientific community for proposing, conducting, or reporting research. It does not include honest error or honest differences in interpretations of judgments of data.

Meanwhile, the National Science Foundation (1991) provided a similar definition:

"Misconduct" means (1) fabrication, falsification, plagiarism, or other serious deviation from accepted practices in proposing, carrying out, or reporting results from activities funded by NSF; or (2) retaliation of any kind against a person who reported or provided information about suspected or alleged misconduct and who has not acted in bad faith.

It is clear from these definitions that "fabrication, falsification, and plagiarism" serve as the underlying elements of scientific misconduct, at least as defined by these federal agencies. While the notion of fabricating or falsifying research findings is foreign to the principles underlying the scientific method, there have been a number of reported instances in which researchers have made up or altered data or otherwise misrepresented the true findings of the study. For instance, in 1994 charges were filed against researchers at the University of Pittsburgh and other institutions involved in a multi-site federally funded breast cancer research study for falsifying information in some patient records. As a consequence, lawsuits were filed, researchers dismissed, and reputations severely damaged. [Subsequent reanalysis of the data excluding the falsified data confirmed the accuracy of the original findings. In fact, the principal investigator has since been exonerated of any scientific misconduct.] A researcher in the Health Education Department at the University of Utah was found responsible in 1999 for falsifying patient signatures and responses to questions during patient interviews for a federally funded research project with indigent patients (*ORI Newsletter* March 1999). As recently as 2000, a South African researcher was dismissed from his university after admitting to falsifying the results of a study on breast cancer. Further examples of scientific misconduct are regularly reported in publications such as the *Chronicle of Higher Education* as well as the *ORI Newsletter.*

The Office of Research Integrity (ORI) (http://63.162.35.7/orinewsite) is responsible for developing policies, procedures, and regulations related to the detection, investigation, and prevention of scientific misconduct in biomedical and behavioral research conducted or supported by the U. S. Department of Health and Human Services (DHHS) or its agencies. Considerable resources to improve the integrity of research and reduce research misconduct are available at the ORI website, including reports documenting incidents of misconduct activities that have been reported.

Severe penalties are usually imposed on those researchers who are found guilty of scientific misconduct. Drowatzky (1996) provides an extensive listing of possible penalties, which may include letters of reprimand, salary freeze, reduction in professorial rank, prohibition from obtaining outside grants, fines, dismissal from university, and referral to legal system for further action. Student researchers caught falsifying research findings could possibly receive a failing grade, be placed on probation, suspended, or even expelled, depending upon the regulations at the given institution. For example, a graduate student in HHP at the home institution of one of the authors of this textbook received a grade of "F" for nine hours of thesis credit and was suspended from school for fabricating data in research undertaken for the thesis requirement. The penalty could have been even more severe.

Plagiarism is frequently recognized as a problem with student papers or reports, but we also see plagiarism by professionals and students alike in scientific writing. Plagiarism is simply the presentation of the ideas or works of others as your own without giving proper credit. The ethical principle to follow here is merely to give proper credit to those whose work you borrow or cite. This is done through appropriate documentation in accordance with the chosen style manual. Sometimes plagiarism is accidental; the writer is either unfamiliar with the rules for correctly paraphrasing or quoting sources, or is careless in recording and citing sources. A number of universities have established websites that provide tips on avoiding plagiarism. Following are two such examples:

Northwestern University: The Writing Place –
www.writing.nwu/tips/plag.html

Indiana University: Writing Tutorial Services –
www.indiana.edu/~wts/wts/plagiarism.html

Authorship is the primary method through which researchers receive recognition for their research efforts. Authorship should be limited to those who have made a significant contribution to the research. In fact, it is generally recommended that the order of authorship be based upon the magnitude of one's contribution to the research. The researcher who is primarily responsible for conceptualizing the problem and developing the research plan is usually listed as first author. Additional authors are listed in order of their contributions. Moreover, all co-authors should have agreed to be listed as such. It is also noted that inclusion of a co-author strictly on the basis of the position of authority they hold (e.g., departmental chairperson) is inappropriate. It is recommended that all issues about authorship be resolved early on in the research process and certainly prior to commencing the publication/reporting phase. Publication of student research undertaken for a thesis or dissertation requirement poses special problems. Our viewpoint is that the student should always be listed as first author; the faculty chair of the thesis or dissertation committee may be included as a co-author, as well as other faculty, depending upon their contribution to the research. The ethical principles published by the American Psychological Association (APA) and the American Education Research Association (AERA) both include standards pertaining to authorship and should be consulted for further information.

The financial support provided by corporations, agencies, and foundations has provided many researchers with the means to conduct research activities and thus further the body of knowledge. Without this support, it is quite likely that the magnitude and quality of research would be different from what we see today. Yet, *sponsored research* poses particular ethical concerns. Who owns the data? Who controls the release of the research findings? Are there limitations placed upon subsequent publication of the results when they are unfavorable to the sponsor? Is it appropriate to withhold sponsorship information when obtaining informed consent? Controversy over matters such as these can often be resolved through contractual agreement with the research sponsor. It is important for the researcher to carefully read such contracts prior to signing and to understand the rights and responsibilities articulated therein. Violation of contractual agreements is not only unethical, it also constitutes a breach of law. A specific standard concerning the ethical integrity associated with sponsored research is included in the ethical standards of AERA.

Summary

The atrocities associated with human experimentation during World War II shocked the world and served as the impetus for the development of ethical codes of conduct for biomedical and behavioral research. Further revelations of scientific misconduct in the United States resulted in federal policies and regulations being formulated that provide ethical guidelines for research involving human subjects as well as animals. As a result, Institutional Review Boards have been established to provide a mechanism for the protection of research participants and to assure compliance with federal policy. Many professional associations have also promulgated ethical standards that serve to guide the research activities of members as well as the disclosure of research findings.

5

Selection of Research Participants: Sampling Procedures

KEY WORDS

Cluster sampling	Probability sampling	Sample	Simple random sampling
Fishbowl technique	Random assignment	Sampling	Stratified random sampling
Multistage sampling	Random selection	Sample size	Systematic sampling
Nonprobability sampling	Representative sample	Sampling unit	Table of random numbers
Population			

OBJECTIVES

While all steps in the research process are important, perhaps the most crucial to a successful investigation are the procedures used in the selection of research participants. The researcher first identifies and defines the population from which information is to be obtained. To study an entire population is difficult, if not impossible, hence the use of the sampling process. Considerations are given to such factors as sample size, how representative of the population is the sample, and the appropriateness of the participants to the various research methods and tests. The process of sampling permits the researcher to generalize the results from a study of the sample to the larger population.

After reading chapter 5, you should be able to

1. Identify and define a population from which a sample of research participants is to be selected.
2. Know how to determine the characteristics of the sample.
3. Know the various methods of selecting samples.
4. Know the various factors that are used to determine sample size.

The needs of the research problem usually dictate the type of participants who will be selected for study. Quite frequently, the research statement of the problem indicates what participants will be used in an experimental or descriptive study. It is imperative that the researcher have a carefully thought-out plan for selecting the participants.

The participants must be appropriate to the methods, techniques, and instrumentation that will be incorporated in the study so they can produce the needed research data. Participants should be selected who may be expected to be available throughout the duration of the study. The number should be large enough to (1) assure reliability of the research results, and (2) permit a reasonable number of participants to be available to produce data in the event of subject mortality (e.g., injury, absence, dropout for any reason).

Obviously, the realities of the research setting and the practical needs of the researcher often affect the subject selection process. A physical fitness study involving children may need a large number of participants, whereas a mountain climbing study on the relationship of nutrition and altitude may involve few participants. A researcher studying selected mechanical aspects in pole vaulting cannot select just any pole vaulter. The objective would be to study the high-level, world-class vaulters; the availability of these athletes is very likely to present a problem for the researcher.

Population and Sample

The term **population** refers to an entire group or aggregate of people or elements having one or more common characteristics. Often, a population is the focus of a research effort. Populations can be made up of people, animals, objects, organisms, institutions, attributes, materials, or any other defined element. We can talk about a population of fitness test scores, organizations, and personality traits. All four-year colleges and universities in the United States, all fourth-grade teachers in Iowa, all adolescents in Battle Creek, Michigan, all NCAA Division III basketball coaches, and all health education majors at the University of Georgia can be referred to as populations. The point is, researchers can define or describe a population any way they choose to suit the particular research purpose. The variable of self-efficacy, for example, could be studied among older Americans, athletes, the mentally disabled, various socioeconomic groups, teenagers, and many other populations.

Populations, then, can be defined in numerous ways. They can be quite large, theoretically infinite, as would be the case of the fitness test of all high school students; or they can be finite, such as the number of dance majors at a particular college. As a general practice, populations are considered finite.

A major reason for doing research is to obtain information that can be generalized to a population of interest. This could be accomplished by studying an entire group, but this is often impractical, if not impossible, to do. For example, if we really wanted to know the physical fitness status of all preadolescent children in the United States, we could fitness test all members of that group. However, this would not be possible in terms of the number of researchers needed to collect the data, the tremendous amount of money needed to finance the project, and the exorbitant time and energy the project would require.

Because it is often difficult, if not impossible, to study an entire population, the process of sampling is undertaken. **Sampling** is the process whereby a small proportion or subgroup of the population is selected for scientific observation and analysis. A **sample,** then, is a small subgroup of a population of interest that is thought to be representative of that larger population. The researcher observes and analyzes certain characteristics of the sample to get an idea of what those characteristics may be like in the entire population. From the information (data) obtained from the sample, the researcher then makes inferences about the population. The mean blood pressure score for a sample of cardiac rehabilitation participants is used to approximate the mean blood pressure for the entire population of such participants enrolled in a rehabilitation program. These statistics, then, are used to estimate the population information (parameters).

The first step in the sampling process is the identification of the target population. Since it is often not realistic to work with the entire target population, it is usually necessary to identify that portion of the population that is available to the researcher, the *accessible population.* This accessible population actually represents the *sampling frame,* or collection of elements, from which the sample is actually taken. Obviously, the accessible population should closely resemble the target population. The researcher then determines the desired sample size (e.g., the number of research participants) and chooses the method of sampling that best meets the needs of the research in terms of feasibility and the ability to select an appropriate sample. Lastly, the sampling plan is implemented and the research participants are selected. It is important to note that the sampling process described here follows a logical, top-down approach, whereby the population of interest is first determined and then the sample is selected. It is all too common for the beginning researcher to use the opposite approach, selecting the subjects first and then trying to retrofit this sample into some population. The recommended steps in the sampling process are summarized below

1. Identify the target population.
2. Identify the accessible population.
3. Determine the desired sample size.
4. Select the specific sampling technique.
5. Implement the sampling plan.

The crucial element in the selection of a sample from a population, is that the sample be **representative,** or similar to, the population on the characteristics being investigated. If a researcher uses just a few health promotion majors to find out what may be true about a very large number of health promotion majors, then it is imperative that the researcher be as certain as possible that the small group of majors is representative of the total population of health promotion majors. Said another way, whatever variable is being studied in a particular population (e.g., attitude, behavior, self-concept, fitness, motivation, etc.) should be present in the sample drawn from that population.

Random Processes

Randomization in sample selection is important to the quality of the research for three reasons: first, to help ensure the representativeness of the sample to the population about which generalizations will be made; second, to show that the researcher was unbiased as to which members of the population were selected for the study; and third, to equalize characteristics among groups in research studies requiring multiple groups, such as experimental and control groups. If each group is representative of the population, the groups will start the research equal in ability, and the research will be safe from criticism about which subjects were selected and placed in each group. Furthermore, random sampling is a basic requirement underlying inferential statistical tests.

Before discussing specific sample selection techniques in more detail, it is important that a clear distinction be made between **random selection** of subjects and **random assignment** of subjects. While both utilize random processes to achieve their goals, the underlying purposes are very different (Drew, Hardman, and Hart 1996). As we have already seen, the purpose of random selection is to select a sample that is representative of the population. This is important for generalizing the results of the study and enhancing the external validity of the study. Meanwhile, the purpose of random assignment is to establish group equivalence by randomly assigning research participants to treatment conditions or comparison groups. It is especially desirable that groups are equivalent prior to the introduction of a treatment condition, thus providing greater confidence in attributing posttreatment differences to the treatment. Random assignment is important to the internal validity of a study, particularly in experimental research. In chapter 7, we provide further discussion of both internal validity and external validity. Since the use of random selection or random assignment procedures will increase your ability to generalize to a population and to reduce the chances of extraneous variables affecting your results, researchers are advised to use randomization procedures whenever possible (Harris 1995).

Sample Selection Methods

There are two primary types of sampling procedures, **probability sampling** and **nonprobability sampling,** each of which has several different techniques. Probability sampling involves using selection techniques wherein the probability of selecting each participant or element is known. These techniques all rely on random processes in the selection of the sample. Examples of probability sampling techniques include **simple random sampling, stratified random sampling, systematic sampling,** and **cluster sampling.** In nonprobability sampling, meanwhile, random processes are not used in the selection of the sample, thus making it impossible to know the probability of selecting a given participant or element from the population. As a result, it is more difficult to claim that the sample is representative of the population, thus limiting the ability of the researcher to generalize the results of the study. Nonprobability sampling techniques include purposive sampling, convenience sampling, and quota sampling.

Probability Sampling

As previously described, probability sampling utilizes random processes or chance procedures to derive the sample. A key characteristic of probability sampling is that every element within the population, more precisely the sampling frame, has a known probability of being selected for the sample. Furthermore, when random processes are used to select a sample it is possible to estimate *sampling error,* or the chance variations that may occur in the sampling process. Sampling error is not indicative of mistakes in the sampling process, but merely describes the inevitable chance variations that occur when a number of randomly selected sample means are computed (Best and Kahn 1998). Although no sampling technique, including probability sampling, can guarantee a sample that is representative of the population, probability sampling is generally recognized as an efficient method of drawing a representative, unbiased, sample from a population.

Simple Random Sampling.   A **simple random sample** is obtained when every individual or element in the population has an equal chance of being selected, and the selection of one person does not interfere with the selection chances of any other person. This process is considered to be bias free because no factor is present that can affect selection. The random process leaves subject selection entirely to chance.

Several different procedures may be used to obtain a random sample—the fishbowl technique, a table of random numbers, and computer-generated random numbers. In the **fishbowl technique,** the names of every individual in a population are written on a piece of paper. The pieces of paper are placed in a bowl, box, hat, or similar container, and the number of pieces of paper corresponding to the number of subjects needed in the sample is drawn from the container one at a time. If we wanted to study 50 students from a population of 300 fourth-grade students, we would place the names of the 300 students in a container. One name at a time would be drawn until the sample of 50 was filled. This technique can be accomplished in two ways. If, after each name is selected, it is put back into the container, the method is called *random selection with replacement.* If the names are not replaced after they are drawn, this is called *random selection without replacement.* There is not a lot of difference between the two procedures when the population size is large, but without-selection replacement does not strictly meet the definition of the random selection process. In the example above, each student has 1 chance in 300 of being selected. If the names are not replaced, the probability of each subsequent name being drawn increases (1 in 299, 1 in 298, etc.). So, if a name is selected, it should be replaced. If it comes up again, put it back into the container. Each person in the population then continues to have the same opportunity, or percentage of chance, to be selected. Despite the statistical correctness of random selection with replacement, most researchers sample without replacement since an individual cannot be used as a subject again after once being selected.

Perhaps a more convenient and sophisticated way to select a random sample, or to assign subjects to groups, is to use a **table of random numbers.** Many tables have

TABLE 5.1	Excerpt from a Table of Random Numbers								
014	801	501	101	536	020	118	164	791	646
223	684	657	325	595	853	933	099	589	198
241	304	836	022	527	972	657	639	364	809
421	679	309	306	243	616	800	785	616	376
375	703	997	581	837	166	560	612	191	782
779	210	690	711	008	427	527	756	534	981
995	627	290	556	420	699	949	887	231	016
963	019	197	705	463	079	721	887	620	922
895	791	434	263	661	102	811	745	318	103
854	753	685	753	342	539	885	306	059	533

been produced in which the numbers (0–9) are randomly ordered. Table 5.1 is an excerpt from a table of random numbers. Such tables are relatively simple to use. Just assign a number to the members of the population, then use the columns of numbers to pinpoint those members of the population who will be selected for the sample.

For a more complete random number table as well as for guidelines for its use, you may wish to consult a basic statistics textbook such as Harris (1995).

There are a variety of computer programs, SPSS among them, that can generate a set of random numbers and greatly aide the sample selection process. Moreover, there are websites available that are specifically designed to assist researchers in randomly selecting research participants as well as randomly assigning them to experimental conditions. One such site is the Research Randomizer, located at www.randomizer.org. Another online service to generate random numbers can be found at www.random.org.

Stratified Random Sampling.   A big help in ensuring a representative sample is the process of *stratification*. This is accomplished by dividing the population into various strata or subgroups, based on some characteristic that is important to control in the study, and then selecting a set number of subjects from each strata. The following is an example from a study of how the high schools in a given state financed the girls' athletic programs.

SCHOOL SIZE		
Small	**Medium**	**Large**
0–499 pupils	500–999 pupils	>1000 pupils

Let's say that there are 400 schools in the state and the researcher decides to study financing practices in a sample of 100, or 25 percent of the schools, and randomly selects that number. There are many more small schools than medium or large ones, and just by luck the selected sample contains 80 small schools, 15 medium schools, and five large schools. The resultant data on how schools in the state finance the girls' athletic programs would probably be unbalanced in favor of the small schools and would not fairly represent the financing strategies of the medium and large schools. This problem could be overcome, or at least minimized, by first stratifying the schools by size, then taking a proportional random number of schools from each stratum. In our example above, there are 250 small schools, 125 medium schools, and 25 large schools. Since the researcher wants a final sample of 100 schools (25%), proportional stratified random sampling (taking .25 $\times$ the number of schools in each stratum) would yield, roughly, 63 small schools, 31 medium schools, and six large schools. Thus, the final sample of 100 schools is quite representative of the total population of 400 schools. Any generalizations or inferences from the sample to the population stand a better chance of being more valid than if proportional stratified random sampling had not been used. While not completely foolproof, this procedure is considered to be the most efficient way to achieve representativeness.

In some studies, however, the primary focus is on the differences among the various strata or subgroups in the population. In these situations, nonproportional stratified random sampling should be used to select equal-sized samples from each stratum, thus making group comparisons easier. If the focus of the research question is on differences among the strata, the researcher should select an equal number of participants (elements) from each stratum; if the characteristics of the entire population are the main focus, proportional sampling is more appropriate (Ary, Jacobs, and Razavieh 1996).

Systematic Sampling.   When some "system" is applied to the selection of research participants, we call the procedure **systematic sampling.** More precisely, systematic sampling involves drawing a sample by selecting every *k*th element from a list of the population, where *k* is a constant representing the sampling interval. For example, in a study of a population of 200 public and private schools in a large city, the researcher obtained an alphabetized listing of the schools from the state's department of education. The researcher then determines there is a need to draw a 20 percent sample from the population, thus 40 schools will be selected. The sampling interval is determined by dividing the population size by the desired sample size: $k = 200/40 = 5$. The starting point would be randomly selected among the first five schools on the list and then every fifth school thereafter would be selected. In another situation a researcher may decide to select every one-hundredth person listed in a telephone directory. In this case, $k = 100$. Another version of systematic sampling is illustrated by a researcher who is situated at a particular location and stops every fifteenth person who passes by and asks each a series of questions. In each of these examples, some "system" was applied to the selection of the sample.

If the listing of the population elements is in random order, which is rarely the case, systematic sampling is a good approximation of random sampling. However, systematic sampling does not strictly satisfy the definition of random sampling and, hence, is not entirely bias free. Once the first element is selected, all the remaining cases in the sample are automatically determined, while others have no chance of being selected. Thus, all members of the population do not have an independent chance of being selected for the sample. In the schools example above, if every fifth school is selected, schools 4 and 6 have no chance of being selected. Subtle biases may also be present in systematic sampling, particular when the population listing is not in random order. Many parochial schools, because their names begin with *S,* cluster together near the bottom of an alphabetized listing. As a result, they would probably not be adequately represented in a sample chosen through systematic sampling.

Systematic sampling is quick, efficient, and saves time and energy. This is particularly true when populations exist on a definitive list or roster. In this instance, it is simply convenient to select every *kth* element of the population, as opposed to using a table of random numbers, which usually is a little more time consuming. It can also be argued that systematic sampling provides for a broad sampling across a population and, therefore, results in a more accurate sample (Sax 1979).

Cluster Sampling.   Also referred to as area sampling, **cluster sampling** is particularly appropriate in situations where the researcher cannot obtain a list of the members of a population and has little knowledge of their characteristics, where the population is scattered over a wide geographic area, and in situations where it is impractical to remove individuals from a naturally occurring group. Cluster sampling is a type of probability sampling in which the sampling unit is a naturally occurring group or cluster of members of the population. Thus, instead of sampling individual members of the population, clusters are selected. Examples of clusters particularly applicable to HHP research include schools, classrooms, city blocks, hospitals, and worksites. Let's say that a researcher wants to survey 1,000 teachers out of a population of 4,600 teachers in 46 schools in a large city. Each school has approximately 100 teachers. If the teachers were selected at random, the subjects in the sample would be scattered all over the city. The expense in time, money, and energy in designing a plan to get information from the 1,000 randomly selected teachers is enormous. The researcher decides to randomly select 12 schools from the population of schools, and then survey all teachers in each school. The teachers in each school comprise a cluster. Allowing for certain factors of subject mortality, the researcher reasonably expects approximately 1,000 teachers to respond. In this example, the random selection is of the schools not of the teachers, who are of interest in the investigation. The schools are the sampling unit because they are what were sampled. Conclusions and inferences are always stated in terms of the **sampling unit.** Since schools are the sampling unit, the mean score of the teachers in a school represents the score for a school, with a sample size of 12, not 1,000.

In general, cluster sampling is more practical and less costly than simple random sampling, but it does hold the possibility of greater sampling error, particularly if the number of clusters is small. Furthermore, if clusters are not of equal size, there is also the possibility of introducing sample bias. An alternative to the cluster sampling procedure described above would be the process of **multistage sampling** which involves successive selection of clusters within clusters. In multistage sampling, the researcher will frequently perform one or more rounds of cluster sampling and then, in the final stage, randomly select elements (research participants) from the chosen clusters. For example, a researcher interested in investigating the health behaviors of high school students in Illinois could not reasonably expect to obtain a listing of all high school students in the state. It is simply not feasible to utilize simple random sampling procedures in this case. However, through the use of multistage sampling, the researcher could first randomly select school districts within the state, then schools within the selected districts, and finally classrooms within schools. If the researcher did not want to utilize all students within the selected classrooms, in a final sampling stage he or she could randomly select students (after all, that is really what we are interested in) from the chosen classrooms.

Nonprobability Sampling

As indicated earlier, if a researcher is to justify generalizations about the population from which the sample is drawn, the sample must be selected at random. The random sample is a chance sample and follows the laws of probability. Some samples do not.

Samples not selected at random are called **nonprobability samples.** Examples are intact classes, volunteers, a typical group, or a typical person. The results of these kinds of samples frequently do not reflect accurately the traits of the population in which the researcher is interested. They may not, then, be representative of the population and can lead to faulty conclusions.

Suppose a researcher wants to study fifth-grade pupils on some physical fitness variable. These students belong to a class made up of four sections of 30 pupils each for a population of 120 prospective subjects. The researcher's plan is to select 30 subjects from the 120 at random. However, the school principal says, "No, the random selection would mean that some pupils from each section might be selected in the sample, and if you indiscriminately pull them out of their respective sections for testing purposes you will disrupt the school schedule. Instead, select just one section, intact, and make arrangements to do your testing before or after the school day." The question is, how representative of the characteristics of all of the fifth graders in the school is this one fifth-grade section? How representative is it of similar fifth-grade populations? The point is, intact or available groups impose a serious restriction on the researcher's ability to generalize the data obtained to the larger population from which the sample was drawn.

The use of volunteers can introduce an element of bias into an investigation. Say a researcher visits four college personal health classes and asks the students to volunteer to be in a study on the sexual behavior and characteristics of undergraduate college men and women. Twenty-five of the 150 students volunteer. How representative are four classes of a population of undergraduate men and women? Maybe the population should be the 150 students in the four classes. How representative of the

150 are the 25? The sample of 25 volunteers may be biased. What caused 25 students to accept the invitation to participate in the study and 125 to decline? The problem with volunteers is that they may be different from the nonvolunteers on the characteristics that are the focal point of the study. They usually possess special kinds of characteristics, which permit them to volunteer and which tend to bias the sample. Similarly, the selection of one individual elite swimmer or one group of elite swimmers, based upon the assumption that they are typical of all elite swimmers, provides for an element of bias also. Selecting subjects in this manner does not permit all elite swimmers an equal chance to be studied; the law of probability, or chance, has not been permitted to operate. To generalize from the "typical" subject to, perhaps, several hundred, would be stretching a point, to say nothing about the limits it would place on the researcher's ability to gain statistical significance when generalizing from the "sample" of one (or one "typical" group) to a larger population.

Purposive Sampling.   With this method, the researcher knows that specific characteristics exist in a certain segment of a population. Since these traits are extremely critical to the results of the investigation, the researcher using *purposive sampling* selects those subjects who contain the characteristics. Biomechanics researchers oftentimes purposely select excellent performers in a sport when they are trying to determine correct kinetic and kinematic parameters. Such factors are found in the top gymnasts, swimmers, basketball players, and other athletes, but they are probably absent in beginners or lower-level performers. Since this selection process is always biased, its use is encouraged only when the research advantages are superior to both the statistical and public relations aspects of bias-free selection (Fox 1969).

Convenience Sampling.   Convenience sampling, as the name suggests, is selecting the research participants on the basis of being accessible and convenient to the researcher. This approach to sampling often involves the use of volunteers and those subjects in existing groups who are handy to the researcher. This could be, for example, students who are enrolled in a class taught by the researcher, fellow graduate students, participants in a health promotion program that is administered by the researcher, or members of a sport team that the researcher coaches. However, volunteers are known to be different from nonvolunteers. Yet, the use of convenience samples in research, particularly that conducted by graduate students, is commonplace. The major problem with a study using this approach to selecting research participants is that the results are not likely generalizable beyond the participants in the study. This does not mean that the study should not be conducted or that the results are not accurate or credible; it simply means that the researcher should be cautious in generalizing the findings. In an attempt to justify the use of a convenience sample, researchers generally attempt to show that the characteristics of the sample are similar to those of the population. Nevertheless, a wise researcher should recognize the limitations of using a convenience sample and point this fact out in the written report of the study.

Sample Size

Often the first question that a beginning researcher asks is, "How many subjects do I need?" **Sample size** is difficult to determine with any degree of certainty. Beginning researchers, particularly students, often believe that a large sample will produce better data and more valid conclusions based upon these data. Regardless of size, the crucial factor is whether or not the sample is representative of the population. A well-selected and controlled small sample is better than a poorly selected and poorly controlled large sample. Sample size is influenced by population size. Fifty subjects out of 100 may be representative, but 50 subjects from a population of 1,000,000 would not be representative.

In the 1936 presidential election, the *Literary Digest Magazine* predicted that the Republican candidate, Alfred Landon, would defeat the incumbent Democrat, Franklin Roosevelt. The prediction was based on responses to the magazine's survey of 10 million United States voters, 2 million of whom responded. President Roosevelt won the election in a landslide, carrying forty-six of the then forty-eight states. While one might say that 2 million respondents is a large sample, it is obvious that the majority opinion of these people did not represent the entire population of eligible voters. The sample was drawn from telephone and automobile registration lists. In 1936, in the depths of a depression, a lot of people did not have telephones or automobiles. Those who did possess them had money and probably aligned themselves with the Republican party. The sample was biased and unrepresentative of the political leanings of most U. S. citizens.

In contrast, George Bush, in 1988 was predicted to be the presidential victor with less than 5 percent of the votes cast. The sample on which the prediction was based was obtained through careful stratification of the voting population on several characteristics previously known to be related to voting practices, followed by proportional random sampling. This sample was unbiased and representative.

The size of the sample does become important in the statistical applications used to analyze the data produced by the sample, and in making inferences from the sample to the population. The power of a statistical test is the probability that the test will reject the null hypothesis when, in fact, the null hypothesis is false. A powerful statistical test is one that can detect even small differences or a small effect. One of the factors that influence the statistical power of a test is sample size. In general, the larger the sample size, the more statistical power generated by the statistic being used. A long-standing convention in experimental research is to consider 30 per group as the minimum acceptable sample size. Another guideline is that sample size never needs to exceed 50 percent of the population. Conducting a prospective power analysis before a study has started can help a researcher determine the sample size needed to detect a difference that is considered important. For more information about statistical power and conducting a power analysis to determine sample size, the interested reader may wish to consult other research and statistics books, such as Thomas and Nelson (1996), Kraemer and Thiemann (1987), and Cohen (1988).

Sample size will also depend on the research approach utilized. Experimental studies will typically employ fewer subjects than will descriptive studies. Samples in experimental research are usually quite "captive" and, depending on the data-collecting demands, result in less subject mortality than in descriptive research. In the descriptive approach, especially when sending survey instruments through the mail, subject mortality, or attrition, can be quite large. The practice in descriptive research is to select a large enough sample so that if attrition does take place (i.e., people fail to return a completed survey instrument or questionnaire), an ample amount of data will still be produced.

Nonresponse in questionnaire studies must not be taken lightly. If 500 questionnaires are sent and only 100 are returned, what does this mean? How representative is the sample of 100 of the larger population from which the 500 prospective subjects were drawn? What selective or systematic factor is operating to cause 400 people to decline the opportunity to participate?

Some years ago at Indiana University, a researcher planned a study of male high school basketball officials. The study was an attempt to determine the physical fitness ability of these men to withstand the demand of officiating basketball games. Included were measures of several fitness variables, one of which was heart rate as determined by an electrocardiographic radiotelemetry heart rate system. The population of male basketball officials in the state at that time was 1,000. The researcher's desire was to select at random 10 percent of the officials, believing that 100 would be a representative sample from which to generalize back to the population of 1,000. So, 100 officials were sent invitations to participate in the study; 12 accepted, 88 declined. If 100 could be representative of 1,000, could 12? Obviously concerned, the researcher wrote to each of the men who declined the invitation in an attempt to ascertain the reason(s) for the declinations. Among the reasons given were: (1) they thought the radiotelemetry device would interfere with their ability to officiate without distraction, (2) they were just too busy, and (3) they could not afford the time to come to the university lab for a treadmill exercise designed to reproduce the demand of running up and down a basketball court to enable the researcher to collect gases. Hence, in this case, the data-collecting procedures operated in a manner that caused subject attrition. The researcher changed his mind about conducting an inferential study and opted for studying the 12 subjects as planned, and then presenting the results as they related to that group using descriptive statistics. It might be added that the study was conducted successfully and contributed to several states increasing the physical fitness standards for officials (Holland 1970).

Probably as important as sample size is the appropriateness with which the sample is selected. Random sampling, as indicated earlier, is the best approach to sample selection because the laws of probability operate in such a way that sampling error in both large and small samples can be estimated. Utilizing random sampling, however, does not guarantee that the sample will be representative of the population. *Sampling error* is the variation due to chance that exists between a population parameter and a sample statistic. This should not be considered a mistake or carelessness in the sampling process, but rather it is the expected random variation that a researcher would expect when using random processes for selecting the sample. Estimates of sampling error give researchers a gauge of the confidence they should place in their findings (Best and Kahn 1998). The selection process, the types of variables being studied, how the data on those variables are collected, the proposed statistical procedures, and elements of public relations may all operate to dictate sample size.

Whenever a sample is used, it is logical to wonder what the results might have been if all of the people in the population had been included. An appropriate sample usually provides a good estimate of what the results would have been. All estimates involve some degree of error; the goal is to minimize that error. The researcher never knows exactly how much error is present, but it can be at least partially controlled by obtaining a sample that is in proportion to the total number of people in the population. Let's say, for example, that a researcher wants to survey parental opinion on whether or not sex education should be taught in the elementary school. The percent of "yes" responses will be determined. The researcher wants to be able to say with 90 percent certainty that the sample percent comes within 5 percentage points of what the findings would be if all of the parents had been surveyed. Although the researcher knows there will be some variation in the percent of "yes" opinions from the sample to the population, if there is high confidence (90%) that this variation is small ($\pm$ .05), faith in the sample percentage increases.

In this example, if 3,000 parents made up the population, the sample would have to include 341 parents. While several attempts have been made to develop a foolproof computational formula for determining the exact size of a sample, none presently exists. However, many statistics books do present various procedures for determining the sample size needed based on the confidence limits set by the researcher. Table 5.2 of this text presents a table that was developed by Krejcie and Margan (1970) for determining sample size. It is based on 90 percent certainty (confidence) that the sample and population percentages do not differ more than .05. Tables for other situations can be found in books devoted to statistics or sampling procedures. In addition, there are numerous resources on the World Wide Web that provide online calculations for determining sample size. The following are examples of such sites:

Sample Size Calculator – http://ebook.stat.ucla.edu/calculators/sampsize.phtm

Creative Research Systems – www.researchinfo.com/calculators/sscale.htm

As we have seen, a variety of factors affect sample size determination. The following guidelines, adapted from Best and Kahn (1998), summarize key considerations for determining sample size:

1. Sampling error is inversely related to sample size. That is, the larger the sample size, the smaller the sampling error and the greater likelihood that the sample is representative of the population.

TABLE 5.2 Determining Sample Size from a Given Population*

N	S**	N	S	N	S
10	10	220	140	1,200	291
15	14	230	144	1,300	297
20	19	240	148	1,400	302
25	24	250	152	1,500	306
30	28	260	155	1,600	310
35	32	270	159	1,700	313
40	36	280	162	1,800	317
45	40	290	165	1,900	320
50	44	300	169	2,000	322
55	48	320	175	2,200	327
60	52	340	181	2,400	331
65	56	360	186	2,600	335
70	59	380	191	2,800	338
75	63	400	196	3,000	341
80	66	420	201	3,500	346
85	70	440	205	4,000	351
90	73	460	210	4,500	354
95	76	480	214	5,000	357
100	80	500	217	6,000	361
110	86	550	226	7,000	364
120	92	600	234	8,000	367
130	97	650	242	9,000	368
140	103	700	248	10,000	370
150	108	750	254	15,000	375
160	113	800	260	20,000	377
170	118	850	265	30,000	379
180	123	900	269	40,000	380
190	127	950	274	50,000	381
200	132	1,000	278	75,000	382
210	136	1,100	285	1,000,000	384

Note: N is population size.
      S is sample size.
* Krejcie, Robert V. and Margan, Daryle W. (1970). Determining sample size for research activities. *Educational and Psychological Measurement,* 30, 607–610. Reprinted by permission.
** Sample size for 90% confidence that the difference in the population and sample percentage is no more than .05.

2. Descriptive and correlational research typically should have larger samples than are required for experimental studies.

3. Sample size should increase as variability within the population increases. In other words, larger samples are needed with a heterogeneous population as compared to a population that is more homogeneous in nature.

4. When samples are to be divided into smaller groups to be compared, the initial sample size should be large enough that the subgroups are of adequate size to make meaningful comparisons.

5. Practical factors such as subject availability and costs are legitimate consider-ations in determining appropriate sample size.

6. The power of the statistical test needed to detect a meaningful effect or rela-tionship is a factor related to sample size determination. The larger the sample size, the greater the statistical power, all other factors remaining constant.

Summary

Sample size is important, but probably not as important as the representativeness of the sample to the population. Data from previous studies in the problem area and from pilot studies can provide the researcher with some indication of how large a sample needs to be in order to produce significant results. A sample of adequate size will be one that permits the study to be sensitive enough to determine a statistically signifi-cant difference if, in fact, it exists, and to be able to properly generalize the results.

Formative Evaluation of Objectives

Objective 1   Identify and define a population from which a sample of partici-pants is to be selected.

1. What difficulties would a researcher encounter if the research idea was to study selected health knowledge concepts in all U. S. seventh-grade children as participants?

Objective 2   Know how to determine the characteristics of the sample.

1. Why should a sample include characteristics that are also in the population from which the sample was drawn?

Objective 3   Know the various methods of selecting samples.

1. What are some of the problems involved in sampling? What methods of sampling are usually applied to obtain an unbiased sample?

Objective 4   Know the various factors that are used to determine sample size.

1. Is accuracy in a research study enhanced by selecting a large sample from a population? Why or why not? How do researchers attempt to procure a representative sample?

Reading and Evaluating Research Reports

6

OBJECTIVES

A published research report is often the culmination of the research process. The ability to read, understand, and critically evaluate research reports is an important expectation of the professional consumer of the research literature. Although the content will differ, developing a familiarity with the general format of a research report is a first step in becoming an informed consumer. The astute reader should be able to judge the content of the various sections and discern the overall quality of the report and the underlying research.

After reading chapter 6, you should be able to

1. Identify the general format of a published research report.
2. Understand the various sections of a research report and the information required within each section.
3. Critique and evaluate a research report.

As previously discussed, each of us is a consumer of research information in one way or another. As our knowledge has advanced, the world in which we live has changed dramatically. Our growth as a society is directly related to the knowledge we have acquired through scientific research. Consider the changes that have occurred just within the last two decades as a result of the invention of the computer and the exponential growth in computing technologies. We are inundated with product research in our everyday lives—whenever we read the newspaper, listen to the radio, watch television, or browse the Internet. As professionals, our programs and practices are shaped by the results of research in HHP. Whether you are a physical education teacher, a school nurse, an exercise specialist, a youth sport coach, or the director of a corporate wellness program, you have an obligation to those you serve to provide appropriate programs and services in an effectual manner. Keeping abreast of the contemporary knowledge in your field is essential. Therefore, as a research consumer, you will undoubtedly have cause to read and evaluate research reports.

A quintessential characteristic of the scientific method is the public disclosure of the findings and the knowledge acquired. Therefore, the culmination of the research process is the disclosure, in one form or another, of the findings of the research study. Frequently, this means a written research report published in a professional journal. A research report is really nothing more than a report summarizing the researchers' activities and the results of the study. Although there may be some variation in terminology as well as in the arrangement of the different sections, almost all published research reports follow a similar format. In general, research reports typically include the following main sections: introduction, methods, results, discussion, and references. The outline shown in table 6.1 illustrates a typical format used in published research reports. In the remainder of this chapter, you will learn more about the content of research reports and you will acquire information to help you evaluate such reports.

Preliminary Information

The **preliminary items** usually include the title, author and organizational affiliation, acknowledgments (if applicable), and abstract.

The title of the research article should be clear and concise, yet accurately reflect the content of the research study. As previously recommended, a title should generally be less than 15 words in length, should identify the key variables, and should provide some information about the scope of the study. Since indexing and Internet searching are tied to the key words of an article, authors should carefully select words for the title.

The authors' names usually appear beneath the article title and, typically, are ordered in accordance with the relative contributions made to the research study. The institutional or organizational affiliation of each author usually appears in a footnote or in a special box located on the first page of the article. In some journals, the highest degree earned, special titles (for example, FACSM, designating Fellow, American College of Sports Medicine), and the current position of each author, are also presented. Moreover, the mailing address or e-mail address of the primary author is usually provided in order to facilitate communication by readers who may have questions or want article reprints.

TABLE 6.1 Typical Contents within a Research Report

- Preliminary Information
  - Title
  - Author and organizational affiliation
  - Acknowledgments (if any)
  - Abstract
- Introduction
  - Background information and literature review
  - Rationale for study
  - Problem statement
  - Hypotheses or research questions
- Methods
  - Participants
  - Instrumentation
  - Procedures
  - Statistical analysis
- Results
  - Presentation of data
- Discussion
  - Conclusions
  - Recommendations
- References
- Appendix (if appropriate)

Authors often acknowledge individuals who have contributed in some way to the research or to the writing of the report. The acknowledgements may include persons who have assisted with the design of the study, with data collection, and/or with **statistical analysis,** or someone who has reviewed the manuscript. In addition, specific acknowledgment should be made of any sponsoring agency or funding source. **Acknowledgments** usually appear in an author's note that is located either at the beginning or end of the article, depending upon the journal. See Example 6.1.

Journal **abstracts,** typically 150 to 200 words long, depending upon the journal, are usually located at the beginning of the article, immediately following the title and authors' names. Quite frequently, abstracts are set in a special type (i.e., italics) or indented to distinguish them from the main article. An abstract is a brief summary of the research study and should include a succinct problem statement, information about the participants and methods used to investigate the problem, a concise summation of

EXAMPLE 6.1
Acknowledgments
From Katz, D. L., Brunner, R. L., St. Jeor, S. T., Scott, B., Jekel, J. F., and Brownell, K. D. (1998). Dietary fat consumption in a cohort of American adults, 1985–1991: Covariates, secular trends, and compliance with guidelines. *American Journal of Health Promotion*, 12(6), 382–390.

Acknowledgments

Support for the RENO Diet Heart Study has been provided by grant #HL34589 from the National Heart, Lung, and Blood Institute of the National Institutes of Health. The authors are grateful to Michaela Kiernen for technical assistance, to Linda Bartoshuk, PhD, for guidance and insight, and to Catherine Sananes Katz, PhD, for critical review of the manuscript.

the findings, and conclusions drawn from the study. According to Huck (2000, 2), "the sole purpose of the abstract is to provide readers with an overview of the material they will encounter in the remaining portions of the article." Inasmuch as an abstract should provide an overview of a research study, it is inappropriate for an abstract to simply state "The results are provided," or "The conclusions and recommendations are presented." Example 6.2 illustrates a variety of published abstracts. It should be noted that not all journals require abstracts. Additional information about abstracts is presented in chapter 15.

Introduction

The **introduction section** normally appears immediately following the abstract and often is presented in published form without the use of a heading preceding the content. The introductory section of an article generally contains two primary elements: (a) background information and (b) a statement of purpose. Some articles may also include the researcher's hypotheses. A well-written introduction section will not only enable the reader to clearly understand the problem of the study, but will also provide critical background literature that helps the reader understand why the author conducted the study.

Typically, the background portion of the introduction acquaints the reader with the problem and establishes the foundation and rationale for conducting the study. The length of this portion of the introduction varies substantially depending upon the nature of the problem being investigated and the amount of related literature. It may be as short as only a single paragraph, but more likely it will be several paragraphs in length. Because of space limitations in most journals, the **background information** does not represent a comprehensive review of literature of the topic being studied, but it should include references to the most important and timely literature. In explaining the underlying basis for their study, authors will often point to gaps in the existing literature, contradictory results or unexpected findings from previous research, and the likely practical benefits to be derived from their study. It is important that the authors make the connection between their study and similar research or published materials.

Abstract [1]

This study assessed the influence of fitness- and health-related goal setting on exercise adherence. Students (N=104) in a community college fitness program were randomly assigned, after stratification by letter grade versus credit only and self-motivation score, to one of three groups: goal setting (GS), reading (R), or control (C). Every other week, the GS group received written goal setting information and strategies, whereas the R group chose fitness-related and health-related articles to read. The C group received no communication during the 16-week intervention. At the conclusion of the study, analysis of variance results indicated no significant differences among the three groups in exercise adherence. Subjects enrolled for letter grade, however, had a significantly greater number of fitness center visits and total hours of activity than those enrolled for credit only (p<.05). Chi square analysis also confirmed that self-motivation was a significant factor (p<.05) in greater exercise adherence. It was concluded that written goal setting strategies, without personal contact, were not effective in improving exercise adherence, whereas letter grade enrollment and self-motivation were significant factors influencing greater exercise adherence.

Abstract [2]

Past studies have shown that electroencephalographic alpha activity increases as people learn to perform a novel motor task. Additionally, it has been suggested that motor performance and learning decline as people age beyond 60 years, and it has been hypothesized that physical fitness may attenuate this decline through its impact on the cerebral environment. This study was designed to replicate past research by assessing changes in alpha activity as a function of learning and to extend past research by examining differences in motor performance, motor learning, and alpha activity as a function of age and fitness. VO₂max was assessed in 41 older (ages 60-80 years) and 42 younger (ages 20-30 years) participants. Participants were randomly assigned to experimental or control conditions, which differed in the amount of practice received. Participants performed trials on the mirror star trace on both an acquisition and a retention day. Results indicated that younger participants performed better and had greater learning than older participants. Fitness was not found to impact either performance or learning. Participants in the experimental group improved more than those in the control group and maintained this difference at retention, which suggests that learning occurred. Associated with these improvements in performance capabilities was an increase in alpha power.

EXAMPLE 6.2
Abstracts
1: From Cobb, L. E., Stone, W. J., Anonsen, L. J., and Klein, D. A. (2000). The influence of goal setting on exercise adherence. *Journal of Health Education,* 31(5), 277–281.
2: From Etnier, J. L. and Landers, D. M. (1998). Motor performance and motor learning as a function of age and fitness. *Research Quarterly for Exercise and Sport,* 69(2), 139–146.

The author(s) will usually state the specific purpose of the study or problem statement near the end of the introduction section, although it could be positioned anywhere in the introduction. It is usually pretty easy to locate the **statement of purpose,** as researchers often use wording such as

- "The purpose of this study was to ..."
- "This study was designed to ..."
- "This investigation sought to ..."
- "The present study explored ..."

The statement of purpose is often only one sentence long, although it could be a couple of sentences, or even a short paragraph. A well-written statement of purpose will enable the reader to identify the key variables in the study as well as understand something about the scope of the study. Examples of purpose statements from published articles are shown in Example 6.3. Although it is becoming less common, authors will occasionally state their research hypotheses in a paragraph immediately following the purpose statement. It is rare today for authors of published articles to state the hypothesis in the null form, preferring instead to specify the research hypothesis, or the predicted outcome of the study. In lieu of stating hypotheses, sometimes authors may provide a listing of research questions that the study proposes to answer. Regardless of the specific format and organization, after reading an introduction section the reader should have a clear understanding of what is being studied and why it is being studied.

Methods

The next major part of most published research articles is the **methods section,** generally identifiable by a section heading titled, *Methods, Methodology, Procedures,* or something similar. Here the author provides a description of the research participants (subjects), research instruments, and procedures for the administration of treatments as well as for data collection. Sometimes the author will also provide information about the data analysis. It is fairly common for each of these parts to be presented as a specific subsection, complete with a subheading, within the methods section of a published research report. The methods section tends to be highly structured and should contain detailed statements explaining the methodology used to conduct the study. Ideally, the entire methods section should be written in such a way that would enable an interested and qualified reader to replicate the study using the same methodology.

Research Participants (Subjects)

Typically, the first part of the methods section is used to describe the **research participants.** This should include information about the target population, the number of participants, and how they were selected. In addition, pertinent characteristics of

Purpose [1]

Therefore, the purpose of this study was to determine the effect of utilizing nasal strips or athletic mouthpieces or both on anaerobic exercise performance.

Purpose [2]

In summary, the present study examined one possible explanation for the severe underrepresentation of women in coaching basketball teams, namely, gender differences in orientations toward coaching as an occupation. The study, based on the theories relating to career choice, posed the following four research questions to be investigated.

1. Do women and men differ in (a) their perceptions of their self-efficacy regarding coaching, (b) their preferences for specific need-fulfilling attributes in an occupation, (c) their perceptions of the extent to which the coaching occupation possesses the need-fulfilling attributes, and (d) perceptions of working hours as a barrier to entry into coaching?

2. Do female participants, grouped on the basis of the gender of the head coach, differ in their perceptions of discrimination as a barrier to entry into coaching?

3. Do the genders differ in their desire to be paid, full-time coaches?

4. What are the relationships between perceived occupational factors (i.e., coaching self-efficacy, valence of coaching, and perceived barriers) and preference for coaching?

Purpose [3]

Resistance training might alter the contractile protein composition in addition to its effects on CSA. It has been reported that lifelong resistance training results in a significantly lower proportion of Type I myosin in skeletal muscle of the elderly (Klitgaard et al., 1990a). To our knowledge, however, no comparable data are available on the influence of short-term resistance training. Therefore, the aim of the present study was to examine muscles of elderly participants after an 8-week resistance-training regimen, using information provided by biopsy sampling to assess the extent of change in selected muscle-fiber characteristics.

Purpose [4]

Therefore, the aim of this study was to investigate running economy, fractional utilization of maximal oxygen consumption and metabolite concentrations, at a steady state absolute workload (16.1 km. h^{-1}) and

EXAMPLE 6.3

Purpose Statements

1: From Thomas, D. Q., Bowdoin, B. A., Brown, D. D., and McCaw, S. T. (1998). Nasal strips and mouthpieces do not affect power output during anaerobic exercise. *Research Quarterly for Exercise and Sport,* 69(2), 201–204.

2: From Everhart, C. B. and Chelladurai, P. (1998). Gender differences in preferences for coaching as an occupation: The role of self-efficacy, valence, and perceived barriers. *Research Quarterly for Exercise and Sport,* 69(2), 188–200.

3: From O'Neill, D. E. T., Thayer, R. E., Taylor, A. W., Dzialoznski, T. M., Noble, E. G. (2000). Effects of short-term resistance training on muscle strength and morphology in the elderly. *Journal of Aging and Physical Activity,* 8(4), 312–324.

4: From Weston, A. R., Mbambo, Z., and Myburgh, K. H. (2000). Running economy of African and Caucasian distance runners. *Medicine and Sciences in Sports and Exercise,* 32(6), 1130–1134.

EXAMPLE 6.3
Concluded

> at 10-km race pace in African and Caucasian groups of runners who are matched for current 10-km performance. In addition, to minimize the potential effects of body mass on running economy, the groups were as closely matched as possible for body mass.

the participants, such as age, gender, grade level, socioeconomic level, ethnicity, and any other characteristics that may have a bearing on the problem being studied should be described. If appropriate to the study, the author should also describe how participants were assigned to comparison groups or treatment groups. It is important that the author carefully describe how the research participants were obtained, including a description of the population, thus enabling the reader to make a judgment about the generalizability of the results. Were they volunteers? Were they randomly selected? What selection criteria were established? What sampling technique was used? Chapter 5 provides a full description of various sampling techniques and the process of selecting research participants. When sampling procedures are not well defined, it is wise to believe that a convenience sample was used. See Example 6.4 for examples of excerpts from published articles describing research participants.

Instrumentation

This subsection of a journal article should contain a description of data collection instruments, materials, and any equipment or apparatus used in the study. Given the diverse nature of HHP research, **instrumentation** may vary substantially. For some researchers, instrumentation is largely a paper-and-pencil variety and may include tests, checklists, scales, inventories, questionnaires, interview schedules, or observation reports. Other researchers, however, utilize specialized equipment for data collection, such as skinfold calipers, timing devices, strength gauges, metabolic measurement systems, cinematographic equipment, and heart monitors, among others. Furthermore, some researchers utilize standardized performance tests, such as sport skills tests or physical fitness tests as their means of collecting data.

Whereas space limitations within the journal may prohibit the actual reproduction of a written instrument in the article itself, authors should provide a complete description of the instrument, including pertinent psychometric properties (i.e., validity and reliability), if available. Similarly, equipment or research apparatus should be thoroughly described, including evidence of its technical properties. Sometimes illustrations or photographs of testing equipment may be used to supplement the written description.

Researchers utilizing published instruments or commercially available equipment often cite manufacturer's specifications or the work of other researchers as the basis of asserting the validity and reliability of the chosen instrument. If the measuring

EXAMPLE 6.4
Methods: Research
Participants
1: From Weiss, M. R.,
McCullagh, P., Smith, A. L.,
and Berlant, A. R. (1998).
Observational learning and
the fearful child: Influence
of peer models on swimming
skill performance and
psychological responses.
*Research Quarterly for
Exercise and Sport,* 69(4),
380–394.
2: From Papaioannou, A.
(1998). Students' perceptions
of the physical education class
environment for boys and girls
and the perceived motivational
climate. *Research Quarterly
for Exercise and Sport,* 69(3),
267–275.

Participants [1]

Children were recruited from community school or nonschool youth programs. Program instructors and parents were asked to identify children who had minimal swimming experience, were fearful of the water, and had low self-confidence. In all, 24 children (18 boys and 6 girls) met these criteria. Their average age was 6.2 years ($SD = .90$), 62.5% ($n = 15$) had taken formal swimming lessons, and they averaged 9.5 ($SD = 11.4$; range = 0 to 40) weeks of swimming lesson experience.[2] Children were matched to group by age and lesson experience, and then groups were randomly assigned to one of three model type conditions: control, peer mastery, and peer coping. All parents provided informed consent prior to study procedures, and children signed an assent form on the first day of the study prior to any swimming skill or questionnaire assessments.

Participants [2]

The 310 adolescents participating in this study were enrolled in six junior high schools ($n = 77$ boys, $n = 64$ girls; M age = 13.5 years, $SD = 1.5$) and six senior high schools ($n = 76$ boys, $n = 93$ girls; M age = 16.5 years, $SD = 1.5$). All physical education classes were coeductional and taught by 12 physical education teachers, 3 male and 3 female teachers in junior high schools and 3 male and 3 female teachers in senior high schools. These schools were randomly selected from the total number of schools in Thessaloniki, Greece, a town with 1 million residents.

instrument is new and specifically designed for the study described in the article, the authors would be expected to go to greater lengths describing the development of the instrument as well as pertinent validity and reliability evidence. The main concern for the author(s) is to establish that the instrumentation used in the study was appropriate for the particular research problem and that it enabled the researchers to collect accurate and credible information. Example 6.5 provides illustrations of instrumentation sections in published articles.

Procedures

The **procedures** portion of the methods section includes a description of data collection procedures as well as experimental treatments and how they were administered. Basically this is a description, step by step, of how the researcher conducted the study. Where was the study performed? What did the subjects do? What did the researcher do? Who collected the data? How long did it take? What safeguards were

EXAMPLE 6.5

Methods: Instrumentation

1: From Amorose, A. J. and Horn, T. S. (2000). Intrinsic motivation: Relationships with collegiate athletes' gender, scholarship status, and perceptions of their coaches' behavior. *Journal of Sport and Exercise Psychology,* 22(1), 63–84.

2: From Kandakai, T. L. and King, K. A. (1999). Perceived self-efficacy in performing lifesaving skills: An assessment of the American Red Cross's responding to emergencies course. *Journal of Health Education,* 30(4), 235–241.

Instrumentation [1]

Intrinsic Motivation

Intrinsic motivation was assessed using a sport-oriented version of the Intrinsic Motivation Inventory (IMI; McAuley, Duncan, & Tammen, 1989). An original version of the IMI was used by R. Ryan and his colleagues (e.g., Plant & Ryan, 1985; R. Ryan, Mims, & Koestner, 1983) as a multidimensional measure of subjects' intrinsic motivation for a specific achievement activity. McAuley et al.'s sport-oriented version of the IMI contains 16 items that assess four components of intrinsic motivation, including interest-enjoyment, perceived competence, effort-importance, and tension-pressure. McAuley et al. reported acceptable psychometric properties for the four subscales.

A fifth subscale was included in the current study questionnaire based on suggestions by McAuley et al. (1989). This additional subscale, labeled *perceived choice,* included four items to assess the degree to which athletes believe they are participating in their sport by personal choice. The four items include the following: (a) "I participate in this sport because I want to", (b) "I would quit this sport if I could", (c) "Working hard in this sport is something I choose to do", and (d) "When my eligibility is up I will quit this sport."

Each item on the IMI is followed by a 7-point Likert-type scale, with response choices ranging from *strongly disagree* to *strongly agree.* Subjects are asked to indicate their agreement or disagreement with each statement by circling the appropriate response.

Instrumentation [2]

Based on a comprehensive review of the literature, a 12-item instrument was developed to assess subjects' perceived self-efficacy in performing life-saving skills and the impact of training on subjects' willingness to act during an emergency and in the presence of noted barriers. The instrument consisted of four demographic items (age, gender, race, and education level) and five background items (level of previous training, first aid requirement for college major or job, reasons for taking the first aid course, field of study, and previous experience in giving first aid and CPR). The instrument also contained questions based on Bandura's self-efficacy model. Efficacy expectations, outcome expectations, and outcome values subscales consisted of three items each. The remaining questions contained three items examining subjects' willingness to perform lifesaving skills in the presence of specified barriers.

EXAMPLE 6.5
Concluded

To establish face validity, items in the survey instrument were constructed based on a comprehensive review of the literature. Content validity was established by distributing the instrument to three national experts in survey research and one national expert on the self-efficacy model. Experts were defined as individuals who were recognized authorities on survey research or the self-efficacy model and who had recently published articles on these topics. Recommendations offered by experts were taken under consideration and appropriate revisions were made to the survey instrument. Stability reliability was assessed utilizing a sample of 25 male and female undergraduate college students who were given the instrument twice, 5 days apart.

provided? The procedures should be presented with sufficient detail and clarity that another researcher would be able to follow the steps described and replicate the study. You might consider this to be the "recipe" for conducting the study.

For experimental studies, this section should also include a description of the research design, clearly identifying the independent and dependent variables, and describing the experimental treatments. It is important that the research design be appropriate to the solution of the research problem and be relatively free of threats to the validity of the study. See chapter 7 for a more thorough discussion of internal and external validity. All studies will include a description of the data collection procedures. These procedures should be appropriate to the research participants and should correctly use the selected measuring instruments. Although not seen in all published research articles, sometimes a description of the **data analysis** procedures will be included here. This approach is typical in theses and dissertations. Otherwise, the data analysis procedures are described in the results section. Examples of procedures sections are shown in Example 6.6.

Results

The **results section** of a published article is where the researcher reports the results of the data collection efforts as well as the outcomes of the various statistical treatments that were applied to the data. If the data analysis procedures were not previously discussed under the methods section, that information would be presented here. For many readers of research reports, the results section is the most difficult part to read and understand because of all the statistical information and numerical data. As a consequence, many readers simply skip over the results section. Yet, in order to become an astute consumer of the research literature, you will need to

EXAMPLE 6.6
Methods: Procedures
1: From Engels, H. J., Zhu, W., and Moffatt, R. J. (1998). An empirical evaluation of the prediction of maximal heart rate. *Research Quarterly for Exercise and Sport,* 69(1), 94–98.
2: From Weston, A. R., Mbambo, Z., and Myburgh, K. H. (2000). Running economy of African and Caucasian distance runners. *Medicine and Science in Sports and Exercise,* 32(6), 1130–1134.

Data Collection [1]

Each participant completed a continuous graded treadmill test using the Bruce protocol (Bruce, Kusumi, & Hosmer, 1973) to determine both HRmax and VO_2max. The treadmill tests were performed under the supervision of specifically trained, qualified medical personnel throughout the day over a collection period of approximately 6 months. During each maximal exercise test, oxygen consumption was measured continuously by open-circuit spirometry using a Beckman metabolic Cart (Beckman Instruments, Schiller Park, IL). A participant's heart rate response was determined electrocardiographically from the V_5 position. For that purpose, electrocardiogram chart paper recordings were obtained during the last 30 s of each completed exercise stage and continuously once a participant signaled that he or she was approaching exhaustion. Individual HRmax was defined as the highest heart rate achieved (15-s R-R interval count), which usually occurred during the last minute of exercise.

Data Collection [2]

Submaximal exercise testing.

On a separate day, subjects returned to the laboratory 3 h after eating. Subjects did not ingest caffeine overnight or before the test. Subjects again warmed up at 14 km. h^{-1} for 5 min. Subjects then completed two submaximal workloads, one at 16.1 km. h^{-1} and the other at current 10-km race pace, with all subjects utilizing the same calibrated treadmill (Powerjog EG30, Birmingham, England). Each workload was undertaken for 6 min separated by a rest period of 5 min. VO_2, V_E, RER, and HR were measured continuously and results averaged over 15-s intervals. Mean values of the last 60 s were designated as steady state values for data analysis. A venous blood sample was obtained exactly 1 min after exercise for each workload for determination of plasma ammonia and plasma lactate concentrations. Samples were immediately centrifuged at 4° C at 3000 rpm and plasma was obtained. Plasma ammonia was assayed spectrophotometrically in duplicate within 2 h (NH_3 kit, Boehringer Mannheim), and plasma was stored for later spectrophotometric analysis of lactate in duplicate (bioMerieux lactate PAP, Boehringer Mannheim).

develop some level of competence in reading and understanding results sections. Chapters 12 and 13 in this textbook describe common descriptive and inferential statistical techniques frequently seen in the research literature. For a more in-depth explanation of the various statistical techniques, readers are referred to basic statistics textbooks such as Harris (1998) or Ferguson and Takane (1989).

The nature of the research problem will determine, to a large extent, the type of statistical technique that is used. We previously saw that research questions generally fall into three categories: descriptive, relationship, and difference. Statistical techniques can also be grouped into these same three categories. Therefore, if the reader of a research article can identify the type of questions(s) being asked, this is a first step in understanding what general category of statistics is required to answer the question. It is important to note that a single research study will usually contain more than one research question; therefore, it is likely that several different statistical techniques will be used within a single study. Consequently, the results section will likely include the outcomes of several statistical techniques.

Results sections should not contain a discussion, explanation, or interpretation of the results (Tuckman 1999). This information will follow in the discussion section. Demographic information about the research participants, if not previously presented in the methods section, is usually presented first, followed by the more substantive findings related to the research questions. Results sections are often organized around each hypothesis or each research question of the study. Most articles, regardless of the type of research, will generally report basic descriptive statistics, such as means, standard deviations, frequencies, and percentages for the key variables. Studies asking relationship questions as well as those asking difference questions will also report correlational statistics and inferential statistics, as appropriate. The use of tables and figures to complement the information reported in the text of published articles is commonplace. Tables and figures should always follow their contextual reference.

While it is impossible to indicate exactly what information should be presented in a results section, some general guidelines may be helpful. Ultimately, the nature of the research problem being studied and the statistical procedures utilized will go a long way in determining the precise content in the results section. In accordance with the recommendations of Tuckman (1999), we suggest that the following elements, if appropriate for the study, should be included in a results section:

1. A brief restatement of each hypothesis
2. An indication of the descriptive statistics used (e.g., means, standard deviations)
3. An indication of the inferential statistics used (e.g., t-test, ANOVA, correlations)
4. Specification of the significance level used for hypothesis testing
5. A brief statement identifying the statistical assumptions examined
6. The anticipated effect size and power of the statistical test used
7. The results of the statistical tests (including t-values, F-ratios, probability levels, and degrees of freedom, if appropriate)
8. The magnitude of the effect obtained
9. An indication as to whether the null hypothesis was accepted or rejected

In qualitative studies, researchers often have notes from interviews or field observations that must be organized and synthesized. Qualitative researchers generally do not have numerical data to report or analyze. Consequently, the results section of a qualitative study takes on a different appearance, one that is largely a narrative presentation of the findings, often supported by the words of the participants, including direct quotations. More information about qualitative research is found in chapter 9 of this textbook.

Example 6.7 presents examples of results sections from various published reports. It is noted that each example represents only a portion of the complete section in the published article. Several examples also refer to tables or figures that have not been reproduced here.

Discussion

The **discussion section** of a journal article contains a nontechnical explanation of the results. Basically, the discussion section is where the author presents the outcomes of the study. Here, the author provides his or her interpretation of the findings, culminating with a conclusion that provides an answer to the research problem. It is noted that some authors may include in the paper a separate section labeled **Conclusions.** The discussion section is often the least structured of the research report, enabling the author to take considerable latitude in the writing. However, if the study was set up to test hypotheses, the discussion section should include a report on the results of each hypothesis test. Tuckman (1999) suggests that the discussion section of a research report serves six major functions:

- **To summarize the findings** – a rather straightforward function is to provide a summary of the major findings in the form of conclusions, thus providing the reader with an overall picture of the results

- **To interpret the study's findings** – the author's explanation or interpretation of what the results mean [note: we would propose that this may be the most important function of the discussion section]

- **To integrate the findings** – an attempt to synthesize the various findings, both expected and unexpected, to achieve meaningful conclusions and generalizations

- **To theorize** – occasionally, a study generates a number of interrelated findings that might serve as the basis for theory development, either as support for existing theory or for the establishment of original theory

- **To recommend or apply** – since results from research frequently have implications for enhancing or altering professional practices, the discussion section provides the venue for making such **recommendations**

- **To suggest extensions** – inevitably, the results of a research study give rise to more questions; the discussion section of a report often includes recommendations for future research

Results [1]

A total of 53 (43%) older adults had dropped out of the exercise program within 4 months. There were no demographic differences found between those who dropped out of the exercise program and those who remained, except for education level. Education level differed significantly between the two groups; a greater proportion of the attrition group reported less than a 12th-grade education ($x^2 = 7.33$, $p < .05$).

Health differences were found between the exercise attrition group and those who completed the program (Table 2). Compared with those who continued in the exercise program, the attrition group reported poorer self-ratings of health ($x^2 = 6.0$, $p < .05$), a greater frequency of not having enough energy to do the things they need to do ($x^2 = 6.57$, $p < .05$), and that they climbed fewer flights of stairs per day. If the PAR-Q scale had been used as an eligibility screening tool, a greater proportion of attrition group individuals would have been considered ineligible for the program, as more of them reported having one or more problems on the revised PAR-Q scale indicating greater health risk ($x^2 = 3.58$, $p = .058$).

Results [2]

Intrinsic Motivation, Gender, and Scholarship Status. To test whether athletes' intrinsic motivation would vary as a function of their gender, scholarship status, and perceived percentage of athletes on scholarship, a 2 x 3 x 2 (gender by scholarship status by scholarship percentage) MANOVA was conducted. The dependent variables for this analysis were the five subscale scores from the IMI (interest-enjoyment, perceived competence, effort-importance, perceived choice, and tension-pressure). The independent variables were gender (male, female), scholarship status (full, partial, none) and perceived scholarship percentage (low: $\leq 70\%$, high: $\geq 75\%$). The descriptive statistics for each group are presented in Table 3.

Due to the nonorthogonal nature of the research design, the significance of the main and interaction effects was tested in hierarchical fashion (Finn, 1974; Tabachnick & Fidell, 1996). This procedure revealed a nonsignificant three-way (gender by scholarship status by scholarship percentage) interaction effect. In addition, the Scholarship Status x Scholarship Percentage interaction, the Gender x Scholarship Status interaction, and the Gender x Scholarship Percentage interaction were all nonsignificant. The scholarship percentage main effect was also nonsignificant. However, both the scholarship status main effect, Wilks's lambda = .94, $F(10, 740) = 2.37$, $p < .01$, and the gender main effect, Wilks's lambda = .97; $F(5, 370) = 2.39$, $p < .04$, were significant.

EXAMPLE 6.7
Results

1: From Prohaska, T. R., Peters, K., and Warren, J. S. (2000). Sources of attrition in a church-based exercise program for older African-Americans. *American Journal of Health Promotion,* 14(6), 380–385.

2: From Amorose, A. J. and Horn, T. S. (2000). Intrinsic motivation: Relationships with collegiate athletes' gender, scholarship status, and perceptions of their coaches' behavior. *Journal of Sport and Exercise Psychology,* 22(1), 63–84.

3: From Spencer, L. (1999). College freshmen smokers versus nonsmokers: Academic, social and emotional expectations and attitudes toward college. *Journal of Health Education,* 30(5), 274–281.

4: From Etnier, J. L. and Landers, D. M. (1988). Motor performance and motor learning as a function of age and fitness. *Research Quarterly for Exercise and Sport,* 69(2), 139–146.

EXAMPLE 6.7
Concluded

Results [3]

The Freshman Survey with tobacco-related questions was completed by 544 first-semester freshmen. Both genders were fairly equally represented, with 305 (56%) females and 232 (43%) males completing the survey (7 students did not indicate gender). Unfortunately, the survey instrument did not include a question about race or ethnicity; however, other sources provided this information about the entire freshman class ($n = 1142$). Eighty-three percent ($n = 943$) of the class was white, 7% ($n = 83$) was African-American, 6% ($n = 69$) was Hispanic, 3% ($n = 29$) was Asian, one was Native American, and 1% ($n = 17$) did not indicate ethnicity.

Sixty-six percent of respondents ($n = 360$) reported that they have never been smokers. Twenty-seven percent ($n = 148$) reported smoking either regularly (more than 1 day per week) or occasionally (1 day per week or less). Specifically, regular smokers were more prevalent ($n = 91$) than occasional smokers ($n = 57$). Among all smokers, 86 (58%) were female, 56 (38%) were male, and 6 (4%) did not indicate gender. Only 7% of respondents ($n = 36$) reported being former smokers. Among current smokers, the average age of smoking initiation was 16 years, with a range of 8-18 years. Former smokers began smoking at age 14 and smoked for 2 years before quitting, on average.

Results [4]

Initial Differences

Demographic data are presented in Table 1 as a function of Age Group, Fitness Group, and Treatment Group. Results showed no significant difference in years of education since high school as a function of Age Group, Fitness Group, or Treatment Group ($p > .05$). There was a significant main effect for Fitness Group on weight, $F(1, 79) = 11.03$, $p < .001$, such that fit participants ($M = 76.03$ kg, $SD = 9.12$) weighed significantly less than unfit participants ($M = 83.86$ kg, $SD = 11.80$). There was also a significant main effect for Age Group on self-reported physical activity level, $F(1, 79) = 13.91$, $p < .001$, such that the scores for the older participants ($M = 11.63$, $SD = 7.51$) were significantly higher than those for the younger ones ($M = 7.09$, $SD = 1.32$).[3] For VO$_2$ max, there was a significant main effect for Age Group, $F(1, 79) = 146.14$, $p < .001$, such that younger participants ($M = 43.05$ ml/kg/min, $SD = 9.15$) were significantly more fit than older participants ($M = 28.30$ ml/kg/min, $SD = 9.82$). Examination of the time interval between acquisition and retention trials indicated that there was not a significant difference as a function of Age Group, Fitness Group, Treatment Group, or the interactions of these variables, $F(1,75) = 0.00 - 2.65$, $p > .05$. Importantly, for the older participants, there was no significant difference in years since retirement as a function of Fitness Group, Treatment Group, or their interaction ($p > .05$).

While each of these functions may not be served in the discussion section of every published research report, it is important to realize the breadth of possible content. It is common for the discussion section to begin with a brief restatement of the research problem, followed by a general statement summarizing the results. This is usually followed with a more detailed discussion of the specific findings. The discussion section generally does not contain the statistical notation and numerical information found in reporting the results, but usually consists of a narrative discussion in which the author summarizes and explains what the results mean, often attempting to explain why the results turned out as they did. In explaining the results, the author attempts to connect the results of the study with appropriate theory, professional practice, and the related literature. The author should be careful to avoid reaching conclusions that are not supported by the results of the study. Moreover, the author should present only implications and recommendations that are based on the results of the study, not on what the author had hoped to be true. Sometimes the author cautions the reader about possible misinterpretations, pointing out the limitations associated with the research. A common error made by researchers as well as by consumers of the research literature is to overgeneralize the results, that is, attempting to apply the findings and resultant conclusions to settings or populations that are not warranted by the study. Generalizability of research findings is discussed in more detail in chapter 7 under the topic "external validity." Example 6.8 provides examples of excerpts taken from discussion sections in published reports. Please note that each excerpt is only a portion of a complete section.

References and Appendix

Following the text of the published article will be a list of **references.** This list includes all books, journal articles, or other sources that were cited by the author. The format of the reference list will vary according to the publication guidelines of the specific journal. Regardless of the style manual specified, every item in the reference list should have been cited in the text of the paper and every source cited in the paper should be included in the reference list. The reference list is an excellent place to attain information about articles, books, or other sources that pertain to the topic under investigation.

     Readers are advised to carefully note the references cited, taking into consideration such factors as the date of publication and the nature of the journal or publication source. For instance, an article in which most of the references are 25–30 years old should be viewed cautiously. While there may be legitimate reasons for a preponderance of old references, an astute reader of the research literature should at least ask the question, "Why?" In addition, a lengthy reference list does not necessarily mean a quality article. Locke, Spirduso, and Silverman (2000) point out that the use of nonselective references may be an indication of poor scholarship and may reflect the inability of the author to differentiate between the trivial and the important in research.

EXAMPLE 6.8
Discussions

1: From Lewis, P. C., Harrell, J. S., Deng, S., and Bradley, C. (1999). Smokeless tobacco use in adolescents: The cardiovascular health in children study. *Journal of School Health,* 69(8), 320–325.

2. From Behlendorf, B., MacRae, P. G., and Vos Strache, C. (1999). Children's perceptions of physical activity for adults: Competence and appropriateness. *Journal of Aging and Physical Activity,* 7(4), 354–373.

3. From Cheatham, C. C., Mahon, A. D., Brown, J. D., and Bolster, D. R. (2000). Cardiovascular responses during prolonged exercise at ventilatory threshold. *Medicine and Science in Sports and Exercise,* 32(3), 1080–1087.

Discussion [1]

This study supports the literature that shows males are more likely to be current users of smokeless tobacco over females[1, 6, 9, 24, 25] and smokeless tobacco use increases with age.[3, 6, 8] However, the ethnic diversity of use found is very different from what is reported in the literature. This study found that Hispanics were more likely to be current users (11.4%) than Whites (4.2%), Blacks (2.1%), or Others (6.8%). Studies have reported Hispanics have a higher prevalence of smoking and using smokeless tobacco than Black or "other" ethnic groups,[6,.8,.25-27] but none of those studies reported higher use in Hispanics than in Whites. Since North Carolina is a tobacco-producing state, perhaps patterns of use are different compared to national samples. This fact makes interpretation of these results difficult and underscores the need for further research on smokeless tobacco use in ethnic minority groups.

Discussion [2]

Competence

As hypothesized, age was the most significant factor in determining the perceived competence of the adults involved in the three physical activities. The main effect for age accounted for 61% of the variance, whereas type of physical activity accounted for 8% and gender accounted for 0%. The results indicate that the older adults were perceived as less competent than the middle-aged adults, who were viewed as less competent than the young adults. These findings support those of Ostrow et al. (1987), who reported that preschoolers' perceptions of motor skill proficiency decreased as the age of the referent person increased from 20 to 40 to 60 to 80 years. Similarly, Kite and Johnson (1988) found in their meta-analysis that measures of competence in older adults were more negatively rated than in young adults. They cautioned that it is unlikely that older people are evaluated more negatively than young people on all dimensions. For example, the elderly might be seen as less competent or physically attractive than young people but might not be seen as less kind, friendly, or satisfied (Deaux & Lewis, 1984). A multidimensional approach that includes physical, cognitive, social, and affective aspects of older adults might be more informative and lead to greater insights in understanding age effects on perceived competence.

Discussion [3]

In conclusion, the results of this study indicate that the cardiovascular responses to prolonged exercise are similar in boys and men. Specifically, the magnitude of cardiovascular drift is similar between boys and men, although

EXAMPLE 6.8
Concluded

there is a tendency for the increase in HR and decrease in SV to be somewhat higher in adults. In addition, the cardiovascular responses during prolonged exercise at VT are similar to previous studies examining prolonged exercise in children and adults relative to VO_{2max}. Therefore, it seems that the cardiovascular responses to prolonged constant-load exercise are somewhat independent of whether the intensity is below or above VT, and thus individual differences in VT may not be a concern during prolonged constant-load exercise, although whether this idea applies to exercise at equal intensities above VT is unclear and worthy of future research.

Some published articles may also include a notes section or appendix at the end of the article. A notes section is a likely place to locate acknowledgments and may be positioned either at the beginning of the article or at the end, depending upon the requirements of the journal. Although less likely to be seen in published articles because of space limitations, appendices may be used to include copies of questionnaires, inventories, tabular information, special materials, or even illustrations of testing equipment.

Critiquing a Research Article

Criteria

The **criteria for critiquing an article** are the same criteria a researcher could apply to a manuscript being developed. Most research books and guides contain a list of criteria for evaluating an article or other research publication. These lists differ to some degree but are generally similar. The majority of the criteria on these lists usually apply to any article or research publication, particularly ones based on experimental research. Due to the variety of research conducted, no article or research publication should be expected to fulfill all the criteria on any list.

Isaac and Michael (1982) present an excellent checklist for evaluating an article (Example 6.9). They also provide a lengthy checklist for items that might be included in a research proposal and a long list of criteria for evaluating a research report, article, or thesis. The checklist for a research proposal is arranged by the typical chapters of a dissertation: (1) the problem, (2) review of related literature, (3) methodology of procedures, (4) findings (analysis and evaluation), and (5) summary, conclusions, and recommendations. Criteria for evaluation of a research report, article, or thesis are arranged under the title of the article or report; the problem, design, and methodology (procedures); presentation and analysis of data; and summary and conclusions.

The authors of this book had an unreferenced list of criteria for evaluating research in health, physical education, and recreation. It is organized similar to the

EXAMPLE 6.9

Checklist for Evaluating an Article—Form for the Evaluation of an Article[1, 2]

Form for the Evaluation of an Article on page 220 in Isaac, J. and Michael, W. B. (1982), *Handbook in Research and Evaluation*. EdITS Publishers, San Diego, CA. Reproduced with permission.

CHARACTERISTIC	COMPLETELY INDEPENDENT (1)	POOR (2)	MEDIOCRE (3)	GOOD (4)	EXCELLENT (5)
1. Problem is clearly stated					
2. Hypotheses are clearly stated					
3. Problem is significant					
4. Assumptions are clearly stated					
5. Limitations of the study are stated					
6. Important terms are defined					
7. Relationship of the problem to previous research is made clear					
8. Research design is described fully					
9. Research design is appropriate for the solution of the problem					
10. Research design is free of specific weaknesses					
11. Population and sample are described					
12. Method of sampling is appropriate					
13. Data-gathering methods or procedures are described					
14. Data-gathering methods or procedures are appropriate to the solution of the problem					
15. Data-gathering methods or procedures are utilized correctly					
16. Validity and reliability of the evidence gathered are established					
17. Appropriate methods are selected to analyze the data					
18. Methods utilized in analyzing the data are applied correctly					
19. Results of the analysis are presented clearly					
20. Conclusions are clearly stated					
21. Conclusions are substantiated by the evidence presented					
22. Generalizations are confined to the population from which the sample was drawn					
23. Report is clearly written					
24. Report is logically organized					
25. Tone of the report displays an unbiased, impartial scientific attitude.					

1. Wandt, Edwin, California State College, Los Angeles
2. Not all of these twenty-five criteria or characteristics are appropriate in the evaluation of a given article.

ones previously mentioned with major headings: (1) problem, (2) report, (3) procedures, methods, and techniques, (4) data, and (5) analysis and interpretation of the findings. A *checklist for evaluating a research paper,* similar in organization to those previously presented, appears in Example 6.10.

Article Critique

Articles in journals associated with well-qualified manuscript reviewers will have few if any faults, since any faults in the manuscript either caused it to be rejected or were corrected before it was published. Also, keep in mind that all researchers and manuscript reviewers have their own ideas concerning how research should be conducted and what are the most important evaluation criteria. Readers of an article often see certain things they think could be improved, but these may just be opinions. It is always easier to criticize the research of others than to conduct the research yourself.

EXAMPLE 6.10
Checklist for Evaluating
a Research Paper

An Outline of a Checklist for a Research Paper

Because of the wide diversity of types of research projects as well as the multitude of approaches that may very well be taken with any single problem, it is not possible to present either an outline or a checklist that would be appropriate for all cases. Nevertheless, the researcher should be able to answer the questions listed below. Obviously, if a question does not apply, it should be disregarded. Those that do apply should merit positive answers by the investigator.

I.   **The Problem**

    1. Does the statement of the problem meet the criteria of being:

        (a) stated in a few sentences?

        (b) clearly stated in both theoretical and operational terms?

        (c) firmly based on a stated theory and/or problem?

        (d) clear on the definitions of the variables that are to be studied?

        (e) based on variable hypotheses?

    2. Has the problem been delimited in such a fashion that it can be pursued realistically?

    3. Has an important problem been selected, the study of which will make a worthwhile contribution to education?

EXAMPLE 6.10
Continued

II.   **The Review of Relevant Literature**

1. Is it apparent that an adequate job was done in sampling the relevant literature on the topic?

2. Were references drawn from recent literature?

3. Is a wide variety of sources represented?

4. Are cited references either quoted sufficiently or interpreted accurately?

5. Have references been organized by topic and/or by date of publication?

III.   **Design, Procedure, and Method**

1. Is the design appropriate to the problem?

2. Was the population studied clearly specified?

3. Were sampling procedures clearly specified and the total sample adequate?

4. If a control group was involved, was it selected from same population?

5. Were the various treatments (including control) assigned at random?

6. Were appropriate statistical procedures selected and the level of significance selected in advance?

7. Were the reliability and validity of the data-gathering instruments and procedures established and reported?

8. Are the limitations of the study acknowledged?

9. Were the treatments and/or methods of data collection described so clearly and completely that an independent investigator could replicate the study?

10. Were extraneous sources of error either held constant or randomized among subjects of all groups?

11. Was the response from the sampled population equal to 80 percent or more?

12. Are the characteristics of the respondents clearly representative of the sample?

EXAMPLE 6.10
Concluded

IV.   **Analysis of the Data**

1. Are the data clearly presented?

2. Is appropriate use made of charts, tables, figures, descriptions, and/or historical narratives?

3. Were all possible comparisons of the data made and reported?

4. Were the statistical assumptions necessary for valid tests of the hypothesis satisfied?

V.   **Interpretation of the Findings and Conclusion**

1. Are generalizations confined to the population from which the sample was drawn?

2. Do the conclusions of the study meet the criteria of being:

    (a) consistent with the obtained results?

    (b) relevant to the problem?

    (c) based on the data?

    (d) justified by the data?

    (e) constructive and free from bias?

    (f) not "stretched" to support a bias?

3. Are implications given for both education practice and for further research ?

VI.   **Summary**

1. Is a concise summary given of the problem, design, methodology, findings, interpretation, and conclusions?

2. Does the reading of this section alone present an accurate overall picture of the study?

VII.   **Bibliography**

1. Are complete references presented for all sources read or referred to in conjunction with the study?

VIII.   **Appendix**

1. Are samples present of all questionnaires, lists, interview forms, letters, and so forth used in the study?

2. Are such materials clearly labeled and lettered for quick and easy reference?

Earlier in this chapter, the parts of a research report were discussed, starting with the title and ending with the references. These parts were discussed from the standpoint of reading and understanding the article. Keep in mind that many articles are written assuming the reader has had at least one graduate-level course in the general area of the research. Further, there are certain terms unique to research writing. Thus, do not be too discouraged if you do not understand all research articles.

If the title of the article does not interest you, it is doubtful you will read further. If you do read the abstract, look for the statement of the purpose for the research study, the subjects and methods used in the study, and the major findings and conclusions.

In the introduction and review of related literature section, look for why the research was needed, a review of articles bearing on the conduct of the study, and a statement of purpose for the study. After reading the procedures and methods section, you should have a good understanding of the type and number of subjects involved and the procedures and methods used in the study. Further, you should feel that the study was well conducted. If you do not feel the study was well conducted, there may be no reason to read further.

Most readers of a research article falling within their area of expertise can understand the information up to the results section. The results section may be difficult to understand if your statistical knowledge is limited or if quite advanced statistical techniques are used. To the best of your ability, determine if the appropriate statistical techniques were correctly applied and, more importantly, whether the results have been accurately stated. The discussion and conclusions section is based on the results of the study. If you do not fully understand the results section, you may have to accept some of the discussions and conclusions not knowing whether they are totally correct; worse yet, you may not understand them. Even if you do not fully understand the results or discussion and conclusions sections, you may find some comfort in the fact that the reviewers of the manuscript found their presentation acceptable. However, the danger remains that, due to lack of knowledge, you may misinterpret the information set forth in these two sections.

The reference section may be of particular interest to you if you want to evaluate the quality of the books and journals cited in the literature review. Also, the references may be valuable to your own research study.

Summary

Professionals working in all fields, including HHP, should have the ability to read, understand, and critically evaluate research reports. Whereas the specific format of a published article must follow the guidelines for the journal in which it is published, a research report generally follows a similar format, usually consisting of the following sections: introduction, methods, results, discussion, and references. The basic content of each of these sections is described and numerous examples are presented to aid the student in developing an understanding of the components of published research report. It is also noted that differences exist between reporting a quantitative study and a qualitative study. Moreover, criteria for reading and critiquing a research report are presented.

Part Two

Types of Research

Research can be classified or typed in a variety of ways. Some authors use a three-classification system: experimental, descriptive, and historical. Other authors use a system with more than three classifications, which essentially splits into more parts the three classifications previously mentioned. Classifications can be developed based on a variety of criteria, such as the methods used, the intended use of the research, and the type of setting in which the research takes place. More than anything else, classifications of research serve as a convenient way of presenting research. Many research studies do not fit neatly under one research classification but have characteristics of several research classifications. The point to remember is that all well-conducted research is good research. There is no hierarchy to these research classifications.

In this book, types of research are discussed under five chapter headings. In chapter 7, "Experimental Research," we deal with a type of research that is traditional and commonly conducted. It is research to find new ways of doing things in the future. In chapter 8, "Descriptive Research," we cover many different research approaches. These also are traditional and commonly conducted types of research to describe the present situation. In chapter 9, "Qualitative Research," we describe a common type of research in the social sciences though a relatively new type of research in HHP. The methods in qualitative research differ considerably from the methods commonly found in experimental research. In chapter 10, "Meta-analysis," we deal with a re-analysis of many research studies already conducted in an attempt to draw conclusions which are supported by many studies. It is a type of research which has become commonly used in some areas of HHP. In chapter 11, "Additional Research Approaches," we consider three other approaches to conducting research and an alternative to research. Historical research describes research conducted to show what happened in the past. It is not a common type of research in HHP but is slowly becoming more prevalent. Epidemiological research is often conducted in public health and physical activity/fitness. Single participant research may be conducted in a variety of areas and is becoming more commonly used in HHP. Creative activities covers activities undertaken in order to create something new and unique, such as a new dance, technique, piece of equipment, or art form. It is a common type of activity as an alternative to research in a department of fine arts but relatively new to HHP.

7

Experimental Research

KEY WORDS

Analysis of covariance (ANCOVA)	Designs	Overrater error	Selective manipulation
Block design	Double-blind study	Physical manipulation	Single-blind study
Central tendency error	External validity	Placebo	Statistical techniques
Covariate	Halo effect	Preexperimental design	True experimental design
Counterbalanced design	Independent variable	Quasi-experimental design	Underrater error
Dependent variable	Internal validity	Research hypothesis	Variate
	Matched pairs design		

OBJECTIVES

This chapter contains information concerning experimental research. You should be familiar with how experimental research is conducted and the major issues in conducting this type of research.

After reading chapter 7, you should be able to

1. Understand what experimental research is and how it is conducted.
2. Know the threats to validity and how to control them.
3. Recognize the types of designs commonly used in experimental research.

Experimental research is a traditional type of research and is conducted in most disciplines. It is virtually the only type of research performed in the sciences. In all cases, experimental research is conducted to increase the body of knowledge in the discipline and to suggest what procedures should be followed in the future. For example, a researcher who compares the effectiveness of two or more teaching or training methods, drugs, or techniques is trying to determine if there is one that is best and should be used in the future. The scientific method discussed in chapter 1 is always followed in experimental research. Finally, experimental research always involves manipulation of the experimental unit (e.g., human participants, animal participants).

Consider the typical methodological study where each group of participants receives a different treatment. The treatment received by a participant has the potential to change (manipulate) the participant. Isaac and Michael (1981) state that the purpose of experimental research is to investigate cause-and-effect relationships by subjecting experimental groups to treatment conditions and comparing the results to control groups not receiving the treatment.

Steps in Experimental Research

In order to conduct a research study in a systematic manner, the researcher should follow a definite, step-by-step procedure, starting with initiating a problem area and ending with dissemination of the research findings. The five Ps, Prior Planning Prevents Poor Performance, really apply here. In chapter 2 a twelve-step procedure was presented. Isaac and Michael (1982) have defined a procedure similar to the fourteen steps that follow.

Step 1   The first step is *stating the research problem,* clearly identifying both the problem to be researched and the purpose of the research. The research should not continue without a clear statement of the purpose because all subsequent steps and the entire conduct of the study are based on the statement of purpose.

Step 2   The second step is *determining if the experimental approach is appropriate.* Experimental research is conducted for the future and involves some manipulation of the participants by applying an experimental treatment. Not all aspects of the research have to be experimental, but the major thrust and conduct of the research is experimental.

It is interesting to note that a study comparing existing groups (e.g., physical fitness differences between boys and girls) is often considered experimental research, but there is no manipulation of the participants. However, if the difference between boys and girls in terms of leisure time pursuits is being studied, the research is more apt to be classified as not experimental. In these two situations, the research will be conducted the same way no matter how it is classified.

Step 3   Step 3 is *specifying the independent variable(s) and the levels of the independent variable(s).* An **independent variable** is used to form the experimental groups and is unaffected by the experimental treatment. The levels of the independent variable are the number of different values it will take in the research study. For example, if four treatment groups are used in a study, the independent variable is treatment, and there are four levels. If the independent variables are training days with three levels and training time with four levels, the design is two-dimensional and each of the twelve groups receives a different combination of the two treatments, as presented in Table 7.1. Group 1 trains three days a week for thirty minutes each training day, while group 12 trains five days a week for sixty minutes each time.

Essentially, it is during this step that decisions are made concerning the basic design of the study.

Step 4   Step 4 is *specifying all the potential dependent variables*. **Dependent variables** are the variables that could be measured during the research study to generate the data for analysis. Scores of participants on these variables are dependent on the treatment they received. One or more dependent variables are identified at this step. The number and type of dependent variables are influenced by the statement of the research problems in step one.

Step 5   Step 5 is *stating the tentative hypotheses*. Experimental research requires a written **research hypothesis** that is either accepted or rejected based on the findings of the research study. The hypothesis is based on personal belief, presently accepted beliefs, and/or what the research literature supports. Since the researcher is supposed to be unbiased as to the outcome of the study and, in many cases, has no special insight as to outcome of the study or present beliefs, the research hypothesis is often one of equality. That is, the research hypothesis states that all groups are equal in ability at the end of the study, or, if a single group is measured before and after the experimental treatment, the hypothesis states there is no change in the ability of the group. However, a research hypothesis of inequality is also common. For example, if the research is comparing a traditional method with a new method and the researcher thinks the new method is better, the research hypothesis will be stated accordingly.

This statement is considered tentative because hypotheses very often have to be modified as the planning of the study progresses. Further, tentative hypotheses need to be established at this early stage because they influence some of the later steps in the research process.

TABLE 7.1 Example Two-Dimensional Design

		MINUTES OF TRAINING TIME PER DAY			
		30	40	50	60
NUMBER OF TRAINING DAYS PER WEEK	3	Group 1			
	4				
	5				Group 12

Step 6   Step 6 is *determining the availability of measures for the potential dependent variables,* which were identified in step 4. These measures must have acceptable validity and reliability. Ideally, these measures already exist and are easily identified based on the researcher's knowledge and/or review of the literature. Often, the researcher will have to modify an existing measure to meet the needs of the study and to make the measure appropriate for the participants in the study. Such modification is acceptable as long as the measure, as changed, remains valid and reliable. Sometimes the researcher will have to develop an entirely new test, instrument, or procedure to obtain the measure for a dependent variable. This is time-consuming since validity and reliability of the new measure must be determined before it is used. If the researcher decides a measure neither exists nor can be developed, the potential dependent variable is eliminated from further consideration.

Step 7   Step 7 is *pausing to consider the success potential of the research.* Based on all steps up to this point, does it seem that the research can be successfully conducted? If the research has little success potential, the project should be dropped before considerable time and energy is invested. Many things can be considered here. Certainly the time, expense, and difficulty of doing the research are concerns, and availability of participants is often a major consideration. The possibilities for establishing the levels of the independent variable(s) (see step 3) realistically and ethically must be taken into account. Also, the availability of measures for the dependent variables influences the success potential of a study.

Step 8   The eighth step is *identifying the full potential of intervening variables.* Variables should be classified into the following groups: (1) should be controlled; (2) can be permitted to vary systematically; (3) can be ignored because of their relationship to variables classified as (1) or (2); and (4) can be left alone. Variables that can affect the outcome of the study must be controlled. Ways of controlling variables are discussed in this chapter. Systematic variables are not a danger to the outcome of the study because they vary in a known manner or in the same manner for all participants and groups in the study. Maturation of the participants is an example. If two variables are highly related, controlling one of them will control the other. Height and weight are an example. Variables that the researcher does not believe can affect the outcome of the study can be left alone. Care should be exercised to make sure that all important intervening variables are identified and that they are not misclassified as unimportant.

Step 9   Step 9 is *making a formal statement of the research hypotheses* and is a refinement of step 5 based on information gained and changes made in the study during steps 6 through 8. Issues related to stating hypotheses are addressed under step 5 and should be reviewed here. The research hypotheses stated at step 9 are important because the execution of the whole study is geared toward eventually providing the researcher with evidence for accepting or rejecting the hypotheses.

Step 10   Step 10 is *designing the experiment.* This is usually a time-consuming step in experimental research because it involves considerable planning and identification of procedures for conducting the study. Even the smallest details of the day-to-day conduct of the study must be carefully considered. Insufficient planning at this step is the downfall of many experimental research studies. Planning for data collection, sample selection, and data analysis all take place at this step. *Before* any data collection takes place, it is important that each research hypothesis be stated and that analysis techniques for all the data to be collected are known to exist. The value of conducting a pilot study at this step cannot be overemphasized.

Step 11   Step 11 is *making a final estimate of the success potential of the study.* It is good to pause before the experiment begins and check whether all stages of planning have been conducted adequately. Are there any aspects of the research study that could seriously limit the quality of the experiment in terms of potential conclusions? Particularly, are the procedures and controls in the potential study going to produce valid results addressing all of the research hypotheses?

Step 12   Step 12 is *conducting the study as planned in steps 1 through 11.* There are likely to be aspects of the study that could be improved, but if the planning of the study has been thorough, no major problems will compromise the quality of the study. During the implementation of the study, constantly verify that the integrity of the experiment is being maintained. This step terminates with the final data collection.

Step 13   Step thirteen is *analyzing the data* according to the data analysis plan. The need for some analysis not in the original plan may arise during the course of the data analysis. This additional analysis is acceptable as long as it does not seem to be an effort to obtain findings in support of what the researcher wants to prove.

Step 14   The fourteenth and last step is *preparing a research report.* This report should, at minimum, contain the procedures used in the study as well as the major findings of the study. The report may be little more than a record of the research that the researcher will later use for reference when the memory of the details of the research is less clear. On the other hand, the report could be as extensive as a master's thesis.

Internal and External Validity

Validity was defined and discussed in chapter 3 in terms of a measurement. Experimental research involves two other important classifications of validity. The first classification is **internal validity.** Internal validity deals with how valid the findings are within, or internal, to the study. Did the experimental treatments make a difference in the study in that the treatments caused the participants in the study to change in ability or are the changes in the ability of the participants due to other factors (see "Threats to Internal Validity" later in this chapter)? If the treatments caused the change in the ability of the participants, then internal validity can be claimed.

The second classification, **external validity,** is the degree to which findings in a research study can be inferred or generalized to other populations, settings, or experimental treatments. Particularly, external validity is concerned with whether the findings for the sample of participants in the study can be inferred to the population they represent and to other populations. In other words, are the findings in the research study unique to the participants in the study, or do the findings apply to other groups? If the findings in a research study can be inferred or generalized to other populations, settings, or experimental treatments, external validity can be claimed. A study using inmates in a prison might lack in external validity. Good internal validity is required to have good external validity, but good internal validity does not guarantee good external validity.

Control of all variables operating in an experimental research study is highly desirable but seldom, if ever, accomplished. The researcher would like all participants to be treated the same in terms of all variables (e.g., sleep, food, exercise) except for the experimental or treatment variable, which is allowed to vary among participants. Too much control can harm external validity, but not enough control destroys internal validity. Having so much control that the research setting is unique or totally removing the research from the setting where it will be applied destroys external validity. Excellent control is possible in prisons and military installations, but findings on participants in these places may not apply to participants in other situations.

Controlling Threats to Validity

Campbell and Stanley (1963) discuss twelve factors that can threaten the validity of an experimental research study. Isaac and Michael (1982) and Van Dalen (1979) also discuss these potential threats in detail. The first eight factors threaten internal validity and the last four factors threaten external validity. Obviously, a researcher tries to control as many of both types of these factors as possible in an experimental research study.

Threats to Internal Validity

History.   History refers to specific things that happen while conducting the research study that affect the final scores of the participants in addition to the effect of the experimental treatment. Suppose that participants participate in an activity or program outside of the research study but that this activity is very similar to the experimental treatment. If this outside participation increases their final scores, it makes the experimental treatment seem more effective than it really is. A second example is the atypical occurrence, such as an epidemic, local disaster, or one-time emphasis on the research topic in the community, that occurs in the lives of the participants during the research study and that affects their final scores.

Maturation. Because they grow older during the experimental period, the performance level of the participants changes and this change is reflected in their final scores. Seasonal changes might also be considered here. Example 1: As young participants grow older during the fifteen-week experimental period, their physical performance level changes no matter what the effect of the experimental treatment. Thus, change in the performance of a treatment group from pretest to posttest may be inflated by maturation. Example 2: Between September when the research study begins and December when the study ends, participants become less physically fit due to less daily activity because they are in school all day and the weather is bad. This loss of fitness counteracts the effect of the experimental treatment. A control group (group receiving no treatment) can be a check on the maturation threat.

Testing. The act of taking a test can affect the scores of the participants on a second or later testing. For example, participants are pretested, then the experimental treatment is administered, and finally the participants are posttested. One reason why participants do better on the posttest is because they learn from the pretest. The pretest is like a treatment. This poses a real problem if the pretest and posttest are the same knowledge or physical performance test. Baumgartner (1969) tested participants with several physical performance tests, retested them two days later, and found that scores had improved from the initial test to the retest.

Instrumentation. Changes in the adjustment or calibration of the measuring equipment or use of different standards among scorers may cause differences among groups in final score or changes in the scores of the participants over time. This suggests that researchers need to check the accuracy of their measuring equipment regularly and frequently and make sure a standard scoring procedure is used. Any difference in the test scores of several treatment groups or change in the test scores of the participants in a group over time (pretest to posttest) must be due to differences among groups or a change in the participants over time and not due to changes in the calibration of the equipment or scoring procedure. Testing equipment and scoring procedures must be held constant for each participant in research environments involving multiple pieces of the same equipment, multiple scorers, or multiple days of data collection.

Statistical Regression. The tendency for groups with extremely high or low scores on one measure to score closer to the mean score of the population on a second measure is called statistical regression. This tendency may be mistaken for experimental treatment effect. For example, a high IQ and a low IQ group are formed. An experimental treatment is applied to both groups for twelve weeks. Then a physical ability test is administered to both groups, and it is found that they are equal in physical ability. This equality may be due to the regression effect or to the treatment effect. Using random sampling procedures to form groups eliminates the threat.

Research studies in which the research question is whether groups that differ in one attribute differ in terms of another attribute may have similar problems. For example, does a population of individuals with disabilities differ from a population of individuals without disabilities in their beliefs concerning use of leisure time? No treatment is applied in this example, so random samples from the two populations are obtained and a score for beliefs about the use of leisure time is obtained for each participant. The finding that the two populations do not differ in their leisure-time-use beliefs is due to the regression effect.

Selection.   The way participants are selected or assigned to groups can be biased. This may result in groups that are not representative of a population, groups that are not equal in ability at the beginning of the experiment, and/or groups that differ at the end of the experiment for reasons other than differences in the integrity of the experimental treatments. Random selection of participants and random assignment of participants to groups usually controls this threat. Thus, following the random sampling techniques outlined in chapter 5 and using sample sizes that are sufficiently large for the research situation will control this threat. When participant selection is a threat it is often due to small sample size per group and/or failure to use one of the necessary alternatives to simple random sampling when required for the research setting.

Experimental Mortality.   This particular threat to internal validity is created with the excessive loss of participants so that experimental groups are no longer representative of a population or similar to each other. Some participant loss is to be expected in a research study, but if many participants of the same type drop out of a group it can considerably change the characteristics of the group and the outcome of the study.

Interaction of Selection and Maturation or History.   The maturation effect or history effect is not the same for all groups selected for the research study, and this influences final scores. This problem may arise when each group is an intact preexisting group rather than a randomly formed group. For example, if the groups differ considerably in age or background, this may affect how they respond to the experimental treatments. Also, if groups start out unequal in ability due to maturation or history, they may not have the same potential for improvement as a result of the experimental treatments.

Also, this applies to disproportional participant loss among the groups. Usually groups are about the same size at the start of the research study, but if at the end of the research study they are considerably different in size, this is a concern.

Threats to External Validity

Interaction Effect of Testing.   This effect occurs when the pretest changes the group's response to the experimental treatment, thus making the group unrepresentative of any particular population and certainly unrepresentative of a population that has not been pretested. There is always the danger that administering a test before the experimental treatment (pretest) changes the participants. For example, the pretest may make the participants more aware of the need to increase their knowledge or performance level, causing them to respond to the experimental treatment more positively than they otherwise would.

Interaction Effects of Selection Bias and Experimental Treatment.   The participants or groups selected in a biased manner react to the experimental treatment in a unique way so they are not representative of any particular population. High IQ or high skill level or metropolitan participants may not react to a particular treatment in the same way as low IQ or low skill level or rural participants and, thus, are not representative of them. If the population is well defined before the sample is drawn, this threat should be minimal. The problem (threat) can easily occur when a convenient group is used in the research and an attempt is made to define a population that fits the group.

Reactive Effects of Experimental Setting.   The experimental setting is such that the experimental treatment has a unique effect on the participants or groups that would not be observed in some other setting. Thus, the results of the study are not representative of any particular population. If any element of the experimental procedure alters the normal behavior of the participants, then the effect of the experimental treatment may be altered and it will not have the same effect on a different group of participants. For example, participants may think the experimental treatment or drug is supposed to cause a change in their behavior or performance, so they react or perform differently for reasons that are not due to the treatment. Participants who react to the researcher in a unique manner provide another example. Conducting the research in a lab rather than in the natural setting is a third example.

Multiple-Treatment Interference.   Multiple-treatment interference is the effect of prior treatments on the response of the participants or groups to a present treatment. This makes their response to the present treatment unique and not representative of the way any other population would respond to the present treatment. This effect can occur when the same participants are used in several related studies. For example, the same high performance level runners are used in three different studies dealing with the physiological responses to running. Are their responses in the third experiment influenced by participating in the two previous studies? Researchers should check on the background and experiences of potential participants to control this threat to external validity.

Types of Designs

Designs are the variety of ways a research study may be structured or conducted. Campbell and Stanley (1963) present the advantages and disadvantages of many types of design in terms of how each controls the threats to validity. They classify designs as being either preexperimental, true experimental, or quasi-experimental. Only a few representative designs are presented here since it is impossible to present all the designs that the reader may encounter.

The **preexperimental designs** are weaker than true experimental designs in terms of control. Preexperimental designs have no random sampling of participants, are usually one group or two unequated groups, control few threats to validity, and have many definite weaknesses. The one-group pretest/posttest design is an example. It requires that a group be tested before the experimental treatment is administered and again after the experimental treatment has been administered. For example, fifty participants are administered an initial (pretest) fitness test. Then the participants are administered the experimental treatment which, in this case, is doing prescribed exercises one hour per day, three days per week for eighteen weeks. Finally, the final (posttest) fitness test is administered. This is the same fitness test used for the pretest. If the group improved in fitness from the pretest to the posttest, the experimental treatment is judged to be effective. But all of the change from the pretest to the posttest may not be due to the experimental treatment. The change could be partially or totally due to the threats to validity of history, maturation, testing, instrumentation, selection and maturation or selection and history interaction, interaction effect of selection bias and experimental treatment, or interaction effect of testing. Only the threats to validity of selection and experimental mortality are definitely controlled in this design. Another example is the use of intact classes. All pupils in one class receive treatment A and all pupils in another class receive treatment B. There is no random sampling of participants or random assignment of participants to treatments, so it is not known if the two treatment groups started the study equal in ability. If the treatment groups are unequal at the end of the study it may be because (1) the treatments were not equally effective, (2) the groups were unequal at the start of the study, or (3) some combination of the two previous reasons.

The **true experimental designs** are recommended over other classifications of designs because they offer good control. True experimental designs always have random sampling of participants, random assignment of participants to groups, and all threats to internal validity controlled. The pretest/posttest control group design is an example. It is an extension of the pre-experimental design just presented. Here, the experimental group is tested before and after the experimental treatment is administered. The control group is tested at the same times as the experimental group, but receives no treatment that changes its ability. Each group is a random sample from a population. Provided the experimental and control groups are equal in ability on the pretest, if the experimental group performs better than the control group on the posttest, the result should be due to the experimental treatment. This design controls the eight threats to internal validity but does not control the interactive effect of testing. Another example is the use of two experimental groups and a control group. From a population some members are randomly assigned to each of the three groups, but all members of the population are not selected as participants. Further, the two experimental and one control treatments are randomly assigned to groups. Assuming the three groups are equal in ability at the beginning of the study, differences among the three groups at the end of the study should be due to differences in the effectiveness of the three treatments.

Many times, the researcher will conduct the research in the setting where the research will actually be applied, but the situation will lack the control required for the true experimental design. The researcher quite often controls the data collection times and who is tested, but does not totally control when and to whom the experimental treatment is administered. Further, random assignment of participants to groups is not always possible. These situations lead to quasi-experimental designs.

The **quasi-experimental designs** are fine as long as the researcher understands what the designs do not control. These designs lack either random sampling of participants or random assignment of participants to groups. Quasi-experimental designs are much better than preexperimental designs. The nonequivalent control group design is an example. It is just like the pretest/posttest control group design except participants are not assigned to groups by using random sampling procedures. Instead, the experimental and control groups are existing groups, like classes or facilities, that are similar in characteristics and may be equal in ability. The pretest will indicate how similar they are before the experimental treatment is administered to the experimental group. This design controls the threats to validity of history, maturation, testing, instrumentation, selection, and experimental mortality; but it does not control threats to validity of the interaction effects of maturation and history, or the interaction effect of testing. Thus, this design does not have as much control as the true experimental design—the pretest/posttest control group design.

Designs have been discussed in terms of how they control the threats to validity. Also, designs can be discussed in terms of their complexity and ability to answer research questions. Simple designs answer one research question and more complex designs answer several research questions. To present various designs in an abbreviated form, X is used to represent a treatment is administered and O is used to represent data is collected. For example, $O_1 X O_2$ indicates that the participants are tested initially (O_1), a treatment is administered (X), and participants are tested once again (O_2). Presented in Table 7.2 are examples of designs ranging from simple to complex. In designs 1 and 2, the research question is simply whether some treatment will cause a change in the scores of a group; design 2 is the better design because it uses a control group. Designs 2 and 3 are both two-group designs but have different research questions. The fourth design is a combination of designs 2 and 3. Design 5 is essentially design 3 extended to three or more groups. Design 6 is presented primarily as a lead-up to design 7. Design 7 is superior to design 6 because more information is obtained in the form of combinations of A and B treatments. The A treatment and B

TABLE 7.2 Example Research Designs in Ascending Order of Complexity

DESIGN	RESEARCH QUESTION	DESIGN*	REMARKS
1	Is treatment effective?	O_1 X O_2 $\quad$ *tested* $\quad$ *treatment* $\rightarrow$ *tested again*	A group is tested before and after a treatment; compare means for O_1 and O_2 to see if O_2 is better
2	Is treatment effective?	O_1 X O_2 O_3 O_4	Treatment group gets X and control group gets no treatment; sometimes O_1 and O_3 not collected; if means for O_1 and O_3 are equal, groups started equal; compare means for O_2 and O_4 to see if O_2 mean is better
3	Which treatment is better?	X_1 O_1 X_2 O_2	One group receives X_1 and another group receives X_2; compare means for O_1 and O_2 to see if equal
4	Is each treatment effective? Which treatment is better?	O_1 X_1 O_2 O_3 X_2 O_4	One group receives X_1 and another group receives X_2; if means for O_1 and O_3 are equal, groups started equal; compare O_1 and O_2 means and compare O_3 and O_4 means to see if treatments are effective; compare means for O_2 and O_4 to see if one treatment is better
5	Which treatment is better?	X_1 O_1 X_2 O_2 X_3 O_3	Same as design 3 but more than two groups; compare means of O_1, O_2 and O_3
6	The two questions are:		
	(1) Which A treatment (A_1, A_2, A_3) is best?	A treatment X_1 O_1 X_2 O_2 X_3 O_3	See design 5; compare means of O_1, O_2, and O_3
	(2) Which B treatment (B_1, B_2) is better?	B treatment X_1 O_1 X_2 O_2	See design 3; compare means of O_1, and O_2
7	The three questions are:		
	(1) Which A treatment (A_1, A_2, A_3) is best?	X_{11} O_{11}** X_{12} O_{12} X_{21} O_{21}	A treatment: Compare means of $(O_{11} + O_{12})$, $(O_{21} + O_{22})$, $(O_{31} + O_{32})$
	(2) Which B treatment (B_1, B_2) is better?	X_{22} O_{22} X_{31} O_{31} X_{32} O_{32}	B treatment: Compare means of $(O_{11} + O_{21} + O_{31})$, $(O_{12} + O_{22} + O_{32})$
	(3) Which combination of the A and B treatments $(A_1B_1, A_1B_2, A_2B_1, A_2B_2, A_3B_1, A_3B_2)$ is best?		Combinations: Compare means for O_{11}, O_{12}, O_{21}, O_{22}, O_{31}, O_{32} See designs 3, 5, and 6
	There are six groups, each receiving one of the six combinations of A and B.		

$$\begin{array}{c|cc} & B_1 & B_2 \\ \hline A_1 & A_1B_1 & A_1B_2 \\ A_2 & A_2B_1 & A_2B_2 \\ A_3 & A_3B_1 & A_3B_2 \end{array}$$

*X = treatment is administered $\quad$ O = data is collected
**X = the treatment for the A B treatment group

treatment in designs 6 and 7 are two different treatments. For example, *A* treatment is three methods of instruction, and *B* treatment is two different number of weeks of instruction. In this example, design 7 is used because combinations of treatments *A* and *B* are possible. However, if *A* treatment is three ways of teaching first aid and *B* treatment is two ways of teaching sex education, the two treatments cannot be combined, so design 6 is used.

A design must control the major threats to validity and allow the researcher to answer the research questions. However, the KISS principle (Keep It Simple, Stupid) should not be overlooked. The design must be adequate but don't make the design any more complicated than it has to be.

Validity in Summary

Two classifications of validity and the threats to each classification have been discussed. In many research studies maximum internal and external validity cannot be obtained due to constraints on finances, time, participants, the research setting, or other resources. The researcher must decide what is most important, internal or external validity, and which threats to validity are more important to control than others.

As indicated earlier in the chapter, good internal validity is required to have good external validity. Campbell and Stanley (1963, 5) indicate that internal validity is the basic minimum for an experimental design. Thus, a research study must be designed in a manner that establishes good internal validity.

A researcher must consider the threats to validity while designing the study. After selecting a tentative design of the study, the researcher should determine which of the threats to validity exist, the seriousness of these threats, and how easy it is to control each threat. It is impossible to generalize to all research situations, but the strategy to follow is to modify the tentative design of the study to control the major threats to validity and those that are easy to eliminate. Minor threats and threats that are hard to eliminate may have to be uncontrolled. This strategy is much harder to accomplish when a major threat is hard to eliminate.

Cook and Campbell (1979) subdivide internal validity into statistical conclusions validity and internal validity, and subdivide external validity into construct validity of cause or effect and external validity. Discussion of statistical conclusion validity and construct validity of cause or effect requires background beyond the scope of this book. Advanced students may appreciate a discussion of the four types of validity.

Methods of Control

Control is vital in experimental research. The researcher wants to control the effect of all variables except the experimental variable. Although ideal, this degree of control is seldom if ever achieved in HHP research. Nevertheless, the researcher must control the effect of the variables that could have a major impact on the study. Control of variables can be obtained in several ways.

The best way to control the effect of variables is by **physical manipulation.** The researcher physically controls all aspects of the participants' environment and experience throughout the experimental period. Thus, the amount of sleep, food intake, drug use, stimulation, stress, exercise, practice, or training is the same for all participants unless one of these variables is the experimental treatment. For example, if each of four groups is being taught by a different method, teaching method is the experimental treatment. The method varies from group to group, but the researcher tries to keep all other variables constant for all groups. Controlling all variables except the experimental treatment is difficult unless the participants happen to be prisoners, military recruits, or animals. The researcher tries to be sure each group receives the designated teaching method without any additional benefit from the method outside the experiment and without opportunity to benefit from the teaching method of another group. Since some variables cannot be physically controlled, the researcher might resort to other control methods.

Selective manipulation is commonly used to gain control and can take many forms. The intent of selective manipulation is to increase the likelihood that treatment groups are similar in characteristics and/or ability at the beginning of an experiment. By selecting only certain participants, the researcher manipulates the treatment groups to gain control. **Matched pairs** and **block designs** are forms of selective manipulation. The population to which the results of the research study are inferred or applied is defined. Accessible members of this population are tested on one or more variables that the researcher wishes to control in the study. Based on this variable(s) participants with similar scores are matched into pairs if two groups are needed or into blocks if more than two groups are needed in the research study. The same number of participants are randomly assigned to each treatment group from each pair or block. This procedure produces groups that start the experiment basically equal in terms of the variable(s) used for matching.

The variable(s) used for matching should be ones the researcher feels must be controlled because the variable(s) can have a major effect on the outcome of the study. Some common matching variables are initial ability, age, height, weight, gender, and IQ.

> *Example 1:* The researcher wants to compare two teaching methods. She believes that gender may influence the effectiveness of a teaching method. So, the researcher assigns twenty boys and twenty girls to each teaching method using random sampling procedures.

This is different from subject pairing as presented earlier because it equates or balances the two treatment groups in terms of gender. If the researcher is willing to match participants based on both gender and IQ, twenty pairs of boys and twenty pairs of girls could be formed with the two participants in a pair basically equal in IQ score. From each pair, a participant is randomly assigned to each teaching method group. The groups are taught by the teaching method assigned to them, and then a test is administered to all participants. Differences between groups are checked based on test scores.

Example 2: The researcher is going to compare three different methods of developing strength in college males. Ninety-eight students are administered a strength test. Based on these initial test scores thirteen blocks with six students of similar strength in a block are formed. Two students from each block are randomly assigned to each group. Participants train for ten weeks with the method assigned their group. Then the strength test is administered again to each participant. Based on this final test score, differences among groups are determined.

Another common form of selective manipulation to gain control is the **counterbalanced design.** These designs require that all participants receive all treatments, but in different orders. However, these designs are limited to situations where it makes sense for participants to receive all treatments. Counterbalanced designs are an alternative to designs where each group receives one of the treatments and differences among groups are examined to see if all treatments are equally effective. Campbell and Stanley (1963) and statistics books like Winer, Brown, and Michels (1991) and Keppel (1991) discuss counterbalanced designs.

A simple example of a counterbalanced design is the comparison of the effectiveness of two drugs, A and B. To conduct the study a sample of participants is randomly drawn from a population. One-half of the participants receive drug A first and drug B later, while the other half of the participants receive drug B, then A. The process sequence is the same in both cases: A drug is administered, the participants are tested to determine the effect of the drug, a period of time passes to allow the drug to wear off and the participants to return to normal, the other drug is administered, and the participants are tested to determine the effect of the drug. Each participant receives a score under both drug A and drug B, so a comparison between the two drugs is possible. If there is an order effect so that the first drug taken influences the response of a participant to a second drug, the order effect is neutralized by counterbalancing.

Sometimes researchers conduct a study using only participants of one rather than both genders, or participants very similar in age or experience rather than more heterogeneous in terms of these attributes. For example, rather than use college undergraduate students as participants, the researcher uses 18- or 19-year-old freshmen. These techniques might be considered selective manipulation.

Often, **statistical techniques** are used to gain control in an experimental research study. Statistical techniques are applied when physical manipulation or selective manipulation of variables is not possible. The researcher knows, at the beginning of the study before the treatments are administered, that the experimental groups differ in terms of one or more variables that must be controlled in the study. If these variables are not controlled, the integrity of the research study is seriously compromised. Sometimes the variables that must be controlled are the same ones that would be used to form blocks in the block design discussed under selective manipulation techniques. In this situation, the research setting is such that the participants are already in groups so a block design cannot be used. The following is an example of this situation.

Treatment groups in the research study very often differ in initial ability. If the groups differ in ability at the end of the experiment, it is not known whether this is due to the initial inequality or difference in effectiveness of the treatments. A statistical technique commonly used in this situation is **analysis of covariance (ANCOVA).** Basically, the ANCOVA technique adjusts the differences among the groups in scores at the end of the study based on differences in initial ability among the groups. If differences among the groups are found after final scores are adjusted, the researcher concludes that all experimental treatments are not equally effective.

In the ANCOVA technique, one or more scores called the **covariates** are obtained at the beginning of the study. Covariates are used to adjust differences among groups in terms of a score called the **variate,** collected at the end of the study. A statistical test of the differences among the groups in terms of the adjusted data is provided as part of the ANCOVA technique. The ANCOVA technique can be used with a variety of research designs and with as many covariates and types of covariates as the researcher desires. Extensive discussion of ANCOVA is found in Huck and Cormier (1996), Winer, Brown, and Michels (1991), Keppel (1991), and Dayton (1970).

In chapter 13 there is a discussion of effect size, statistical power, and design sensitivity. Some of this discussion relates to the issue of control.

Common Sources of Error

Many possible sources of error can cause the results of a research study to be incorrectly interpreted. When error is present, the outcome of the study is not totally due to the experimental treatment. These sources of error are more specific than the threats to validity discussed earlier in the chapter. All sources of error are not a concern in every research study. Those sources of error discussed in this section of the chapter do not cover all potential sources.

Hawthorne Effect

This source of error is named for a research study that was conducted at the Hawthorne Electric Plant in the 1920s. It was observed that having a group of workers participate in a research study caused them to feel special so they acted differently from the typical worker. The research study was conducted to determine how changes in the working environment would affect productivity. Results of the study showed that productivity increased no matter whether the change in the working environment was supposed to increase or decrease productivity. This points out that participants in an experiment may perform in an atypical manner due to the newness or novelty of the treatment and because they realize that they are participating in an experiment. This suggests that, as much as possible, the participants should be unaware that they are participating in an experiment and also unaware of the hypothesized outcome of the study. Particularly in studies comparing new and traditional methods (e.g., teaching, training), the researcher does not want the new method to seem superior to the traditional method due to the Hawthorne effect.

Placebo Effect

The participants in an experimental treatment may believe the treatment is supposed to change them so they respond to the treatment with a change in performance. In a typical study to determine the effect of a drug, participants are pretested, administered the drug, and posttested. The researcher wants any change in the performance of the group from pretest to posttest to be due to the drug and not due to the fact that the participants think the drug is effective. In this example, the researcher has a second group (control group) that goes through the same procedure (pretest, drug, posttest) as the experimental treatment group, except the drug the control group receives is a **placebo,** a drug that can have no effect on the participants. Assuming the experimental and control groups were equal in pretest scores and that the psychological response to a drug is the same for both groups, superiority of the experimental group in posttest scores is due to the positive effect of the drug.

In some studies the experimental group receives a treatment and the control group receives nothing. This seems like a poor research technique since the control groups should be receiving some placebo if psychological response to a treatment is to be the same for both groups. The treatment for the control group should be one that cannot affect the test score used to compare groups at the end of the study.

"John Henry" Effect

In studies with an experimental group and a control group, the control group knows it is not supposed to be better than the experimental, so it tries harder and outperforms the experimental group. This might be called the "Avis effect" after Avis Cars—we are number two, but we try harder. Of course, there could be a reverse "John Henry" effect where the control group gives up. It is also possible for the experimental group to improve due to the treatment and for the control group to improve due to the "John Henry" effect, thereby making the groups equal in performance at the end of the study. Again, it seems better to keep the design and expectations of the study unknown to the participants if possible.

Rating Effect

Several kinds of rating errors can occur. The **halo effect** is the tendency to let initial impressions or ratings of a participant or group influence future ratings. Where **overrater error** and **underrater error** occur the researcher tends to overrate or underrate participants. Finally, there is **central tendency error** where the researcher tends to rate most participants in the middle of the rating scale. Also, these rating errors can occur when participants are asked to rate statements about beliefs, practices, or problems (see chapter 8). For example, each participant rates each of twenty-five statements about health practices on a 1-to-5 scale, with 5 being important and 1 being not important.

Rating errors can be minimized by not looking at previous ratings. Also, a rating scale with 4 (e.g., excellent, above average, below average, terrible) to 7 (e.g., very strongly agree, strongly agree, agree, neutral, disagree, strongly disagree, very strongly disagree) well-defined different values can minimize rating errors. Rating errors can be minimized if the researcher develops the rating process properly.

Experimenter Bias Effect

The bias of a researcher can affect the outcome of the study. Experimenter bias may influence methodology, treatment, and data collection. This bias is often in favor of the experimental treatment the researcher believes is best.

Some people believe the researcher should not be involved in administering any of the treatments or collecting any of the data in methodological studies where each group receives a different method, such as teaching or training, over many weeks. This brings up an interesting dilemma when there are two or more groups in a methodological study. Should the same person administer the methods to all groups, or should different people administer the methods? If the same person administers all methods, the study could be criticized because the person may have biases and may not be equally effective with all methods. If different people administer each method, the study could be criticized because all people may not be equally effective with their methods. So, the situation is a no-win situation (similar to a "heads I win, tails you lose" coin flip). None of this discussion addresses whether the researcher is administering any methods. In many studies the researcher does not have a choice who administers the methods, but if choices exist the researcher selects the best procedure for the research setting. Usually the researcher is involved in administering the treatments and collecting the data because it is the researcher's study and there is no one else to do these tasks.

When possible, the researcher keeps the participants unaware of the purpose of the study and of their role in the study in order to eliminate any possible participant-caused error. Specifically, the participants are unaware of whether they are receiving the experimental or control treatment. This study is referred to as a **single-blind study.** The research setting and procedures used in many studies often preclude the single-blind study. When both the participants and those conducting the study (administering treatments and collecting data) are unaware of the purpose of the study and the way in which participants are grouped, the study is referred to as a **double-blind study.**

Participant-Researcher Interaction Effect

Do participants respond better to researchers of the same gender, do they respond better to researchers of the opposite gender, or does it make any difference? It is reasonable to assume that, in some research settings, gender of the participants and researcher is influential and therefore contributes to error. What is important in any study is that the difference among groups in the research study and the effectiveness of the treatments in the study are not due to a participant-researcher interaction. The participant-researcher interaction effect should be minimal if the researcher functions with all groups in the same professional manner.

Post Hoc Error

This type of error is introduced by assuming a cause-and-effect relationship between two variables when such a relationship does not exist. For example: More people die in bed than any other place; therefore, beds are dangerous.

Measurement in Experimental Research

Experimental research almost always requires measuring the participants involved with some test or procedure. Thus, questions like, What tests or procedures are available?, How are the reliability and validity of these measures determined?, How are these tests or procedures administered?, commonly arise. Guidance in answering these questions is often found in measurement books. Researchers collecting physical performance data should consult measurement books in physical education and exercise science like Baumgartner and Jackson (1999). If using some paper-and-pencil test or instrument to collect data, researchers might read measurement books in education and psychology such as Thorndike et al. (1991). Two excellent measurement books in health, which also contain considerable information on measurement in research, are Green and Lewis (1986) and Sarvela and McDermott (1993).

The newest tests, procedures, and techniques may not yet be in the measurement books, so they must be found in the research journals. Measurement specialists tend to conduct research dealing with improving or developing measurement tests, procedures, and techniques. Some researchers in all areas do measurement research on occasion.

Summary

Experimental research is characterized by participant manipulation with a treatment and tight control of the variables that operate in the research study. The potential variety of types of experimental studies is endless. For this reason, techniques for conducting experimental research are specific to the experimental study, and only topics common to all experimental research were addressed in this chapter.

Formative Evaluation of Objectives

Objective 1 Understand what experimental research is and how it is conducted.

1. What is the purpose of experimental research?
2. What is the importance of "control" in experimental research?
3. In experimental research there always is a hypothesis. What are some other things that always occur in experimental research?

Objective 2 Know the threats to validity and how to control them.

1. What are five common threats to the validity of research in your area?
2. What are the three most common techniques used in your area to control threats to the validity of the research?

Objective 3 Recognize the types of designs commonly used in experimental research.

1. What are two experimental research designs commonly used in your area?
2. What are the advantages of an experimental research design with a control group in it?
3. What are the advantages of a repeated measures design (pretest-posttest)?

8

Descriptive Research

KEY WORDS

"After the fact" research	Cross-sectional approach	Norm referenced	Semistructured interview
Closed-ended item	Longitudinal approach	Open-ended item	Structured interview
Completion item	Multiple choice item	Percentile rank	Unstructured interview
Criterion referenced			

OBJECTIVES

This chapter contains information about descriptive research. You should become familiar with the various types of descriptive research and the techniques commonly used in conducting descriptive research.

After reading chapter 8, you should be able to

1. Identify the common types of descriptive research.
2. Identify techniques commonly used in descriptive research.

Whereas in the last chapter we found that experimental research focuses on the future, descriptive research is oriented toward the present. Descriptive research is conducted to describe a present situation, what people currently believe, what people are doing at the moment, and so forth.

Descriptive research is a broad classification of research under which many types of research are conducted. Some people mistakenly believe that experimental research is the only approach. Others mistakenly think that descriptive research is easier to conduct than experimental research. Any type of research is good if it is conducted properly, and all research is demanding. For the study to be conducted well, the researcher needs to have some formal training and practical experience in the research area. It is foolish to try to conduct a research study in physics without sufficient formal training. Likewise, it is an error to try to use on elementary school-aged children the same techniques that are used on adults.

Descriptive research is conducted by collecting information and, based on this information, describing the situation. Descriptive research can, but does not have to, include a research hypothesis. Consider a study in which 10,000 high school seniors are selected from a population and surveyed as to whether they smoke tobacco, and 38 percent indicate they do. The researcher reports that 38 percent of high school seniors in the population smoke tobacco. Using the same research procedures, the researcher could have hypothesized prior to conducting the study that 30 percent of high school seniors in the population smoke tobacco. In this case, the researcher reports the 38 percent and whether the research hypothesis is accepted or rejected.

Descriptive research is commonly conducted in physical education and may be the predominant research approach in health, recreation, and sports management. It is an approach commonly used in dance, as well. Descriptive research is conducted in kinesiology and exercise science, but not as commonly as in the other disciplines mentioned.

Types of Descriptive Research

The types of descriptive research are briefly described in this section to provide a general awareness of and broad appreciation for them. The types of descriptive research discussed are survey, developmental, case study, correlational, normative, observational, action, and ex post facto.

Survey

Survey research is the most common type of descriptive research. It involves determining the views or practices of a group through interviews or by administering a questionnaire. The questionnaire may be administered to a group by the researcher or mailed to the members of the group for them to complete and mail back to the researcher. Survey research will be discussed in detail later in this chapter.

Developmental

Developmental research usually deals with the growth and development of humans over time. For example, what are the growth and developmental changes each year from age 6 to age 18? More accurately, what are the growth and developmental attributes of each age group? Other developmental research might examine how organizations or professional groups develop over time.

There are two approaches to developmental research. One is the **longitudinal approach** in which a group is measured and observed on a regular basis for multiple years. For example, twice a year from age 6 to age 18 a large group of children is fitness tested. Based on this information, fitness standards are developed for each age level. The problem with this research approach is that it takes many years to complete, and it is difficult to keep track of the participants over the many years that the study lasts. However, such studies are tremendously valuable. Presently, many epidemiologists wish there were more fitness data available on middle-aged adults as children—to be able to answer questions concerning how fit children need to be in order to be fit as adults. As valuable as longitudinal studies may be, they are not a good choice for master's theses or doctoral dissertations due to the vast length of time involved.

The other approach to developmental research is the **cross-sectional approach.** Taking the earlier example of developing fitness standards for age groups with the cross-sectional approach, large samples of each age group are tested at the same time, and standards for each age group are developed. The assumption underlying this research approach is that each age group is representative of all other age groups when they will be or were that age. If this assumption is true, cross-sectional research will yield the same results as longitudinal research, but in a shorter time period. Cross-sectional research cannot always answer questions that longitudinal research answers. The earlier question by epidemiologists about fitness in children as an indicator of fitness in adults can be answered only with a longitudinal study.

Case Study

Case study research typically involves studying a person or event in great detail and describing what is found. A study of the training techniques or performance techniques of a highly skilled athlete is an example of a case study. It is assumed that less-skilled performers should use techniques of the highly skilled. A study of the way the Boston Marathon is organized and conducted for use as a model for how to organize and conduct a marathon is another example of a case study.

Being highly organized and very systematic in collecting the information needed to write the report is vital in this research approach. Essential to case study research is preparation by looking at literature on how to conduct case study research and at actual case studies for the techniques used.

Correlational

The purpose of correlational studies is to determine if a relationship exists between variables. The statistical techniques used are correlation and regression (discussed in chapters 12 and 13). To determine if a relationship exists between two variables, each participant must be measured on both variables. For example, to determine if a relationship exists between time spent practicing a task and ability in performing the task, a practice time and task ability score must be obtained for each participant. If the data analysis shows that the longer a participant's practice time, the better the participant's task ability score tended to be, the researcher concludes that a relationship exists and that practicing a task is beneficial.

Usually the variables in a correlational study are not ones that the researcher tries to manipulate as in an experimental study. In the previous example, the researcher just determined how much each participant practiced and how well each participant performed the task. Many correlational studies deal with the relationship between a participant classification variable (e.g., height, weight, gender, age, income, education) and a variable of interest to the researcher. For example, what is the relationship between age and beliefs concerning use of leisure time?

Sometimes correlational studies involve three or more variables, and the purpose of the research is to determine how well one of the variables can be predicted by some combination of the other variables. For example, how well can college grade point average be predicted by high school grade point average and SAT scores?

Correlational studies can be conducted to try to explain why participants differ on a variable. This is a regression approach to a correlational study. Why don't all dancers execute a dance move with equal skill? Part of this difference in ability among dancers is explained by differences in amount of training, percent body fat, flexibility, and leg length to body height ratio. Wouldn't it be interesting to find that the leg length to body height ratio explained much of the difference among dancers in executing a move and that ability had little to do with things like amount of training, percent body fat, or flexibility?

Normative

Norms are standards of performance. The purpose of normative research is to develop performance standards. Performance standards are developed on a large representative sample from a population; these standards then are applied to other samples from the population.

Standards can be **norm referenced** or **criterion referenced.** The majority of standards have been norm referenced, but this discussion will consider normative research contributing to the development of either type of standard. Norm-referenced standards are designed to rank order individuals from best to worst and are usually expressed in **percentile ranks.** Test scores commonly achieved are presented in charts; for each test score there is a percentile rank indicating the percent of the participants in the norming group who scored below that test score. Standards published with most physical fitness tests prior to 1980 and many other nationally distributed tests are norm referenced. An example of norm-referenced standards is presented in table 8.1. Measurement books such as Baumgartner and Jackson (1999) detail how to develop norm-referenced standards.

TABLE 8.1 Example of Percentile Rank Norms for a Ten-Point Test

TEST SCORE	0	1	2	3	4	5	6	7	8	9	10
PERCENTILE RANK	3	8	15	30	42	55	65	74	80	91	100

Criterion-referenced standards are a minimum proficiency or pass-fail standard. Drivers license test standards and Red Cross lifesaving and first aid certification standards are criterion referenced. Many physical fitness tests now have criterion-referenced standards. For example, if the criterion-referenced standard for passing the written drivers license test is 70 percent, the examinee must answer at least 70 percent of the test questions correctly to pass. Any percentage from 0 percent to 69 percent is failing, and any value from 70 percent to 100 percent is passing.

Observational

This is research where the data are observations of people or programs. For example, five days a week for eighteen weeks a researcher observed a community recreation program and wrote down everything he observed. At the end of the eighteen weeks, the researcher wrote a report based on those recorded observations.

With this type of research, data collection and analysis is quite time consuming and involves considerable technique. Formal training and practical experience are necessary before this type of research can be attempted.

Observational research has gained in popularity within HHP since 1980. It is discussed in detail in chapter 9 (Qualitative Research).

Action

Action research is conducted in the natural setting where it will be applied. Thus, it lacks some of the control possible with other types of research, but the results of the research are certainly correct for the setting. Action research is always conducted to try to find an answer to a problem that exists in the natural setting. Practitioners who constantly strive to do a better job are actually performing an informal type of action research. An example of action research could be the testing of a new approach to interest students or adults in starting a fitness program. Isaac and Michael (1982, 56–58) contrast formal research, action research, and the casual approach to solving problems; they characterize action research as less precise and demanding than formal research, but superior to the casual approach.

Ex Post Facto

Ex post facto research is research conducted using data that were generated before the research study was ever conceived. It is **"after the fact" research,** looking for relationships or explanations for certain things that presently exist by looking at data from the past. For example, looking at differences between heavy drinking and non-drinking 18-year-olds based on information kept on file about these individuals over the last eight years is ex post facto research.

Isaac and Michael (1982) present a thorough discussion of this research method, also referring to it as causal-comparative research. Best and Kahn (1989) warn that just because two variables are related does not mean that a cause-and-effect relationship exists, with one variable causing an effect on the other variable. Several research books in education (Wiersma 1991; Van Dalen 1979; Best and Kahn 1989) discuss this research approach in detail.

Survey Research

Survey research is the most common type of descriptive research performed in the Health and Human Performance (HHP) area. For this reason, survey research is discussed further in this section of the chapter. The information presented in chapter 3 under "Measurement Techniques in HHP" and "Questioning Techniques" should be reviewed at this time. Particularly the information concerning scaling techniques (rating scales, semantic differential scales, and Lickert scale) and structured questionnaires applies to the discussion at this time concerning questionnaire construction and use.

In survey research, information concerning opinions or practices is obtained from a sample of people, representing a population, through the use of interview or questionnaire techniques. This information provides a basis for making comparisons and determining trends, reveals current weaknesses and/or strengths in a given situation, and provides information for decision making.

As with most types of research, information obtained by a survey has limitations. Survey information reveals, at best, what the situation *is,* not what the situation *should be.* Surveys that deal with behaviors or attitudes do not reveal the factors that cause or influence the behaviors or attitudes. Further, a survey cannot be used to secure all the information sometimes needed for decision making. Surveys are quite often limited by the sample used and the information obtained. Finally, the information obtained may be inaccurate or misinterpreted.

The many survey methods and techniques used with them make it impossible to discuss all methods and techniques in detail. The author's intent in this section of the book is to provide an overview of the methods and to discuss some of the more common techniques. Books are available on the survey method and the techniques involved with it. Sudman and Bradburn (1988) have written a practical guide to questionnaire design. Sage Publications (1996) and Lawrence Erlbaum Associates (2000) list in their catalogs many excellent publications dealing with survey research, survey construction, phone interviews, personal interviews, attitude measurement, and much more.

Preliminary Considerations in Planning a Survey

As in all types of research, the objective in planning the survey is to try to ensure that the data collected will be pertinent to the research question or problem. Survey research is performed no more easily or quickly than any other type of research. Sufficient training and experience in doing survey research, plus considerable planning, is necessary.

One consideration is whether the survey method is the most appropriate way to investigate the research problem. Survey research can be very time-consuming and financially expensive, so estimates of the time and cost should be made early in the planning stage. Finally, survey research can be conducted by phone interview, personal interview, administered questionnaire, or mailed questionnaire; planning should involve consideration of which survey method is best.

Survey Methods

Phone interviews are not often used by researchers in HHP as the primary data collection method. Personal interviews are becoming more prevalent. Administering a questionnaire to a group of participants is a technique commonly used in the field. However, the mailed questionnaire to a sample of participants is the method more often used than any other.

Phone Interview. Marketing research, a form of survey research, and product sales commonly take place over the phone. Why do people in marketing research always call you at dinner time? Because you are likely to be home and probably have not been home all day. This is a phone interview technique: Call when people are home and are probably willing to talk to you. Don't call at 3:37 A.M., although people are usually home. When the phone is answered, the caller has about ten seconds to say something to get the person's attention, or the individual is likely to hang up. This is also a technique: What questions do you ask the person, and in what order do you ask the questions? How long can you hold a person's attention on the phone? Ask questions that require a short answer, and plan how to record the person's answers. So, there is considerable planning and technique in doing a phone interview. Much of the planning and technique for doing a phone interview is the same as that for doing a personal interview.

What are the advantages of a phone interview over other survey techniques? Phone interviews are quick and inexpensive when the sample is spread over a wide geographical area. But the method does not allow for very many questions to be asked, and recording the answers may be difficult. Talk to the survey researchers in business and sociology on campus who do phone interviews. Read the literature on phone interviews. Many of the educational research books address the topic. Babbie (1992) discussed phone surveys and noted that not all people have phones and listed numbers. This may bias phone survey results. However, Babbie indicated that random-digit dialing overcomes this problem and that this technique has gained popularity.

Personal Interview. In the personal interview the researcher meets with each member of the sample, and based on their conversation, the needed information is obtained. If the sample is small and accessible, this is a feasible technique. When the information the researcher desires cannot be collected by asking a series of questions on paper (questionnaire), the personal interview must be used. For example, an interview is probably necessary to obtain information from a senior citizen about how things were fifty years ago.

What are some things to consider if the personal interview is selected as the data-gathering technique? One issue is how to contact potential participants for an interview time. Another is the decision whether to use a **structured interview** (asking each participant the same specific questions), a **semistructured interview** (asking each participant the same general questions), or an **unstructured interview** (just letting the conversation develop). The decision is dependent on what information the researcher needs, whether questions can be formulated in advance, and what the participant is comfortable with or will tolerate. Still another decision is how to record the information provided by the participant. Tape recording the interview may be best because every word is permanently saved. An alternative is to take notes during the interview. Both approaches may be unacceptable to the participant or be so intimidating that the participant will not be open or totally truthful with the researcher. A sufficiently experienced or skilled interviewer may be able to just talk to people, and then write everything down after the interview is over and the participant is no longer present. The point is, personal interviews require much more planning and technique than many people realize.

Some of the advantages of the personal interview are completeness of response, ability to clear up misconceptions, opportunity to follow up responses, and increased likelihood that the respondent will be more conscientious with the interviewer present. Isaac and Michael (1982) favor the structured interview because it requires less training of the researcher and is more objective than the unstructured or semistructured interview. They also present some guidelines for interviews. Other useful references for those who desire additional information are Wiersma (1991), Rubin (1983), Henderson (1991), Babbie (1992), and Borg (1987).

Administered Questionnaire.   For a variety of reasons, the majority of survey research conducted in HHP uses a questionnaire as the data-gathering technique. A questionnaire is a series of questions or statements on paper. Each participant is given a copy of the questionnaire. The participant responds to the questionnaire and then returns it to the researcher. If the researcher can meet with the participants, the questionnaire will probably be administered to all the participants at one time or to several groups of participants at several times. However, the most prevalent procedure is to mail or distribute the questionnaire to the participants, who complete the questionnaire on their own, and then return it to the researcher. Since the majority of procedures are the same no matter whether the researcher administers the questionnaire or distributes it for completion, the majority of information about questionnaires is discussed in the section on distributed questionnaires. Information specific to administered questionnaires is presented here.

If the researcher is unable to get the participants together at one time or in several groups to administer the questionnaire, the researcher may as well distribute the questionnaire. Often, a researcher seeks permission to administer a questionnaire to an intact group such as a class, school, agency, or exercise program. The other possibility is to organize the participants so they come together in one or more groups to complete the questionnaire. In either case, a room or facility must be secured for administering the questionnaire. The facility must be large enough to easily accommodate the largest possible group and conducive to completing a questionnaire (i.e., is quiet, contains desks or tables providing a writing surface, has adequate seating, etc.). Some thought should be given to whether pencils and other materials need to be provided. Certainly, what to say to the participants about the purpose of the questionnaire and how to complete it needs to be planned. How to pass out and receive back the questionnaires has to be thought through. The larger the group, the more important these plans become, particularly if the researcher has access to the room or facility for only a limited amount of time. A common pitfall is to think that a questionnaire that typically takes forty-five minutes to complete can be administered in sixty minutes. All participants will not arrive on time, giving the verbal directions and distributing and receiving the questionnaire will take time, and some participants will take more than forty-five minutes to complete the questionnaire.

Distributed Questionnaire.   When the sample is geographically spread or cannot be brought together as a group, the distributed questionnaire is used. Distribution may be by mailing it to the participants or putting it in their mailbox at work, by handing it to the participants in class or at work or in some location where they gather, or by having another person distribute the questionnaires for you in classes or on job sites. This will include some planned procedure for having participants return the completed questionnaire to the researcher. Researchers distribute more questionnaires by mail than by any other method.

Good questionnaire research requires considerable planning and technique and is not something that just anyone can throw together quickly. Professional pollsters and marketing research experts conduct outstanding questionnaire research. Graduate students often do a poor job with questionnaires due to lack of knowledge and sufficient planning.

Everyone receives many questionnaires in the mail each year. The good ones are often completed and returned; the poor ones usually go in the trash. By way of example of the latter, the author once received a poorly xeroxed copy of a questionnaire. One question asked, "Do you belong to TAHPERD?" First, was the question referring to the Tennessee or Texas Association of Health, Physical Education, Recreation and Dance? Second, why would a person living in Georgia belong to either one? The questionnaire was a xeroxed copy of one that another researcher had developed for use in Tennessee. The questionnaire went in the trash.

The following discussion of questionnaire research assumes that the questionnaire is distributed and returned by mail. Questionnaire development, format, distribution, return, and examples are treated separately.

Questionnaire Development.   Questionnaires are used for a variety of purposes, and very often the purpose dictates the type of items (i.e., question or statement) used in the questionnaire. So, item type is one decision to be made in questionnaire development. An item is classified as **open-ended** if participants have the freedom to respond however they choose. For example, the question "Why did you enroll in this adult fitness program?" is open-ended. A second type of item is **completion;** the subject fills in the blank. For example, "What is your age in years to the last year?" is a completion item. The third type of item is **multiple choice** or **closed-ended;** the possible responses to the item are provided and the participant selects the most appropriate response(s).

Following are two examples of a closed-ended item:

1. Select the response below that best reflects your feelings about the research course you are presently taking.

   1. Great   4. Below average

   2. Above average   5. Terrible

   3. Average

2. Of the vehicles listed, check the ones you own.

   _____ 1. Car   _____ 4. Motorcycle

   _____ 2. Truck   _____ 5. RV

   _____ 3. Jeep   _____ 6. Van

Commonly, questionnaires are used to determine opinions or attitudes. Here is an example:

Indicate your degree of agreement or disagreement for each of the following items.

1. Being the best in a group is very important to me.

   1. Strongly agree   3. Disagree

   2. Agree   4. Strongly disagree

Each item must be carefully written so it is easy to understand and not ambiguous. This takes considerable time if done correctly since the questionnaire must be read and edited several times. Rules and hints on writing knowledge tests generally apply here. The reading level as well as the attention span of the participants must be considered. Directions for responding to the questionnaire must be presented at the top of the first page of the questionnaire. An example question and response are often provided right after the directions. If the questionnaire is supposed to cover a content area or be all-inclusive, then care must be taken to develop items that cover the necessary area.

Reliability and validity of the questionnaire must be determined *before* it is used in the research study. Validity is the degree to which the questionnaire measures what it is supposed to measure. Just because you developed the questionnaire does not make it perfect. Validity is usually estimated by a jury of experts. The jury should have representation from content experts, questionnaire construction experts, and questionnaire use experts. Hopefully, the jury will find the questionnaire to be well constructed, covering the necessary content, and ready for use. Based on the input from the jury, the questionnaire may be revised and evaluated by the jury again, depending on the extent of the revisions.

Reliability is consistency of response. The researcher wants to be assured that the responses of the participants to the questionnaire would not be different if the questionnaire were administered to them at some other time. As ideal as it might be to administer the questionnaire to some participants on two different days to check for consistency of response, this is rarely done. Instead, researchers put several pairs of items in the questionnaire with items in a pair either similar or opposite. Items 6 and 33, below, provide an example of paired opposite items.

6. I like candy.

   1. Agree

   2. Disagree

33. I don't like candy.

   1. Agree

   2. Disagree

The questionnaire is administered and the responses to paired items are examined to see whether they are as expected. No matter whether the questionnaire is administered on two different days or on one day with paired items, an intraclass R can be obtained as an estimate of reliability, either for each item administered twice or for each pair (see chapter 14 or Baumgartner and Jackson 1999).

The goodness of the questionnaire should be determined before it is used to collect the research data. This is always the case with the validity of a questionnaire just discussed. Some researchers determine reliability using data from the research study. The problem with this is that if the reliability is poor, it is too late to make changes in the questionnaire to improve reliability. Unreliable data are no good, so all unreliable data should be discarded.

As discussed in chapter 3, a pilot study is the best solution to this possible problem. The questionnaire is administered to a small number of individuals similar to the participants who will take part in the research study, and the reliability for their data is determined. As part of the pilot study, it is a good idea to keep track of such things as how long it takes individuals to complete the questionnaire, whether the questionnaire appears to contain any ambiguous items, and any other factor that could affect the successful administration of the questionnaire. Based on the pilot study, the questionnaire is revised as needed.

Questionnaire Format.   The appearance and layout of the questionnaire is as important as the content. The questionnaire must be professional in the way it is typed, and in the quality of the paper and reproduction, or people will not complete it. Items need to be arranged in rows or columns for a neat appearance, ease of completing the questionnaire, and ease of data entry into the computer, if necessary, for analysis. Demographic information such as age, gender, education, and income are often requested on the questionnaire. Since questions about age and income sometimes irritate subjects, demographic questions should be placed at the end of the questionnaire. Irritating questions at the end of a questionnaire are often left blank, but if they appear at the beginning of a questionnaire it may cause the entire questionnaire to go into the trash. In fact, any controversial item should be placed at the end of the questionnaire for the same reason (e.g., "Have you gained a lot of weight in the last five years?").

Answers to closed-ended items that will be computer analyzed need to be numerically coded. Participants should be asked to check the appropriate item or circle the appropriate number.

Example:

Poor format

What is your gender? _____

Good format

Circle the number for your gender.

1. Female   2. Male

or

Check the number for your gender.

_____ 1. Female

_____ 2. Male

Closed-ended items are preferable to completion items. Also, it is better to provide choices in the form of nonoverlapping intervals rather than specific values, particularly on items that may have a large number of different values, for which the participant may not know the exact value, where the researcher does not need the exact value, or which may irritate the participant.

Example:

Poor format

What is your income? _____

Good format

What is your income?

_____ 1. less than $12,000

_____ 2. $12,001 to $18,000

_____ 3. $18,001 to $27,000

_____ 4. $27,001 to $40,000

_____ 5. more than $40,000

Inform the participant whether one answer is desired or whether multiple answers to an item are desired (see the earlier example on vehicles owned, p. 195). This is particularly important when the data are going to be computer analyzed, because sufficient space must be allowed to accommodate all answers. When multiple answers are possible, each answer choice is treated as if it were an item: A one (1) is entered into the computer if that answer is checked, and zero (0) if it is not checked.

Questionnaire Distribution. The biggest concerns with distribution are controlling the cost of getting the questionnaire to the participants and trying to obtain a high rate of questionnaire return. The researcher can influence both. For example, the fewer the pages in the questionnaire, the less expensive it is to mail and the shorter it looks to the participant, the more likely that it will be returned. Generally, there is a tendency to have too many items on a questionnaire. No matter what the number of items, reproduce the questionnaire on both sides of the page and use the smallest readable print size. Even the weight of the paper used can sometimes influence mailing rate.

The researcher is expected to provide a self-addressed stamped envelope for returning the questionnaire. Failure to do so will almost certainly decrease the rate of return. To minimize the postage on the return envelope, ask participants to respond to all closed-ended items on a standardized answer sheet rather than on the questionnaire and to just return the answer sheet. Standardized answer sheets are often an efficient tool for organizing the data to be entered into a computer. However, if groups are not familiar with standardized answer sheets, their use will decrease questionnaire return rate or result in such poorly erased or completed answer sheets that data will be lost.

A good mailing list is an essential component of distributing a questionnaire. Lists are not always highly accessible. Lists with the name of a person rather than a title (e.g., "department head") are generally desirable. However, if the questionnaire is going to the person presently in the position and there is considerable turnover in the position, a title may be better than a personal name. Check into the advantages and disadvantages of bulk mail in comparison to first and second class mail in terms of cost, speed of delivery, and forwarding, because considerable cost reduction is possible with bulk mail.

Researchers can do a number of things to try to improve the percentage of questionnaires returned. To give some idea of the extent of this problem, the expected rate of return is 50 percent; perhaps an 80-percent return may be expected from professional participants who have an interest in the questionnaire results; but only a 10-percent return is likely when surveying the general public. For this reason researchers tend to send out enough questionnaires to ensure a desired number of returns. However, a small percentage of returns makes the goodness of the results questionable. Are the participants who returned the questionnaire really a representative sample of the target population? Would the results have been different if more people had returned the questionnaire? It is important to motivate people in every way possible to return the questionnaire. A cover letter with the questionnaire explaining why the study is being conducted and its importance to humanity will improve the return rate. A cover letter signed by an influential person also increases the return rate. Offering to share the results, giving money, a catchy saying ("a penny for your thoughts," and enclose a penny), all help to motivate people to return the questionnaire.

Sending the questionnaire out at a time when people are likely to have time to complete and return it is good strategy. Sending questionnaires to coaches in the middle of their season or to anyone just before Christmas is not wise. Also, one to three follow-up letters sent at two- to three-week intervals after the first mailing, reminding people to return their questionnaire, increases the percentage of returns. Having participants put their name on the questionnaire before they return it makes follow-up easier and is to the advantage of the researcher. However, some participants will not return the questionnaire or will not be totally truthful in completing it if they have to put their name on it. If there are any highly personal items on the questionnaire or any items dealing with illegal activities, do not request the participant's name on the questionnaire.

Example:

How often do you smoke pot?

1. Weekly
2. Monthly
3. Several times a year
4. Never

Law enforcement agencies have been known to confiscate questionnaires dealing with illegal activities. Generally, it is better not to ask for names on questionnaire returns unless you really need them.

Questionnaire Return.   Most survey studies require the use of a computer to analyze the volume of scores. A fifty-item closed-ended questionnaire returned by 350 participants generates 17,500 scores. So, when questionnaires are returned, scan them to be sure they are ready for data entry. Even if names are on the questionnaires, give each questionnaire an identification number, enter that number and questionnaire data into the computer, check the information for data entry error, and then destroy the questionnaire. Of course, open-ended questions must be analyzed by hand.

Anticipate that some items on some questionnaires will not be answered because participants will accidentally skip or decline to answer certain items. This is acceptable as long as only a few items on each questionnaire are left blank and it otherwise seems that the participant completed the questionnaire accurately. Some researchers put items on a questionnaire to check for accuracy of participant response and reject those questionnaires that fail the accuracy check. For example, a drug use questionnaire includes a long list of drugs and requests participants to check the ones they use. Kerosene is on the list of drugs and a participant checks it; the questionnaire is rejected. Unexpected responses to open-ended items are sometimes found. The same drug use questionnaire contained this item: "Is there a big drug problem on campus?" One participant responded, "No!! You can get it anywhere." The questionnaire was not rejected.

Attitude scale questionnaires usually check for accuracy by stating some items positively (e.g., Smoking is okay.) and some items negatively (e.g., Drinking alcohol is evil.) to produce a varied response to items within participants. In this case, a researcher rejects the returned questionnaire if visual inspection shows that the majority of the items are answered with the same response; it appears that the participant just checked answers without reading the items.

Questionnaire Examples

I. *Poor format*

Listed are activities taught in the physical education department. Please check the activities you have taken at the university. If you check an activity, then please check the skill level you presently have in the activity. "B" is beginner, "I" is intermediate, and "A" is advanced.

		SKILL LEVEL		
ACTIVITY	**TAKEN**	**B**	**I**	**A**
Archery				
Bowling				
Golf				
Dance				
Swimming				
Tennis				

NOTE: This is a poor questionnaire because much space is wasted, and there is no numerical coding of responses.

Improved format

Listed are activities taught in the physical education department at the university. Please use the following code to indicate your status for each activity.

CODE: 0—Did not take activity

1—Took activity; presently have beginner level skill

2—Took activity; presently have intermediate level skill

3—Took activity; presently have advanced level skill

_____ Archery		_____ Dance
_____ Bowling		_____ Swimming
_____ Golf		_____ Tennis

II. _May I have about five minutes of your time?_

I need your assistance.

This is my dissertation research. The purpose of the study is to determine what faculty members think are important attributes in a department head. Using the scale shown below, please rate the importance of each attribute of a department head. Then return your ratings in the enclosed addressed, stamped envelope.

Importance Rating Scale

Not Important At All							Extremely Important
	1	2	3	4	5	6	7

Attributes

_____ Friendly

_____ Professional

_____ Organized

_____ Good looking

III. _Using the key below, rate each task by putting an "X" in the face that best represents your feeling._

KEY ☺ I know that I have the ability to perform the task.

☻ I am not sure that I have the ability to perform the task.

☹ I know that I don't have the ability to perform the task.

1. How do you feel about your ability to dribble a ball without your opponent getting it away from you? ☻ ☹ ☺

2. How do you feel about your ability to do a front roll? ☹ ☻ ☺

Note: This questionnaire can be scored 3–2–1 from smile to frown; the faces follow no pattern from item to item; faces can be used with young children.

IV. *What are the four biggest problems in our discipline today?*

Note: This is an open-ended question because the researcher does not know all the problems and probably does not have enough space on the questionnaire to list all the problems.

V. *What was your undergraduate degree major?*

VI. *An example of a questionnaire is presented in Example 8.1.*

Note: It is not the content but the form of this questionnaire which is important.

EXAMPLE 8.1
Example Questionnaire

The AAHPERD Fitness Tests Opinionnaire

The American Alliance for Health, Physical Education, Recreation, and Dance (AAHPERD) presently distributes the Youth Fitness Test (used by the President's Council on Physical Fitness and Sport) which was introduced in 1957 and the Health Related Physical Fitness Test which was introduced in 1980. AAHPERD must decide whether to continue to distribute the two tests, combine the two tests into one test, or discontinue one test. Numerous groups and committees have given AAHPERD their recommendations. However, public school physical education teachers have had very limited input on this important issue. This is your opportunity to make your views known. What AAHPERD does will influence what fitness tests are available to you in the future.

Funded by: Georgia Association for Health, Physical Education, Recreation, and Dance

Endorsed by: American Alliance for Health, Physical Education, Recreation, and Dance; State Consultant for Physical Education, Georgia Department of Education

This opinionnaire should take less than 15 minutes to complete. Please complete each question and return it today in the stamped, self-addressed envelope.

Thank you,

Dr. Ted Baumgartner
The University of Georgia

EXAMPLE 8.1
Continued

For your information, the Youth Fitness Test is considered a motor fitness test (fitness to participate in physical activities). The Health Related Physical Fitness Test is considered a fitness test for healthy living (throughout life). The items in these two tests and what each item is supposed to measure are presented below:

Attribute Measured	Youth Fitness	Health Related
Cardiorespiratory endurance	Distance run	Distance run
Abdominal strength	Sit-ups	Sit-ups
Arm and shoulder-girdle strength	Pull-ups or flexed-arm hang	
Leg power	Standing long jump	
Body composition		Skinfolds
Flexibility (of lower back and hamstrings)		Sit-and-reach
Speed	50-yard dash	
Agility	Shuttle run	

1. Are you aware of the Youth Fitness Test (due to college classes, reading, workshops, etc.)? (circle number)　1. Yes　2. No

2. Have you administered the Youth Fitness Test within the last three years? (circle number)　1. Yes　2. No

3. Does your school or school system require that you administer the Youth Fitness Test on a regular basis? (circle number)
   1. Yes　2. No

4-a. If you were given the choice, would you administer the Youth Fitness Test on a regular basis? (circle number)　1. Yes　2. No
   3. I do not have enough information about the test to decide.

4-b. If you answered *no* above, circle *one* or *more* reasons why you do not plan to use the test. (circle number(s))

   1. Too time-consuming　　2. Too unfamiliar
   3. Lack of equipment　　　4. Not in line with program objectives
   5. Not sufficiently motivating　6. Not valid
   7. Not enough space　　　8. Other (specify) _____
   _____

5. Are you aware of the Health Related Physical Fitness Test (due to college classes, reading, workshops, etc.)? (circle number)
   1. Yes　2. No

EXAMPLE 8.1
Continued

6. Have you administered the Health Related Physical Fitness Test within the last three years? (circle number)   1. Yes   2. No

7. Does your school or school system require that you administer the Health Related Physical Fitness Test on a regular basis? (circle number)   1. Yes   2. No

8-a. If you were given the choice, would you administer the Health Related Physical Fitness Test on a regular basis? (circle number)
   1. Yes   2. No
   3. I do not have enough information about the test to decide.

8-b. If you answered *no* above, circle *one* or *more* reasons why you do not plan to use the test. (circle number(s))

   1. Too time-consuming   2. Too unfamiliar
   3. Lack of equipment   4. Not in line with program
                                      objectives
   5. Not sufficiently motivating 6. Not valid
   7. Not enough space   8. Other (specify) _____
                                      _____

9. Do you administer some kind of fitness test in your physical education program at least once a year? (circle number)

   1. Always   2. Usually
   3. Seldom   4. Never

For each fitness test item listed below, please indicate if you feel the item should be part of a fitness test battery. (circle a number under *Yes, No,* or *No Opinion*)

	YES	NO	NO OPINION
10. Distance run	1	2	3
11. Sit-ups	1	2	3
12. Pull-ups (boys)	1	2	3
13. Flexed-arm hang (girls)	1	2	3
14. Skinfolds	1	2	3
15. Standing long jump	1	2	3
16. Sit-and-reach	1	2	3
17. 50-yard dash	1	2	3
18. Shuttle run	1	2	3

Finally, we would like to ask a few questions to help us interpret the results and to give you a chance to make comments and suggestions.

1. Is your school located in a rural or urban area? (circle number)
   1. Rural   2. Urban

EXAMPLE 8.1
Concluded

2. What is the student population of your school? (circle number)
    1. 0–100   2. 101–500   3. 501–1,000
    4. 1,001–1,500   5. Over 1,500

3. What is your school called? (circle number)

    1. Elementary school   2. Middle school/Junior high school
    3. Senior high school   4. Other (specify grade levels) _____

4. What percent of your teaching time is spent teaching physical education, *not* health education or other subjects? (circle number)
    1. 0–20   2. 21–40   3. 41–60   4. 61–80   5. 81–100

5. What is your age? (circle number)
    1. 20–29 years   2. 30–39 years
    3. 40–49 years   4. 50–59 years   5. 60 years or older

6. What is your gender? (circle number)   1. Female   2. Male

7. What is the highest degree you hold? (circle number)
    1. Bachelors
    2. Bachelors plus 25 quarter (17 semester) hours of graduate credit
    3. Masters
    4. Masters plus 15 quarter (10 semester) hours of graduate credit
    5. Specialist
    6. Doctorate

8. Are you usually (presently or the majority of the time) a member of the Georgia Association for HPERD (GAHPERD) and/or the American Alliance for HPERD (AAHPERD)? (circle number)

    1. No, neither organization   2. Yes, GAHPERD
    3. Yes, AAHPERD   4. Yes, both organizations

9. Is there anything else you would like to tell us with regard to fitness testing? If so, please use the space below.

Questionnaire Summary.   Research using a questionnaire as the data-gathering instrument is quite common in HHP. Considerable information has been presented concerning construction and use of a questionnaire. For people who will seldom use a questionnaire, it may be too much information. But for people who will use a questionnaire in their research, it is probably not enough information. A number of excellent sources are available for those who desire more information. All of the following are enlightening: Isaac and Michael (1982, chap. 4); Wiersma (1991, chap. 7); Best and Kahn (1989, chap. 6); McMillan and Schumacher (1984, chap. 6); Rubin (1983, chap. 10); Tuckman (1988, chap. 10); and Neutens and Rubinson (1997, chap. 6). Books specific to survey methods and mail surveys such as Babbie (1990), Dillman (1978), and Weisberg and Bowen (1977) are excellent sources.

Summary

This chapter has discussed the purpose of descriptive research and the many types of descriptive research. At a minimum, the student should now have an understanding of why descriptive research is conducted and some of the common types of descriptive research. Students who may conduct or consume descriptive research should have a basic understanding of each type of descriptive research. This chapter was an introductory overview of descriptive research. Considerably more expertise is required to actually conduct a descriptive research study or knowledgeably critique the descriptive research of others than can be gained by reading this chapter.

Formative Evaluation of Objectives

Objective 1   Identify the common types of descriptive research.

1. What are three types of descriptive research commonly conducted in your area?
2. What are several types of descriptive research commonly conducted in HHP?

Objective 2   Identify techniques commonly used in descriptive research.

1. What are four techniques commonly used in descriptive research in your area?
2. When using a questionnaire in a research study, what are five things to do that will increase the likelihood of a successful study?

Qualitative Research* 9

Confirmability
Core variable
Credibility
Critical theory
Dependability
Ethnographic research
Feminist theory
Field notes

Field research
Focus group interviews
Grounded theory
Inductive
Interpretation
Interview schedule
Key informants

Member checks
Naturalistic inquiry
Nonparticipant observers
Participant-observers
Phenomenology
Probes
Reflective field notes

Structured interviews
Symbolic interaction
Thick description
Transferability
Triangulation
Typology
Unstructured interviews

OBJECTIVES

After reading chapter 9, you should be able to

1. Define qualitative research and its most frequently used synonyms, such as ethnography, naturalistic inquiry, and field research.
2. Outline differences between qualitative and quantitative studies.
3. Identify major theoretical frameworks in qualitative research.
4. Outline the general process for conceptualizing a qualitative study, framing the research question, collecting and analyzing data, and writing up a research report.
5. Describe the features of trustworthiness of qualitative data, including credibility, transferability, dependability, and confirmability.
6. Identify questions that can be used to evaluate the quality of a qualitative research article.

*This chapter was written by Judith F. McLaughlin, Department of Health and Kinesiology, Georgia Southern University.

The inclusion of a separate chapter on qualitative methods in research methods texts in health and human performance (HHP) areas is a rather recent phenomenon. It reflects an increased appreciation for the fact that some research problems are best answered using qualitative methods. A tutorial appearing in *Research Quarterly for Exercise and Sport* (Locke 1989) served to introduce qualitative methods to its readership, and entire issues of such journals as *Health Education Quarterly* (Steckler, McLeroy, Goodman, McCormick, and Bird 1992) have been devoted to the subject. Workshops on qualitative methods are common occurrences at national HHP conventions, and textbooks on qualitative research, especially in leisure studies, have been published (Henderson 1991).

When there is a need to understand the context of a phenomenon, or a desire to learn the subject's (or respondent's) perspective, qualitative methods can help the researcher generate detailed descriptive data using **naturalistic inquiry.** The term "naturalistic" in qualitative research denotes being in the natural environment or gathering data on natural behavior. There have been significant numbers of qualitative research studies conducted in HHP since 1980. A variety of problems and questions are addressed in these studies, including questions about teaching and educational organizations, program evaluations, organizational policies such as those to prohibit smoking, and the meaning of such concepts as health, leisure, and movement, to name only a few. The settings in which these studies occur are both domestic and international and include communities, schools, gymnasiums, clinics, and worksites.

The purpose of this chapter is not to provide a primer on the methods and techniques of qualitative research. The terminology itself has no agreed-upon usage, and there is some confusion and disagreement among researchers about appropriate vocabulary and terms. Neither is the chapter designed to be a definitive overview of the philosophy of the paradigm (or research approach), because there is considerable variety in the theoretical perspectives used by qualitative researchers in a number of fields including anthropology, sociology, psychology, and education. Rather, the purpose of this chapter is to describe qualitative perspectives and methods commonly used in HHP and to provide illustrative examples to which the student can refer for further information.

Introduction

Qualitative research is a relative newcomer to education. Until very recently, traditional research methodology in HHP was mostly positivistic-quantitative, objective, deductive, inferential, confirmatory, and outcome-oriented (Cook and Reichardt 1979). This is because these fields have been dominated by the predictive power of the natural science model of scientific inquiry, with less emphasis on historical, philosophical, interpretive, and other social science methodologies. Consequently, randomized field experiments using quantified observations were considered ideal, and most researchers devoted most of their attention to experimental designs and the quantitative methods associated with them.

By the early 1980s, there was growing dissatisfaction with the traditional methods among some researchers, particularly for program and curriculum evaluation. For example, conventional experimental designs were difficult to operationalize into program designs in the field, and they were often unable to detect unexpected positive and negative program outcomes. Curriculum evaluators were sometimes unable to explain why a particular curricular innovation worked, just that it did. Thus researchers in HHP turned to methods used by social scientists that could detect unexpected processes and outcomes, and could be modified according to field conditions.

In addition, some of these researchers began studying phenomena in the natural environment, from the perspective of participants themselves. For example, Griffin (1983, 1984, 1985) conducted a series of studies focusing on student participation in physical education. She developed **typologies,** or categories, of boys' and girls' participation patterns, providing an understanding of behavior styles in the physical education class. More recently, Langley and Knight (1996) explored the practical knowledge of an experienced, senior adult tennis player to determine how he built a successful playing style that maximized his performance while exploiting the limitations of his opponents. Blinde and McCallister (1999) explained the experiences in sport and physical fitness activity of women with disabilities in terms of the gender dynamics that influence their decision to participate or not, while Henderson and Bedini's (1995) study explored how women with mobility impairments experienced physical activity and leisure. Both studies highlighted the need to consider and improve opportunities for physical activity for this group.

These researchers and others used a number of social science concepts, theories, and methods that have generally been grouped under the broad term of *qualitative research.* This type of research refers to the techniques of observing, documenting, analyzing, and interpreting attributes, patterns, characteristics, and meanings of specific, contextual features of phenomena under study (Leininger 1985). Qualitative research methodology has been referred to as holistic, inductive, dynamic, subjective, humanistic, exploratory, and process oriented (Cook and Reichardt 1979).

The Nature of Qualitative Research

The term *qualitative research* is an umbrella term referring to several research traditions and strategies that share certain commonalties. There is an emphasis on process, or how things happen, and a focus on attitudes, beliefs, and thoughts—how people make sense of their experiences as they interpret their world. The researcher is the primary research instrument, and the researcher's insight is the key instrument for analysis. Qualitative strategies enable the researcher to record and understand people in their own terms. Research questions are not framed by delineating variables or testing hypotheses, but most often come from real-world observations, dilemmas, and questions (e.g., Why is this program working well in one school, but not in another?). The data collected consist of detailed descriptions of people, events, situations, and conversations. Depth and detail are revealed through direct quotations and careful descriptions of behavior. This material is usually supplemented by other data such as analysis of official documents, memos, records, photographs, and interviews with additional persons in order to cross-check and fill information gaps. Qualitative researchers collect data through sustained contact with people in their natural settings. They do not consciously intervene in any way or take action to change the situation under investigation. Data are analyzed **inductively;** the researcher builds concepts, explains processes, and develops hypotheses, rather than beginning with hypotheses and analyzing them deductively as in quantitative research. As situations and dilemmas arise during the research process, the investigator records self-reflective field notes about these situations because they may influence data analysis.

Qualitative research is the term most commonly used in HHP to refer to this type of study, but several other terms are often used to describe the study of people, systems, and phenomena in their specific contexts. **Ethnographic research** is sometimes used synonymously with *qualitative approach,* although others use the term to denote a specific type of qualitative research, directed at observing and describing human society and culture (Vidich and Lyman 1994). Some researchers, particularly anthropologists, deplore the use of the term ethnography for anything other than long-term participation in and description of a culture, but its use as a synonym for qualitative research in other fields, particularly education, is widespread. Qualitative research is frequently called naturalistic inquiry and **field research** because data tend to be collected in the field by people engaging in and observing natural, ordinary, everyday behavior (Denzin and Lincoln 1994). The exact use of these terms and others such as *interpretive, ecological,* and *descriptive* vary among individuals, disciplines, and settings with no consensus at present. Throughout this chapter we use *qualitative research* and *qualitative methods* as if these terms were agreed-upon and universally understood, but no such implication is intended.

Differences between Qualitative and Quantitative Studies

Both quantitative and qualitative research operate under assumptions that serve as the foundation of their methodologies. While researchers tend to subscribe to one method or the other in formulating their studies, it is important to note that many of the assumptions of both exist along a continuum (LeCompte, Preissle, and Tesch 1993). However, for practical reasons, it is helpful to dichotomize the two paradigms in order to compare and contrast them. Major differences between the two paradigms are listed below (Bogdan and Biklen 1997; Merriam 1997):

1. The quantitative paradigm uses experimental and quasi-experimental designs and statistical techniques to collect numerical data on a representative population sample. The qualitative paradigm applies anthropological and sociological research methods to understand relevant social phenomena. Data are in the form of words and phrases, and samples tend to be small and nonrandom.

2. The focus of quantitative research is on quantity (how much, how many). The goal of a quantitative investigation is hypothesis testing, prediction, or confirmation. Research is focused on outcomes, and the reliability of measures (e.g., scales, tests, surveys, or questionnaires) is stressed. The focus of qualitative research is on quality (the nature of something; its essence). The goal of qualitative research is hypothesis generation, understanding, or discovery. Research is focused on eliciting an "insider's" view of the group under study, and the researcher is the primary instrument for data collection and analysis. The primary role of the researcher is to be responsive to the context, or situation, to observe, and to ask open-ended questions to determine how people make sense of their lives.

3. Design characteristics of quantitative studies are predetermined and structured. In contrast, qualitative study design characteristics are flexible, evolving, and emergent. Procedures and methods often change with the situation.

4. Researchers using quantitative methods distance themselves from the people they are studying in order to maintain objectivity. Qualitative researchers are actively involved with their subjects, immersing themselves in a culture by observing people and their interactions, participating in activities, and asking questions.

5. Quantitative researchers use methods that provide factual, reliable data at the end of the research study that are usually generalizable to a larger group (population). Qualitative methods generate richly detailed data about the group being studied and provide contextual understanding. Results are not generalized to a reference population, although findings can often be applied as an explanation for the behavior of other groups.

Both the qualitative and quantitative paradigms have weaknesses, which to a certain extent are compensated for by the strengths of the other. Qualitative and quantitative researchers have attempted to justify the use of their methods by finding fault with the other. In reality, whether one uses the methods of the qualitative or quantitative paradigm depends on the nature of the research question; in general, questions that ask "who," "what is," "when," and "where" are likely to be answered by using quantitative techniques. Questions that ask "how," "what," and "why" may be more suited to qualitative methods. The research tools of each method are superior to the other under different circumstances. Some studies have several research questions and employ both quantitative and qualitative methods (see Ennis, Ross, and Chen [1992], for example).

Theoretical Frameworks in Qualitative Research

Theory can be confirmed or generated through qualitative studies by providing a strategy for collecting, describing, or explaining data (Henderson 1991). The function of theory is to give order and insight so that theory and research guide each other

(LeCompte, Preissle, and Tesch 1993). The organizing framework used will take the researcher in a particular direction. Several theoretical frameworks from different disciplines provide guidance for qualitative studies, and five of the most commonly used perspectives are described here. For a comprehensive review of other theoretical perspectives, consult Henderson (1991) and LeCompte, Preissle, and Tesch (1993).

Symbolic Interaction

The **symbolic interaction** perspective has influenced the research of sociologists and anthropologists since the turn of the century, and is used by qualitative researchers as a basis for interpretive research. It assumes that all human experience is mediated by **interpretation** (Blumer 1969), and it suggests that people do not act according to predetermined responses, but rather they interpret meaning and define things through interaction with others. It is based on three premises: (a) that individuals act toward phenomena according to the meaning those things hold; (b) that the meanings are derived from social interactions with others; and (c) the meanings are adjusted according to the individual's interpretation of those interactions (Denzin 1992). Through participant observation, the researcher focuses on how these interpretations lead to behavior in situations they are studying. How individuals interpret some phenomenon, how important or unimportant it is, the words used to describe it—all are indications of how people impart meaning to objects, people, and events, and this in turn determines how people act. For example, West (1989) used a symbolic interaction perspective to study what physical activity meant to fourth graders from diverse cultural backgrounds. Through participant observation and interview, she determined that competence, commitment, excitement, compliance, and social status were significant in the children's perceptions of self. These perceptions determined the degree of involvement in physical activity, and were defined and redefined by social interaction with the teacher and with other children. Thus, for the children in this study, the opportunity to enhance quality of life through physical activity was facilitated, restricted, or denied through this social interaction. The study generated hypotheses about the success or failure of physical activity that can be further tested using quantitative methods.

Phenomenology

The goal of **phenomenology** is to describe and clarify subjects' experiences without any previous assumptions as to their meanings. The researcher attempts to gain entry into the conceptual world of their respondents (Geertz 1973), working very hard to bring no preconceived ideas about that world to the study. The concept of phenomenology has influenced the work of sociologists for a century and today offers an important framework for interpretive research. Phenomenologists often use no interview schedule, preferring to maintain maximum flexibility to pursue information in whatever direction appears to be appropriate. Most questions derive from the immediate situation, allowing the interviewer to "go with the flow" (Patton 1990). As Wilson

(1977, 249) states, "those who work within this tradition assert that the social scientist cannot understand human behavior without understanding the framework within which the *subjects* interpret their thoughts, feelings, and actions." The strength of this perspective is that it allows the researcher to be highly responsive to individuals and situations. By not assuming they know what things mean to the people they are studying, they often gain extraordinary insight into events and interactions. A weakness is that interviews can be lengthy and may occur over a long period of time.

Williamson's (1990) study of how physical education teacher educators (professors) perceive their relationship with public school professionals (physical education teachers) used a phenomenological perspective. No list of specific questions was used when interviewing participants; instead, over three separate interviews, participants shared their thoughts about the experience of being a teacher educator in physical education. The study revealed professors' awareness of an implicit hierarchy between themselves and school teachers that created a social barrier to collaborative relationships. Based on the perspectives, Williamson was able to make recommendations to overcome the perceived dissonance.

Grounded Theory

Grounded theory is more of a framework for *developing* theory than a theoretical perspective itself. Developed and refined by Glaser and Strauss (1967) and Glaser (1978), grounded theory is a sophisticated form of data collection and analysis that uses comparison as an analytic tool to generate concepts and hypotheses. These concepts and hypotheses are interrelated and grouped to form a whole, much as one constructs a picture shaped from parts individually collected and examined. Parts grouped together form a **core variable,** most often a social process; the analysis then traces the emerging process to identify its stages, dimensions, and characteristics. The final goal is middle-range theory in a specific content area such as pain management. The theory is identified as "grounded" because it emerges from the categories of data. It is particularly useful in areas that lack theoretical development and where there is little previous research.

An example of grounded theory research is Ingram and Hutchinson's (2000) study of the reproductive and mothering experiences of HIV-positive women. The authors sought to explain and understand how the women defined their lives with HIV and how they acted in relation to their beliefs and realities. Through their analysis, they revealed mothering to be a priority in the women's lives, keven as they struggled with the physical and emotional ravages of HIV and with the social ambivalence directed at them as mothers. They identified the "double bind", or conflict inherent in their situations as the study's core variable, and suggested that professionals who are attuned to the double bind can be more effective in providing counseling and coping suggestions.

Morgan and Laing (1991) used a grounded theory perspective to clarify the relationship of the concepts of grief and role strain in spouses (caregivers) of persons with Alzheimer's disease. One group's process of grief was described using core variables of "coming to terms," where the spouse exercised such strategies as accepting, letting go, minimizing, protecting, normalizing, adjusting, and preparing. Another group's process of role strain was described as "hanging on," where strategies used by spouses were resenting, organizing, venting, delegating, and ignoring. These two groups emerged during the data analysis process; the nature of the couple's previous relationship was the strongest predictor of the group to which the spouse would later belong. McLachlan (1992), in a study of how family leisure is constrained in families who have a child with Down syndrome, used both phenomenological theory and grounded theory to generate a conceptual framework illustrating the leisure constraints.

Critical Theory and Feminist Theory

These two theories are concerned with the relationship between the researcher and those with whom studies are being conducted. The roots of **critical theory** are in neo-Marxism; as a research perspective it is concerned with the political beliefs of both the investigator and subjects, the purpose of which is to discover what should be done to improve the world of those being studied (Reason and Rowan 1981; Graham 1991; Henderson 1991). Empowerment and emancipation are possible results of the research, often precipitating social action on the part of both researcher and participants. Bain's research project (Bain, Wilson, and Chaikind 1989) of empowerment of a group of overweight women involved in an exercise program is an example.

Feminist theory has influenced qualitative research in the last decade. Because the qualitative paradigm is concerned with feeling and emotion as well as experience, qualitative methods are attractive to feminists who study women's experience from a woman's point of view. Feminism is used as a framework for a qualitative approach in Dixey's (1987) study of women's leisure, which examined why the game of bingo was such an important activity to a group of working class women. As the reasons emerged from the analysis, it became clear that the context in which the activity took place reflected their roles as women. Similarly, Dempsey's (1990) study of women's leisure activity in a rural community demonstrated the relationship of the men's power and how women and their activities were excluded and defined as inferior.

Methods in Qualitative Research

The Process of Qualitative Research

Although the particular theoretical perspective used in the research study will influence the way data are collected, analyzed, and interpreted, the following is a general guide to the process of qualitative research studies. Keep in mind, however, that even the most carefully planned study can end up being designed in the course of its execution. The finished report is the result of hundreds of decisions made during the research, as unanticipated contingencies interrupt data collection and analysis, as data having nothing to do with the original research questions are collected, and as unexpected findings stimulate new ideas to explore. Thus, a research outline often turns out to be a tentative plan. The following hardly constitutes a recipe for doing field research, but rather is a suggestion for ingredients. The stages are not necessarily sequential but often blend together as the phenomenon to be studied is conceptualized and as data are collected and analyzed.

Conceptualizing the Research.   Ideas for study come to qualitative researchers as they ponder interesting, curious, or puzzling phenomena, which they observe, discover, or stumble across (Marshall and Rossman 1999). This leads to further observation, discussion, and reading, and is the first step in formulating the research question or questions. Studies of physical education classes, school health curricula, leisure program administration, organizational climate, and high school coaches begin with an observation of some phenomenon in its natural context and a desire to observe and record what happens. A plan begins to form from hunches. Some plans are more structured than others, and the particular research tradition from which the researcher is working, as well as the researcher's previous experience, affects how the study is conceptualized. Intuition about the importance of the problem, a feeling of "how interesting it will be to learn about this!" often play an early role. Typical questions at this stage are "What specific approach should I take?" and "What kind of data will I collect?" Ideas about how to gain access to the desired research setting also start to form.

Framing the Research Question(s).   The researcher does not begin with a hypothesis to test. Qualitative research starts with observations in the real world that merge to form ideas and give rise to such questions as (1) What does the term "leisure" mean to people? (2) How do leisure patterns change over the course of life? (3) Why is a curriculum not working in this school, even though it is considered highly effective and is nationally respected? (4) What happens to elite athletes or dancers when they suffer a career-ending injury? (5) What is life like for a well-known high school or college coach? (6) What is different about the participants in a health promotion or adult fitness program who finish the course as opposed to those who drop out? Qualitative research questions usually begin with "what," "why," and "how." Most likely, initial research questions will be wide-ranging inquiries that will be refined and reworked as the research unfolds. In a cross-cultural study of the self-care behavior of Danes and Americans with multiple sclerosis (McLaughlin and Zeeberg 1993), for example, the original questions were phrased around whether Danes use alternative therapies to manage their symptoms and promote their health away from the physician. The underlying rationale for the question was based on the fact that Denmark is a social welfare state and all health care is provided for by the government, theoretically negating the use of other kinds of health care. As the study progressed it became clear that Danes used a variety of self-help and self-care strategies including self-medication. Additional questions were framed to learn why this occurs, since cost was not a factor. Thus, the approach of qualitative research is one of discovery, rather than the testing of *a priori* explanations and hypotheses.

Collecting Data.   Qualitative researchers utilize the data collection strategies of direct observation, focused interviewing, document analysis, photographs, and supportive quantitative data. A strategy is chosen that will most clearly reveal the perspectives of the persons under study; the goal of the researcher is to produce **"thick" description,** a term coined by Geertz denoting the richest, most comprehensive description possible (Geertz 1973).

Direct observation.   The researcher usually spends extensive periods of time in the natural setting of the participants, observing the events, processes, and activities in which they are involved. The degree to which the researcher takes part can range anywhere from complete observation to complete participation, but most often falls somewhere between the two extremes. Those who become involved in the social system of the setting have the advantage of familiarity with the environment and developing participants' trust; in this role, researchers are called **participant-observers.** Anthropologists who go to a new country, begin to learn the language, and participate in the culture are an example. Researchers who study aspects of the organizations in which they work also fall into this category, but they must exercise caution in negotiating the thin line between involvement in the daily setting and remaining detached enough to observe the process without bias. **Nonparticipant observers** enter the setting as outsiders to observe events and behavior. They are removed from the social process and must find **key informants**—individuals who are especially knowledgeable about what goes on and who are willing to talk with the researcher and provide explanations. Nonparticipant observers must find ways to negotiate and gain access to the setting, as well as earn the trust of participants. Both observers collect **field notes,** the rough, sometimes unorganized, record of the world they are studying. Field notes are the written accounts of what the researcher sees, hears, experiences, and thinks about in the course of collecting data in a qualitative study (Bogdan and Biklen 1997). Field notes are the detailed log of the developments of the study, providing the rich description upon which analysis is based. These notes can be portraits of participants, reconstructions of conversations, descriptions of the setting, and accounts of particular events and activities. Experienced qualitative researchers write notes down as quickly as possible, at least in outline form; then, they transcribe the notes *the same day* while ideas and details are still fresh.

Researcher's written observations of their own behavior, along with their hunches, insights, and revelations are called **reflective field notes.** Since the researcher is the measuring instrument, reflective field notes are used to document efforts to reduce bias, observed effects of the researcher on the setting, and anything else that might affect the data being gathered (for an in-depth analysis on the method of writing field notes, see Bogdan and Biklen [1997]). These notes may appear as a paragraph in the final manuscript, serving as an audit trail to help the reader judge the quality of the research.

Focused interviewing.   Methods of interviewing, too, range on a continuum from formal **structured interviews** to informal, casual **unstructured interviews.** Formal interview structures so rigidly controlled that respondents cannot tell their stories in their own words fall outside the range of qualitative interviewing. Qualitative structured interviews usually employ an **interview schedule,** a guide consisting of a list of open-ended questions flexible enough for the researcher to note unexpected responses and proceed with further exploration. Interview guides are particularly useful in multisubject and multisite research for gathering comparable data.

Casual interviews are often used in observational studies when the researcher needs clarification about what is happening or wishes to document feelings. Some studies, however, use interviewing, including open-ended interviewing, as their main data collection device. For example, the phenomenological researcher encourages respondents to talk generally about the area of interest, probes to expand on topics the respondent brings up, and focuses on issues of interest to the respondent; the subject thus defines the content of the interview. Qualitative researchers select structured or unstructured interviewing based on their research goal. Frequently, both types of interviewing are used at different stages of the same study.

Interviewing requires an ability to put respondents at ease, a skill that requires patience and practice (see Rubin and Rubin [1995] for a comprehensive guide). Most interviews begin with small talk, then progress to an explanation of the study, a discussion and signing of the informed consent form, and an overview of the way the interview will proceed. Gorden (1975) noted the importance of the opening question in a focused interview:

> There are several important and unique functions of the opening question. It may be broad enough to delineate the entire topic of the interview, or it may select a single point of departure. In either case, it should be clearly connected with the explanation of the interview so that the respondent is immediately aware that the interviewer is pursuing the stated purposes. If possible it should ask for information which is relatively easy for the respondent to give so that there is no chance of ego threat at the outset. The opener may also begin with a point on which the respondent feels particularly qualified to speak, thus appealing to his need for recognition. A well-phrased question might also demonstrate sympathetic understanding of the respondent's problems. (p. 279)

The use of **probes** conveys the researcher's interest in the respondent's statements. They also establish a basis for follow-up with further specific and focused questions in pursuit of the respondent's insights on the social process. Probes include such phrases as "That's interesting, tell me more about it," or "What do you mean by that?"

For short interviews, some researchers rely on memory and wait until later to write down answers. This allows for a very informal conversation with little distraction, but data can be easily lost or distorted. A comprehensive record of the interview can be created by taking notes or using a tape recorder. Taking notes can provide an adequate record, but it can slow the interview down and be distracting to both interviewer and respondent. Tape recording provides a complete account, but makes some respondents uncomfortable enough to inhibit their answers; some individuals refuse to give permission to tape record, and transcription of tapes can be time-consuming and expensive. Researchers who rely completely on tape recording are sometimes horrified to find that the interview is lost because the machine did not work properly. On occasion, the most useful information is obtained after the recorder is turned off.

In some cases it is desirable to interview groups of people to obtain insights into group perceptions, language, and beliefs. Known as **focus group interviews,** they are conducted by a skilled facilitator who guides discussion about topics that are important to the group being studied. Focus groups stimulate participants to freely express their beliefs, feelings, and needs, and are increasingly used in studies about sport. Gould and his colleagues (1999) conducted focus groups with eight Atlanta U.S. Olympic teams, four of which met or exceeded performance expectations and four teams that did not. They found that teams that met or exceeded expectations participated in resident training programs, experienced crowd and family or friend support, used mental preparation, and were highly focused and committed. Teams that did not meet expectations experienced planning and team cohesion problems, lacked experience, faced travel problems, experienced coaching problems, and encountered problems related to focus and commitment. Their descriptions could help Olympic coaches and athletes better prepare for future Olympic games.

Document analysis.   The researcher is the main producer of field notes and transcripts, but information produced elsewhere can also provide useful data. Bureaucratic agencies such as schools and health agencies produce written reports of internal and external communication that can help the researcher understand how the agency or school is defined by its workers and provide potential insight into internal rules and regulations. Documents such as newsletters, news releases, students' records, minutes from meetings, codes of ethics, and philosophy statements offer insight and understanding into the "official" perspective of the agency or school.

On occasion, personal documents written by respondents can also yield useful information. Intimate diaries and personal letters sometimes turn up in the course of interviewing or observation. Often a respondent will volunteer that the documents exist. These materials can be especially valuable in clarifying what respondents have experienced.

While historians depend heavily on documents, qualitative researchers are more likely to use them to augment information gained from observation or interviews. In profiling a teacher, for example, a journal of the teacher's early experiences can prove invaluable in gaining insight into the teacher's perspectives.

Photographs and videos.   Researchers use photographs to learn how people interpret their world. They are often available at schools and agencies in the form of newspaper releases and yearbooks, and can provide a useful sense of people no longer present, offering a historical rendering of the setting and participants. They may be helpful in adding to the evidence when used with other data. Researchers also take photographs and video recordings in the research setting. They can simplify the collection of factual information and serve as a record of events; they can give an idea of how people use a space such as a playground. Photographs and videos taken in the field can be a way to help the researcher remember detail, such as room layouts or classroom members. Showing a photograph to respondents can stimulate their insights and serve as a source of data.

Supportive Quantitative Data.   Quantitative data such as attendance counts, numbers of athletic injuries, achievement scores, and epidemiological data can be useful to the qualitative researcher. Such data can suggest trends of increase or decrease, provide descriptive information about the population, and be extremely useful in exploring the perceptions of respondents by asking whether respondents agree or disagree with the information presented. Most qualitative researchers use quantitative data in their studies to explore the context of the setting and the people.

Triangulation (LeCompte, Preissle, and Tesch 1993) is the process of cross-validation among researchers, research methods, and data sources. Cross-checking across different methods such as observations, interviews, and physical evidence contributes greatly to the study's validity. Flaws of one method can often be overcome by using another method; through cross-checking, events and processes for which data is insufficient can be clarified. For example, statements about program participation can be checked against records, or observations in a gymnasium can be clarified by interviewing instructors.

Triangulation among data sources assesses the accuracy of statements from such sources as administrators, students, and faculty. In constructing explanations, agreement among data sources helps ensure the adequacy of the analysis. If data are inconsistent, cross-checking is necessary to determine whom to believe. Triangulation among researchers involves checking the findings of other researchers who are taking similar measures at the same time, or following up a finding with another researcher to confirm it (Miles and Huberman 1994).

However one chooses to collect primary data, it is important to clearly state the researcher's role, because it is one aspect of gaining entry into the field. For example, if the role selected is one of a nonparticipant observer, officials at the research site will want to know exactly what this will involve (e.g., attending formal and informal meetings with respondents, being in the room with classroom activities, conducting casual interviews with students, and examining records and files). Since gaining entry to the field in most cases requires formal permission to conduct the study, most qualitative researchers write proposals that spell out exactly what data will be collected, how confidentiality of data will be handled, and how the setting stands to benefit from the results of the study. Maintaining good field relationships is crucial, and the researcher should attend to building trust and confidence.

Analyzing Data.   Qualitative researchers begin analysis of data almost immediately, and it proceeds along with data collection. Transcripts of conversations or written observations are examined to generate a tentative coding system from which categories of phenomena are derived. When a category is formed, all the incidents and conversations that appear to fit are compared. New categories are formed from old ones when some incidents initially coded for the old one do not fit. Once major categories are in place, the researcher then searches for trends and differences and inductively begins to synthesize explanations and phenomena. Explanations are checked and cross-checked for accuracy and understanding, and are modified to support new information. The researcher usually continues to observe or interview until no new information for codes and categories is obtained, that is, until the data are "saturated" (LeCompte, Preissle, and Tesch 1993). For a basic, helpful guide to data analysis, see Bogdan and Biklen (1997).

Qualitative researchers often use computer software programs to help interpret and manage the large amounts of text data they obtain. As cassette tapes with data are transcribed, the sentences are typed directly into the software using a word processor, or they can be transferred from another word-processed file using the "copy/paste" function of the word-processing program. Field notes, open-ended survey responses, and other text based documents can also be entered as data. Segments of data that are of interest to the researcher can then be marked with code words in order to look for patterns and meaning. The software is a tool that assists the researcher with the construction and testing of explanation, as well as relating theory to data. Examples of popular programs are *The Ethnograph* (1998) *NU*DIST* (1998), and *Nvivo* (1998). For more information about using computers in qualitative research, see Fielding and Lee (1993).

Writing Up the Research. Spradley (1997) asserts that what qualitative researchers do when they write their study is a translation. This is shaped by the evidence the researcher has collected and is supported by the words of the respondents. Papers are often written in first person and in active voice. No formal conventions are used to establish truth in a qualitative research paper (Bogdan and Biklen 1997). The task of the writer is to convince the reader of the plausibility of the presentation by quoting respondents, presenting short sections from field notes, and explaining triangulation methods. Alternative explanations, points of view of a minority of respondents, and problems in the study are frequently included to help the reader determine the accuracy and truthfulness of the research. Although the discerning reader will often have questions about the study, a well-written manuscript allows a reader who may not know anything about the phenomena to "see" it through the researcher's explanations and supporting data.

Trustworthiness of Qualitative Data

Qualitative studies are often criticized for their lack of "rigor," for making suggestions rather than reaching conclusions, and for lacking reliability and generalizability. Qualitative researchers tend to think about rigor differently than quantitative researchers, but qualitative studies can be rigorous. Lincoln and Guba (1985) suggest that qualitative data can be evaluated in terms of its "trustworthiness," and that the features of trustworthiness parallel the terminology of quantitative data, including internal validity (credibility), external validity (transferability), reliability (dependability), and objectivity (confirmability).

Credibility (or internal validity) in qualitative studies is largely controlled by the researcher. Because researchers may not know initially what they want to measure, perfect validity is theoretically impossible since it is difficult to know if measurement is appropriate (Henderson 1991). In qualitative studies, internal validity is related to the emerging theory, and findings should be credible if grounded theory corresponds to observations. To improve credibility, qualitative researchers (1) provide quotes and descriptions that support the conclusions; (2) use corroboration and triangulation techniques; (3) document data with extensive field notes; and (4) use **member checks,** or have study participants comment on the conclusions.

Transferability (or external validity) in qualitative studies is concerned with the degree to which the individuals studied are representative of individuals to which results might be generalized (Henderson 1991). There is much debate over whether qualitative results can or should be generalized, but qualitative researchers tend to think of transferability in terms of *kinds* of people or units that are examined, rather than *number* of people or units studied. Some researchers think of findings as working hypotheses or theoretical frameworks that can be transferred to other studies (Guba and Lincoln 1981). Transferability can be heightened by (1) careful explanations of the research setting and individuals; and (2) providing thick descriptions of data.

Dependability (or reliability) of qualitative data can be thought of as the closeness of fit between what researchers record as data and what actually occurs in the setting (Kirk and Miller 1986; Henderson 1991). There are those qualitative researchers who believe that reliability can be achieved similarly to the way it is achieved in quantitative studies (LeCompte, Preissle, and Tesch 1993). Others suggest that replicability is not important in qualitative studies because variables are not controlled (Marshall and Rossman 1999). There are a number of things that can be done to increase dependability: (1) carefully document the research plan, especially any changes in the plan that occur; (2) triangulate the methods used; (3) triangulate researchers to gather other data interpretations; and (4) document the researcher's role.

Confirmability (or objectivity) suggests that data are factual and reliable. The objectivity of qualitative studies that are factual and that report the differences in information collected in the study can be assessed by other researchers. Confirmability can be increased by (1) being clear about observations in the final report, and (2) providing several explanations for observations (Henderson 1991).

Judging the Merit of a Qualitative Research Article

While qualitative studies were once presented mainly in book format, they are now likely to appear as studies in research journals. A survey of these journals reveals very little standardization in research reports as yet. Style of reporting varies with the type of study and can range from the well-known format of most quantitative studies to "the creation of an evocative form whose meaning is embedded in the shape of what is expressed" (Eisner 1981, 6). Some qualitative research is so lacking in focus that it appears to have no design. Without standardized criteria on which to rely, the reader may have difficulty judging the quality of the study presented. The following questions have been compiled to assist the reader and provide guidance in evaluating the "quality" of a qualitative research article (LeCompte, Preissle, and Tesch 1993; Chilcott 1987; Smith 1987; Lincoln and Guba 1990; Wolcott 1990).

What are the study's goals? Purpose?

Are the research questions stated?

Why was this particular research setting chosen? How was entry obtained? How long and how regularly was the researcher involved in the setting? Is the setting described in sufficient detail to communicate a concrete picture to the reader?

What is the period of time of the study?

What evidence does the researcher provide for having obtained trust and rapport with the participants?

Is the researcher's role identified (participant-observer; observer; interviewer)?

Who actually collected the data?

Does the researcher report the use of a theoretical perspective? If not, can it be inferred?

How were respondents selected (convenience sample [available subjects]; theoretical sample [selected subjects by plan]; snowball sample [subjects named by other subjects])?

Is demographic information on respondents presented?

Is generalizability of the data addressed?

How does the researcher support the accuracy and truthfulness of the report (participant verification; comparable studies from supporting literature; triangulation of methods, data, researchers)?

How was data collection accomplished (note taking, tape recording, videotape)?

If interviews were used, what kind were they (structured, unstructured)? When during the study did the interviews take place? How is interview material combined with other data in the study?

Are direct quotations from participants used?

How does the researcher account for possible bias (reflective field notes, discussions with interested colleagues)?

What analytic strategies did the researcher use?

Is the researcher using a participant or personal approach to meanings (*etic* = external, perspective of the observer; *emic* = internal, participants' categories)?

How does the researcher support the stated conclusions? Does the researcher present negative evidence?

Does the report generally make sense (orderly, effective, logical)?

The reader should be able to answer the majority of the questions. The credibility of the results in qualitative studies depends in large part on the researcher's ability to demonstrate value and trustworthiness. This is why qualitative reports explicitly "tell" the reader a great deal about data collection methods and research conditions, including decisions to alter strategies, doubts, and concerns. Some recent articles include a paragraph written by one or more participant(s), particularly if they disagree with the researcher's conclusions; this honest difference of opinion is presented to help readers decide for themselves with regard to the study's credibility (Lincoln 1991).

Uses and Applications of Qualitative Data

Researchers in HHP conduct qualitative studies for a variety of reasons and audiences. An increasing number of qualitative studies have been conducted for purposes of making practical decisions about and improvements in programs, curricula, and practices. Program evaluation research has increasingly involved a qualitative component. Participant interviews and observations can add richly illustrative information to heighten understanding of the evaluation report. Qualitative methods can provide unique and valuable data about the motivations of participants, their adherence to health and fitness regimens, and their reasons for low participation rates in health promotion and adult fitness regimens, or, alternatively, high adoption rates by others. For example, Steckler, Eng, and Goodman (1991) combined quantitative and qualitative evaluation strategies to evaluate a health education workshop on combating childhood communicable diseases in Nigeria. Using focus groups and participant observation, they were able to improve the workshop's content and methods, and the program has been disseminated to other countries.

Qualitative research is also useful in pedagogy, the evaluation of curricula and teaching. Hastie and Buchannan (2000), through observations and interviews of students and a teacher, developed an improved hybrid model of Sport Education and teaching of personal and social responsibility (TPSR) called Empowering Sport, a curriculum model that included sport skill competence, social responsibility, and personal empowerment. Ennis and her colleagues (1999) used participant observation and interviews in their evaluation of the Sport for Peace curriculum and found that the curriculum's structures fostered shared responsibility for learning, trust, respect, and a sense of family, creating a class community more conducive to engagement and participation. Ennis and Chepyator-Thomson (1990) used qualitative methods to examine the learning styles of field-dependent children within a movement curriculum. Their observations enabled them to recommend changes in teaching styles to help field-dependent children function more analytically. A large curriculum evaluation project used naturalistic methods to explain results obtained quantitatively (McLaughlin et al. 1992). A randomized control trial of a high blood pressure curriculum for sixth graders revealed that comparable families diffuse information about hypertension differently. A qualitative investigation revealed profiles of "high transfer of information" and "low transfer of information" families, as well as typologies of the children and parenting styles, enabling changes to be made in the curriculum. Maatz-Majestic and Tapp (1992) used qualitative methods to explore strategies used by college students to avoid problems associated with alcohol and to study their definitions of responsible use. Health educators can use this information to develop more effective prevention strategies, because the study points out the need for specific and targeted messages in teaching about responsible decision making in the use of alcohol.

Qualitative methods can be used as a preliminary step to questionnaire or survey instrument design. Interviews with a sample of the survey population one wishes to study can provide insights into the meanings of such concepts as health, wellness, fitness, or leisure, thus enabling the construction of more reliable and valid instruments. Additionally, when researchers wish to study the continuum of behaviors of a population and little is known about a phenomenon, qualitative interviews can help reveal these many behaviors. In a study of self-care behaviors and multiple sclerosis, the researchers wanted to survey persons with multiple sclerosis regarding coping strategies, but the self-care actions that people took to manage symptoms, reduce depression, and promote well-being had not been systematically studied. Qualitative interviews with a sample of respondents uncovered a variety of behaviors for the management of multiple sclerosis and resulted in an inventory with items grounded in the perspectives and experiences of the population of interest (McLaughlin and Sliepcevich 1985). Qualitative research has always included basic work, and its explanatory powers ensure its application to programmatic, curricular, and action research.

Summary

The purpose of this chapter has been to present an overview of the process of qualitative research. Obviously, qualitative methods are not equally easy for all to use; it will be particularly appealing to those who enjoy interviewing and interacting with others. The best way to become a better qualitative researcher is to practice, and many universities now offer courses in qualitative design and research. Qualitative methods offer exciting options for HHP researchers asking questions about complex human issues in programs, behavior, and curricula.

Formative Evaluation of Objectives

Objective 1   Define qualitative research and its most frequently used synonyms, such as ethnography, naturalistic inquiry, and field research.

    1. Are there any differences among the four terms—qualitative research, ethnography, naturalistic inquiry, and field research?

    2. Which terms are used most frequently in your experience?

Objective 2   Outline differences between qualitative and quantitative studies:

    1. List the major differences between qualitative research and quantitative research regarding the following:

a) form of the data
b) sample size
c) focus of the research
d) role of the researcher
e) study design characteristics
f) researcher's involvement with subjects
g) generalizability of findings

2. Upon what major consideration does the decision to use quantitative or qualitative methods depend?

Objective 3   Identify major theoretical frameworks in qualitative research.

1. What is the importance of "interpretation" to the theory of symbolic interaction?

2. What are the goals and strengths and weaknesses of phenomenology?

3. How are interview questions derived in phenomenology?

4. Define grounded theory, and describe the final goal of this theory.

5. Compare and contrast critical theory and feminist theory.

Objective 4   Outline the general process for conceptualizing a qualitative study, framing the research question, collecting and analyzing data, and writing up a research report.

1. Why does one's original research outline often end up being a tentative plan in qualitative research?

2. Where does the qualitative researcher get ideas for study?

3. Give an example of a typical qualitative research question.

4. Compare and contrast the following data collection strategies:
   a) direct observation
   b) focused interviewing
   c) document analysis
   d) photograph and video analysis

5. Ask a qualitative researcher how he or she used triangulation in his/her study. What is the advantage of triangulation?

6. If you are planning a qualitative study at a fitness center in a corporate workplace, what are some things you could do to assure and maintain good field relationships?

7. What is meant by data "saturation"?

8. What is the major task of the author when writing a qualitative research paper? How does it differ from a quantitative research paper?

Objective 5　Describe the features of trustworthiness of qualitative data, including credibility, transferability, dependability, and confirmability.

1. Define "trustworthiness." What is your opinion of comparing quantitative and qualitative studies in terms of rigor?
2. What can one do to increase the credibility, transferability, dependability, and confirmability of qualitative studies?

Objective 6　Identify questions that can be used to evaluate the quality of a qualitative research article.

1. Use the list of questions to evaluate a given qualitative research article.
2. Why is there so much emphasis on research conditions, data collection strategies, and analysis in qualitative research articles?

Meta-Analysis 10

KEY WORDS

Meta-analysis   Effective size

OBJECTIVES

In this chapter, we present information concerning the meta-analysis approach in research. You should become familiar with this approach and the terms and techniques used with it.

After reading chapter 10, you should be able to

1. Understand why the meta-analysis approach is utilized.
2. Know how the meta-analysis approach is conducted.

Introduction

Meta-analysis is a relatively new approach in HHP research. Although used in disciplines outside of HHP since the 1960s, it was seldom utilized or discussed in HHP until the 1980s. The tutorial on meta-analysis by Thomas and French (1986) certainly brought the meta-analysis technique to the attention of many people in HHP. **Meta-analysis** is the reanalysis of the results from a large number of research studies in an effort to draw conclusions which are supported by many research studies. Thus, meta-analysis is much more than a review of related literature, as a part of an experimental or descriptive research study; it is the major thrust of the research study since it is the research approach.

Let's take a situation where the meta-analysis approach might be used. The question to be answered is whether warm-up is necessary before participating in physical performance activities. A large amount of research has been done on this topic. The results of the research are inconclusive; some point towards yes, some no. There are so many research studies to consider that it is impossible to read and keep track of all the information; you can't see the woods for the trees. Based on all of this research it is impossible to say whether warm-up is or is not necessary before participating in physical performance activities. Furthermore, if we examine the available research more carefully, we will find that the various studies differ in terms of the way the research was conducted. Some studies were conducted to see if warm-up was beneficial for participants to obtain their best score, while other studies dealt with the effects of warm-up on injury prevention. Some studies were conducted on high performance level athletes and other studies were conducted on novice performance level individuals. Further, some studies were conducted with physical performance activities requiring quick maximum exertion movements for a short period of time (like sprinting), while other studies were conducted with physical performance activities requiring slow submaximal exertion movements for a long period of time (like distance running). In addition, participants in these research studies varied in age (from 14 to 35 years) and in gender. Also, some research studies were conducted with large numbers of participants while other studies were conducted with three to five participants. In some research studies, a small difference was noted between warm-up and no warm-up; in other studies a large difference was noted. Do you give the same importance to both outcomes? Last, but not least, some research studies were conducted with excellent procedures and some research studies were conducted with marginally acceptable procedures. Do you give the same weight to both classifications of studies? What is the big picture here? The results obtained in a single research study may be dependent on one or more of the things just mentioned, and when all the research studies are considered, no conclusion can be drawn as to whether warm-up is necessary. It is much like mixing apples and oranges and getting fruit salad.

With meta-analysis the results from available research studies are reanalyzed and, if necessary, allowances are made for the variables that need to be controlled because they may influence the findings in a research study. In the earlier example, these variables could be training level of the participants, type of physical activity, age, and gender. Further, studies judged to have too small a number of participants and/or marginally acceptable procedures may not be used in the meta-analysis. Certainly, meta-analysis is not using all of the research studies available and counting the number of research studies which support each position of a research question. Meta-analysis has definite procedures with systematic steps which assist the researcher in drawing defensible conclusions. It is an approach where the information from a large number of research studies can be handled in an economical manner, minimizing the chance that the volume of information will overwhelm the researcher and subjective judgments will cause the researcher to draw incorrect conclusions. Presently, meta-analysis studies are commonly conducted in many different areas in HHP to synthesize the results from a large amount of research available on a topic.

The meta-analysis approach can be studied from the standpoint of using it in your research or understanding it when another researcher uses it. Obviously, to *use* meta-analysis in your research requires more knowledge than is required in simply understanding the meta-analysis approach when used by another researcher.

In the Department of Exercise Science at the University of Georgia, a meta-analysis course is taught and, in many universities, such a course is taught in HHP departments, in educational psychology departments, and elsewhere. A class seems to be the best way to learn about the meta-analysis approach. Books like Rosenthal (1991) are written about meta-analysis techniques. A discussion of meta-analysis may be included in some research books. Thomas and Nelson (1996) devoted a twenty-two-page chapter to the topic. Neutens and Rubinson (1997) devoted one page to the topic, in a chapter on analyzing and interpreting data. Tutorials in research journals and books (Thomas and French 1986; Dattilo 1992) and reading research articles in which meta-analysis is used are valuable in learning about the meta-analysis approach. A strategy in learning about the meta-analysis approach might be to read a short overview, like a book chapter or tutorial, concerning the meta-analysis approach to get a general knowledge of the approach and then read a research article in which the meta-analysis approach is used. Following this, if there still is an interest in and/or need to learn more about the meta-analysis approach, taking a meta-analysis course or reading a book dealing with the meta-analysis approach would be advantageous. The approach in this chapter is to provide a brief nontechnical overview of the meta-analysis approach so that you can understand it when another researcher uses it in a research study.

The first chapter in the Rosenthal (1991) book is a good introduction to the meta-analysis approach. Many of his other chapters are somewhat mathematically oriented. However, for the serious reader, his book is an excellent source. In chapter one he states that meta-analysis may be used to compare results from several research studies or combine results from many research studies. No matter whether the intent of the meta-analysis is to compare or combine research study results, the calculation of **effect size** is basic to the meta-analysis approach.

Effect Size

In chapter 1 of this text, the concept of conducting the research on a sample selected from a population was introduced. In chapter 13 dealing with inferential data analysis techniques, using information from a sample to estimate a population effect will be discussed. As presented in chapter 13, a sample is selected from a population and information obtained on the sample is used to estimate population information or effect. For example, if one sample from the population received training method A and another sample received training method B, and based on a statistical test, training method A was found to be superior to training method B, the researcher would infer that, for the population, training method A is superior to training method B. Although based on the statistical test, the researcher concluded that training method A is superior to training method B, there is no guarantee that the difference between the two methods is large enough to be of practical importance. If the sample who received training method A are 10 pounds stronger than the sample who received method B, that may be a practical difference, but if the difference is only .5 pounds, this is not a practical difference. An effect size is calculated in an attempt to estimate whether a difference is a practical difference. Effect size (ES) can be calculated in a variety of different ways depending on the research design and the intent of the research. Here is a common way of calculating ES:

ES = [mean score of Group A − mean score of Group B] / [standard deviation for one group or the standard deviation for the combined (pooled) groups].

For example, if the mean score for sample A is 75 and the mean score for sample B is 65 and the pooled standard deviation is 10, ES = [75–65] / [10] = 1.0. Cohen (1988) states that an effect size less than .20 is small, around .50 is medium, and greater than .80 is large. Thus, in the example, the ES of 1.0 is large and the difference (75–65) is probably a practical difference.

The inferential statistical test that a researcher uses to determine whether two samples differ in mean score is influenced by sample size (n). As sample size increases, the difference between the means to have a significant difference decreases. The sample size does not influence ES.

With the meta-analysis approach, an effect size is calculated for each research study used, so the same measurement or indicator is used for each research study when comparing or combining them. Thus, with the meta-analysis approach, each research study is like a human participant in experimental or descriptive research.

For example, a meta-analysis was conducted to determine if an exercise program was effective in increasing fitness. The researcher suspected that the number of weeks of exercise training would be an influencing factor and that there would be a large difference among studies in the number of weeks of exercise training. So, he analyzed effect size by classifications of weeks of exercise training. Ninety-eight of the 121 identified research studies were used in the meta-analysis. His findings were as follows:

Weeks of Training	Number of Studies	Effect Size
Less than 6 weeks	15	.01–.21
6–9 weeks	28	.19–.63
10–17 weeks	42	.51–.94
More than 17 weeks	13	.58–1.17

Mean ES = .61

In this example, if the analysis had not been conducted by weeks of training, the effect size would have been .61, which is medium size; whereas, from the analysis by weeks of training, large effect sizes were found, indicating practically significant differences. Further, if the meta-analysis had not been used, the researcher might not have been able to make any sense out of the 98 research studies.

As noted earlier, effect size can be calculated with a variety of different formulas. The formula presented where the difference (d) between the mean performance of two samples is used can have several different denominators, depending on the research design. Also, the d-formula is the one commonly used. However, there is another effect size procedure using a correlation coefficient (r). Correlation is introduced in chapter 12. Each procedure for calculating effect size has advantages and disadvantages. When reading meta-analysis studies you will find some where a correlation coefficient was used for effect size.

Steps in Meta-Analysis

As noted earlier, meta-analysis is often used within HHP, in many different areas. In some areas, you will see fewer meta-analysis studies than in other areas. If there are not many research studies available on a topic, there may not be enough research studies and/or a need to conduct a meta-analysis. Also, if the information needed to conduct a meta-analysis (means, standard deviations, correlation coefficients, and so on) is not published in research studies, a meta-analysis will not be possible. For example, this information is typically not published in a qualitative research study. As with all research approaches, a meta-analysis must be conducted in a systematic and carefully planned manner. The meta-analysis is only as good as the research studies and techniques used.

Step 1: Using several different literature search techniques, data bases referenced in chapter 2, and so on, compile a list of all research studies pertaining to the research topic for the meta-analysis. You might find, on the topic, a review article that has a large bibliography. Probably the review article contains only good research studies selected by the knowledgeable author of the article. In addition, some earlier meta-analysis articles on the topic and/or on a topic similar to your topic could yield a large list of references.

Step 2: Make a basic list of things that must be in any research study before you review the studies extensively. Probably you will have a large number of research studies and there is no reason to extensively review a research study if later you will not use it in the meta-analysis. If there is not enough information in the research study to calculate effect size, there is no reason to extensively review the research study. If the knowledge base for the meta-analysis topic is changing rapidly, you might decide to not review any research study that is more than ten years old. This decision might be the correct decision, but it might be perceived as an incorrect decision in that it eliminates any older classic studies and/or limits the generalizability of the meta-analysis study. Research studies not published in research journals or in books based on the research might be excluded from the meta-analysis. Theses and dissertations are unpublished and usually harder to obtain than research journal articles. Some researchers believe that if the research was good, it has been published in a research journal—which suggests that unpublished research is not to be trusted. Again, excluding certain research studies may or may not be the correct decision.

Research studies with small numbers of participants, maybe less than thirty, might be excluded, in that the research findings may be unique to the participants. Of course, it would be nice to review only good research conducted by knowledgeable people and published in good journals.

Step 3: Review each research study carefully, taking good notes concerning the basic information (author, research article title, journal name, journal volume and pages, date the issue of the journal was published), the number and type of participants in the research study, the type of treatment(s) applied to the research participants, the length of time of the study, the quality of the procedures used in the research study, the findings, and the information needed for calculating effect size. Moderator variables are factors which influence the relationship between two variables or effect size. If the relationship between two variables or effect size is not the same for males and females, gender would be a moderator variable. Moderator variables need to be identified and coded at this step. You must have the expertise to evaluate whether a research study was well conducted, because you don't want to use weak research studies in the meta-analysis. Keep a list of research studies reviewed and a list of research studies not reviewed, so you don't go back to a research study twice. It is important to get the necessary information in a research study the first time and apply the same standards to all research studies. A purpose of meta-analysis is to remove subjectivity as much as possible.

Step 4: Make decisions concerning what studies will be used in the meta-analysis and whether moderator variables like gender, age, physical or health characteristics will be considered in the meta-analysis. It is important here, as in step 2, to list the criteria used for *not* using a research study in the meta-analysis and to apply the criteria equally to each research study.

Step 5: Do the meta-analysis, calculating an effect size for each research study used. Summarize the effect sizes for all the research studies used and/or for each classification of participants in the research studies (moderator variables). Some researchers look at the spread in the effect sizes and/or the distribution of effect sizes to determine whether a moderator variable (s) need to be considered. If there is a large spread in the effect sizes and/or the distribution of effect sizes does not resemble a normal (bell-shaped) curve, this may suggest that the influence of a moderator variable (s) should be considered. Probably there should be at least five research studies for each level of a moderator variable. For example, if gender is the moderator variable, at least five research studies with males and five research studies with females are required. Probably this does not suggest that a meta-analysis study could be conducted using ten research studies. One of the purposes of meta-analysis is to synthesize the information from a large number of research studies. Often a moderator variable has more than two levels and there will be considerably more than five research studies for most levels.

Step 6: Write a report or journal article manuscript based on the meta-analysis. An extensive description of what was done in steps one through five is vital. The reader of the research report must know exactly what was done in the meta-analysis study in order to interpret and accept the results. In a study by Dishman and Buckworth

(1996), the authors listed the sixty-two sources referenced in the body of their article and the 127 research articles used in the meta-analysis. If this is allowed in a research journal, it is a desirable feature in terms of offering a complete report and a service to future researchers.

Computer Program

Conducting a meta-analysis becomes more demanding as the number of research studies analyzed increases and as the influence of moderator variables is considered. The use of a computer program to do most of the organizing and computing for the meta-analysis is desirable. Often a computer program is more accurate with computations and provides more information than a person conducting a meta-analysis by hand. The DSTAT program (Johnson 1993) is excellent. It comes with a very comprehensive manual. The program accepts data in a variety of different forms and provides a variety of different values. The sections of the manual are literature review tactics, conducting a meta-analysis review, general program operations and installation, calculation of effect size, management of effect size, analysis of effect sizes, and tutorial. In addition, the manual has an appendix where formulas used in the calculations are presented, as well as a list of references. Schwarzer (1991) has a program called Meta 5.3 which is shareware and follows the Rosenthal (1991) book closely. The program is commonly used.

Selected Meta-Analysis Studies

Dishman, R.K. and Buckworth, J. (1996). Increasing physical activity: A quantitative synthesis. *Medicine and Science in Sport and Exercise,* 28(6), 706–719.

Their research intent was to clarify the literature in the area. They conducted a meta-analysis of 127 studies that dealt with the effect of various interventions on increasing physical activity in people. Effects were expressed as correlation coefficients (r) and examined as they varied according to selected moderator variables.

Criteria for including a study and that the studies occurred between 1965 and August, 1995 were reported. The authors reported how many studies were excluded. All their methods are well explained. The mean effect was moderately large, r = .34. Effects for each moderator are reported in a table.

The many analyses which can be conducted as part of a meta-analysis are presented in this study. This is an example of using a correlation coefficient as the effect measure. The authors used a computer program called Meta. A bibliography for the 127 research studies used in the meta-analysis is provided. This study is a good example of how to conduct and report a meta-analysis.

Payne, V.G. and Morrow, J.R. (1993). Exercise and VO2max in children: A meta-analysis. *Research Quarterly for Exercise and Sport,* 64, 305–313.

Studies examining the ability of children to improve maximal oxygen uptake (VO2max) have yielded inconsistent findings. The researchers examined the effects of four moderating variables on the VO2max of children. Sixty-nine studies were located and twenty-eight met the criteria for inclusion.

The authors provided a brief overview of meta-analysis and cited references to studies in human performance where meta-analysis was utilized. They indicated that three computer searches were used to locate research studies. The criteria for including a research study were presented. Effect size (ES) was calculated for each study. Considerable differences in mean ES were found between contrasted groups formed by using the four moderating variables. Effect sizes of .35 to .94 were found. The authors found that the experimental design, cross-sectional or pretest-posttest, for a research study had an influence on the outcome of a study.

This article is easy to read and understand. It is an example of using ES. A bibliography for the twenty-eight studies used in the meta-analysis is provided. This article is a good example and could be read and understood by a person just starting to learn about meta-analysis. Note, Payne, Morrow, Johnson, and Dalton (1997) conducted a meta-analysis of resistance training in children and youth which the interested researcher might read.

Criticisms of Meta-Analysis

Meta-analysis is not the final answer. It only suggests what to do and what to control in a research study. It may be the combining of good and bad studies. It may be the combining of studies with small and large sample sizes. The research participants in the studies combined in the meta-analysis may vary too much in age and gender; or the study may vary too much in research setting, research methods used, and so on, to trust the findings of a meta-analysis. If there is a difference across moderator variables, but the moderator variables were not manipulated in the studies, then an inference concerning cause and effect cannot be made. Thus, a meta-analysis may be an unidentifiable mix applying to nothing specifically. Clearly, without a definition of the research issue and the population of interest before conducting a meta-analysis, this could be a criticism. There were some criticisms of meta-analysis based on methodological/statistical issues but generally these issues are now addressed in the literature in general and in the literature summarized in books like Rosenthal (1991).

Summary

The meta-analysis approach has been introduced and described. Students should realize that meta-analysis is an accepted research approach when reading the research of others and considering conducting their own research. Students should be able to evaluate the quality of a meta-analysis study conducted by another person and know some of the basic issues and procedures if they are considering conduct-ing a meta-analysis study. Finally, students must realize that they must learn much more than is presented in this chapter about meta-analysis if they are going to use the meta-analysis approach in a research study.

Formative Evaluation of Objectives

Objective 1   Understand why the meta-analysis approach is utilized.

1. What are several reasons for conducting a meta-analysis?
2. What can be accomplished with a meta-analysis which probably can't be accomplished with other approaches?

Objective 2   Know how the meta-analysis approach is conducted.

1. What are the major steps in conducting a meta-analysis?
2. What are some mistakes to avoid in conducting a meta-analysis?
3. What are some steps or procedures which are unique to the meta-analysis approach?

11

Additional Research Approaches

OBJECTIVES

This chapter contains information concerning three additional research approaches and an alternative to research. You should become familiar with each of them and the terms and techniques used with them.

After reading chapter 11, you should be able to

1. Understand what each of the three research approaches are and how they are conducted.
2. Understand the issues involved with creative activities and why they are an alternative to research.

The research approaches discussed in this chapter may not be as commonly used as the approaches discussed in chapters 7–10. The research approaches discussed may be used more often in one area of HHP than in another. Additional research approaches are presented for two reasons. One, you need to know the research approaches available to you as a researcher so that you select the best one for use in your research study. Two, you need to be aware that there are a variety of research approaches and appreciate all of them when reading the research of others. The potential problem is that if all the research you have ever encountered is experimental or is qualitative, you begin to think that it is the only research approach and all other approaches are not research. Often several research approaches are used in a research study. No matter what the research approach, if the research was conducted with good procedures, it is good research.

Three additional research approaches are discussed in this chapter: (1) historical, (2) epidemiological, and (3) single participant. In addition, creative activities as an alternative to research are discussed. The historical approach is a traditional one although not commonly used in HHP research. The epidemiological approach has possible uses in a variety of disciplines and situations related to health and disease. The single participant approach is another approach which is not new but not commonly used in HHP research. The creative activities as an alternative to research is traditional in the arts, and dancers in HHP do creative activities. Both the historical approach and creative activities were presented in the first and second edition of this book.

HISTORICAL APPROACH

The Nature of Historical Research

Using the historical approach, the researcher endeavors to record and understand events of the past. In turn, interpretations of recorded history help to provide better understanding of the present and suggest possible future directions.

Historical researchers, like those conducting experimental and descriptive research, are interested in discovering facts, trying to get at truth. While historians do make observations, they do so through the eyes of other people, those who witnessed a historical event or who wrote about it. Historical studies, like all research studies, involve the collection of data. These data are verified and interpreted following specific standards and then are presented as a report deemed acceptable after critical examination by others.

Historical research is important in HHP. These fields have a common past. A thorough study of the past can lead to an understanding of what each field in HHP has inherited and now serves as its roots. Each field has a history and a heritage from which its depth, tradition, and even its present is derived. History repeats itself. Why we do certain things today is based on what has happened to us in the past. What data may exist concerning the origin, growth, and development of the HHP disciplines? What problems were present and how were they solved? What societal and cultural pressures have affected HHP? What movements have come and gone? Which movements have remained and what form do they now take? Who were the pioneer leaders in each field of HHP? What were their contributions? If all of HHP was once under the umbrella of Physical Education, what was the genesis of the separation into what are now many well-defined fields of study? Who were some of the individuals responsible for the separatist movement? What are the historical justifications for changing the name *Physical Education* to *Kinesiology?* What trends, events, and relationships have dictated this name change?

In seeking data to answer these and other critical questions concerning past HHP history, we will discover that events occurred, ideas surfaced, and people came and went. More importantly, however, a study of the past can let our professions know how they have been shaped by it. What HHP is and what it might become in the future depends largely upon the impressions professionals hold about what HHP used to be and how it developed to the point where it is today. The historical approach is oriented to the past and the researcher seeks to cast light on a question of current interest by conducting an intensive study of material that already exists. Historical research can pull all the information in many scattered sources together in one source. Historical research can put on paper what lies in the memories of older people who were present at historical events. If it is not recorded, the information is lost when these people die. Information from individuals who have for many years attended the Masters Golf Tournament in Augusta, Georgia, can shed much light on that historic event and, in fact, the history of golf in the United States.

It frequently is the case in historical research that the collected data cause us to construct new interpretations of an event or person based on the information gained as a result of study. The assassination of President John F. Kennedy, the matter of whether or not President Zachary Taylor was poisoned, and the origin of the game of baseball are examples of past events whose interpretation has been altered based upon new data. Other historical research is more dramatic and gets higher visibility in seeking to find material not presumed to exist. A good example is the discovery of the Dead Sea Scrolls in 1947 by a group of Bedouins (Best 1981). This was an exciting happening, but such occurrences seldom take place.

Data Control and Interpretation

Historical research differs from other scholarly work because its subject matter, the past, is difficult to capture. This, in turn, makes interpretation of the past unique and difficult. Historical researchers, like those in experimental and descriptive research, utilize data. However, the researcher of history encounters problems with data that are different than those of the other approaches as Fox (1969, 407) pointed out:

1. These data already exist and new data cannot be generated, only found.
2. These data cannot be controlled in the same way they are controlled in the other research approaches.
3. Whatever data are found must be analyzed without clarifying the questions being asked.

In experimental research, for example, we often are concerned about the possible effects of extraneous and intervening variables and we try to control them. This is not possible in historical research. Many factors may have affected the historical data, but the historian can exercise no control over these factors. Typical of the factors that might have affected a document or event are memory, politics, censors, greed, jealousy, ulterior motives, ideology, ego, bias, and discrimination. Thus, historical researchers are faced with two problems in the development of their data. The researchers lack the basic elements of control necessary to produce data of the kind and form they wish, and then they must apply some frame of reference to the data if those data are to be meaningful (Fox 1969, 407).

The historical researcher cannot interpret words and events by using present day terminology. All interpretations must be done according to the meanings of that time. The researcher's task is to take information from a given time period and examine and interpret it from within the societal and cultural perspectives of that period. The meaning of words and use of terms change with time. Using the term *sports medicine* in interpreting the meaning of some athletic training event of fifty years ago would be improper because that term, while in vogue now, did not exist in 1942. Even the term *athletic training* would have to be used in the context of that time and not the way we interpret it today. It is important that the researcher becomes saturated with the educational, political, economic, environmental, and cultural habits of the period being studied. The better the researcher's background knowledge of the time period being studied, the better will be the interpretation of the facts and the more reliable the final report.

Sources of Historical Data

To provide data about the past, the historian must obtain considerable reliable information. To obtain this information, the researcher will consult two categories of material: **primary sources** and **secondary sources.**

Primary Sources

Primary source material consists of original documents or remains of documents and physical artifacts, or people who can provide eyewitness evidence where there is no intervening account of an event between its occurrence and its use by the historical researcher. A primary source is connected directly to the event; it is firsthand information.

Primary sources are of the utmost importance. "They are the basic materials of historical research" (Van Dalen 1959, 471). The historian always tries to obtain original material. The use of secondary kinds of informational sources when the primary ones are available constitutes a major mistake in this research approach.

Secondary Sources

Secondhand accounts of historical happenings, hearsay evidence, for example, constitute secondary source material. An interpreter is placed between the researcher and the historical event. This person is not tied directly to the event and, consequently, is not an eyewitness. Typical secondary sources are textbooks, newspapers, abstracts, almanacs, encyclopedias, and bibliographies. It should be noted that a source can be primary in one situation and secondary in another. This is particularly true in the case of textbooks and newspapers. Textbooks in recreation and park administration are normally considered a secondary source. However, if they are used to determine the depth and breadth of the content of such books, they are considered to be primary sources. Stories and written materials change and get taken out of context when repeated or rewritten over time. The good historical researcher has little faith in secondary sources, though they should be studied and checked out for correctness. Sometimes the lack of primary sources will lead the researcher to secondary sources, but this is the exception rather than the rule. In general, a secondary source cannot be depended upon to yield historical truth.

Evaluating Historical Data

Historical data, once gathered, must be critically evaluated to determine whether or not it can be considered as fact and, consequently, as historical evidence. This is a difficult and complicated procedure as the researcher attempts to determine such factors as authenticity, genuineness, worth, and accuracy.

External Criticism

The researcher uses **external criticism** to determine the authenticity, genuineness, and validity of the source of the data. Many questions are asked about the author, the time and place in which the document was written, the prevailing conditions of the era in which it appeared, and whether or not the document was a hoax or a forgery. Is the document on the concept of the right-to-life genuine? Did Dr. Jones really write the right-to-life paper? If he did write it, was he competent? Was he a truthful person? What motives did Dr. Jones have when he came out strongly against abortion and birth control devices and substances? Did his religious beliefs influence his stance on the concept? On what scientific studies did he base his stand? Is this Dr. Jones's original piece of work or a duplicated version?

In applying external criticism, researchers use several methods as pointed out by Neutens and Rubinson (1997, 210):

1. Physical and chemical tests of parchment, paper, cloth, wood, ink, paint, or metal are used to determine the age and authorship of a data source.
2. Tests of signature, script, handwriting, spelling, and type are used to check authenticity.
3. Consistency in language use, in knowledge and technology of the time period, and documentation are observed closely.

Historians today also enlist the aid of the computer in the authentication of historical data. Such was the case in November 1985 when the manuscript of a poem was discovered. The poem languished unnoticed in the Bodlein Library at Oxford University for 230 years. The poem, a love lyric of nine stanzas, was attributed to William Shakespeare. In an attempt to authenticate the poem as Shakespeare's creation, computer concordance was used. This technique reviewed all of Shakespeare's work and told exactly how often and in what context he used every word he ever wrote. Shakespearean scholars were immediately active with their criticism. Many agreed that the poem was too awful to be genuine and that the quality of lines like "Star-like eyes win love's prize when they twinkle," cast serious doubts about Shakespeare's authorship. They thought the poem was unconventional, that the rhythm was clumsy and the rhymes forced, and the style was utterly unlike Shakespeare's early style. One expert, quoted in an article that appeared in the *Bloomington Herald-Telephone,* 8 December 1985, doubted the poem's authenticity and added this comment, "It is something that a hack of some ability would write."

Internal Criticism

Internal criticism assesses the meaning of the content of the document. Interpretations are made to determine the value of the historical data, and the document or event is closely examined to establish its accuracy and worth. Did the event actually occur? If so, did it take place as it was described? How consistent is the writer's account with other reports about the same event? In the right-to-life example, one would seek to determine if Dr. Jones's statements were representative of health, medical, and historical facts. He may have been the true author of the document, but he may have twisted the truth, either accidentally or on purpose. Many of the statements may reflect bias and prejudice, thus negating the accuracy and value of the account. The author's motives for writing a document or describing an event should be carefully examined. It should not be surprising that the writings of medical science researchers and tobacco company researchers differ with regard to the effects of smoking on health. Have the environmentalists taken liberty with the truth when they produce scathing literature concerning the "facts" of human destruction of the environment? Whether the historical event took place is usually quite easily established, but affirming that it happened *as described* is often difficult. In most instances two or more independent sources, preferably primary ones, are needed to verify a historical fact.

Historical researchers, then, use both types of criticism, but especially that of internal criticism. It must be applied to documents, events, and published and unpublished studies in an attempt to avoid conclusions that may end up being quoted and requoted widely, disseminating a great deal of false information over a long period of time.

Oral History

Oral history research is conducted through taped interviews with individuals who are in a position to be able to recall their involvement and perceptions of various events and movements. Much excellent historical data has been obtained by interviewing people who have made contributions to the fields of HHP. Since 1985, the Oral History Research Center at Indiana University has conducted interviews with current and retired faculty members. Data were gathered from the current faculty members on their perceptions of issues as broad as the quality of life of today's professor, as well as more personal concerns regarding rewards and recognition, research and teaching, and strategies and opportunities for career development. Interviewing retired faculty will add a historical dimension enabling the origins of today's academic priorities and problems to be traced and preserving the memories of those who came before.

There are many ways to handle interviews and the information they provide. For oral history purposes, these seem to be the major considerations:

1. All taped oral history needs to be written down and preferably edited by the person who provided the account.

2. When using the interview technique the content should be written from the researcher's notes, verbatim as much as is possible.

3. The questions asked and how they are asked are most important. Leading questions should not be asked. The researcher should aim to draw out the individual's personal views and feelings, avoiding any tendency respondents may have to say what they think the interviewer wants to hear.

4. Interviewing can be tiring for the person interviewed. Several sessions with the same person may be necessary, but should last no longer than about one hour.

5. Let the person to be interviewed know in advance what topics will be covered so that some preparation can be made.

6. The person conducting the interview should have read the literature concerning the topic(s) about which questions will be asked.

In analyzing data from oral sources, a strict application of external and internal criticism should be observed. Information provided by the oral source can be very subjective and opinionated. Some people have a tendency to embellish past events to make a better story. With older people, memory can be a problem. The researcher should make every effort to maintain historical standards, at the center of which is objectivity, when evaluating the data and writing the oral history report.

Biographical Research

Biographical historical research presents yet another avenue for the professional in a field of HHP to gain further insight into the background of that field. Studying the life, career, and contributions of former leading scholars, teachers, coaches, administrators, dancers, health educators, and recreators can provide a better understanding of the philosophies and movements that are the foundation of current thought and activity in the Health and Human Performance arena. Nevins (1938, 349) stressed biographical study because it "humanizes the past and enriches personal experiences of the present in a way that history can seldom do." Appropriately, the subjects of biographies have been leaders with outstanding professional credentials, their legacies preserved through careful and objective evaluation of their contributions to their respective fields. At the same time, the heritage of each HHP field will be kept and maintained.

Biographical research emphasizes the use of primary source materials and applies external and internal criticism to evaluate the data. Grosshans (1975) completed an excellent biography on Delbert Oberteuffer and his contributions to the fields of health and physical education. Besides extensive personal interviews with Oberteuffer, she talked to his family members, childhood friends, fellow students, professional colleagues, and former employees. In determining the worth of the data obtained from these individuals, Grosshans applied questions originally formulated by Van Dalen (1964), such as:

1. Was the position, location, or association of the contributor favorable for observing the conditions he reported?
2. Did emotional stress, age, or health conditions cause the contributor to make faulty observations or an inaccurate report?
3. Did the contributor report on direct observation, hearsay, or borrowed source material?
4. Did the contributor write the document at the time of the observation, or weeks or years later?
5. Did the contributor have biases concerning any person, professional body, period of history, old or new teaching methods, educational philosophy, or activity that influenced his writing?
6. Did the contributor contradict himself?
7. Are there accounts by other independent, competent observers that agree with the report of the contributor?

The biographer encounters many of the problems typical of most historical research. The following list represents some of the items that can become problematic in a biographical study:

1. Faulty memory of the primary source people.
2. Inability to interview a primary source person of great potential value.
3. Failing to discover a potentially strong primary source person or document.
4. Responses of a living subject of the biography could be biased and could color those of other primary source people.

Hypotheses in Historical Research

Historical studies do not always begin with a hypothesis. If the researcher has no reason or basis for predicting what may or may not be found, then the study will be hypothesis-free. More frequently, however, the researcher develops hypotheses about what the historical data are expected to show. In a 1978 study of the influence that L. B. Sharp, an early leader in the American outdoor education movement, had on the lives and careers of selected educators and youth leaders, Piercy (1978, 3) hypothesized that (1) there is evidence of Sharp's influence on these educators and leaders, and (2) the educators and leaders consider Sharp's personality to be a major asset in his ability to lead. If the gathered evidence supports the predictions, they thus are confirmed. However, they are rejected if the evidence refutes them.

Hence, hypotheses are formulated in an attempt to explain historical phenomena. The goal in testing these hypotheses is to extend our knowledge base concerning historical events, people, and occurrences. Historical research must teach.

Historical Research in HHP

Interest in historical research in HHP has flourished in recent years. In each associated field a group of scholars is devoted to the cultural history of that field of study. Physical education developed a sport history discipline that led to the formation of the North American Society for Sport History (NASSH) in 1973. The publication outlet for sport scholars is the *Journal of Sport History*. An increasing number of sport historians are producing a large body of accurate and insightful work. Many of these researchers reside in major universities offering graduate HHP programs through which students can pursue advanced degrees in history. The curricula for these degrees include courses in history, anthropology, sociology, psychology, and philosophy to collectively provide a broad background for quality historical research.

Great strides have been made in recent years by health education and recreation educators to increase interest in historical research. Each field maintains archives and holds symposia dealing with historical research. The majority of historical studies conducted by HHP graduate students have been sport history reports, biographical sketches of leaders, and treatments of the historical development of agencies, organizations, and athletic conferences. A major and continuing limitation for graduate students interested in engaging in historical research has been a lack of sufficient time to complete a historical project. It is difficult to predict in advance just how long the project will take. The search for new data could take years, and the development of concepts and insights in relationship to the data takes additional time. Graduate students, in most instances, do not have the financial resources to permit them to spend an indefinite period completing a degree. Hence, many graduate students in HHP, while they may be interested in history, opt to do experimental or descriptive research projects which usually consume less time than historical work. The fields of Health and Human Performance offer a wide range of topics for historical research. Following is a brief list of varied topics that have been studied by professionals, including students, in those fields:

1. *A Century of Women's Basketball* (Hult and Trekell 1991).
2. "Hanya: Portrait of a Pioneer: The Story of Dancer/Choreographer Hanya Holm" (Andrews and Drake 1991).
3. "George Warren Donaldson: His Professional Philosophy, Influences and Contributions to Outdoor Recreation" (Stoner 1990).
4. "Prized Performers, but Frequently Overlooked Students: The Involvement of Black Athletes in Intercollegiate Sports in Predominantly White University Campuses, 1890–1972" (Wiggins 1991).
5. "A History of Intercollegiate Soccer in the United States of America" (Baptista 1962).
6. "The Origin and Development of Adapted Physical Education in the United States" (Bishop 1963).
7. *"Out of Many, One: A History of the American College of Sports Medicine"* (Berryman 1995).

EPIDEMIOLOGICAL APPROACH

Epidemiological research is conducted in many disciplines. In HHP, researchers in public health and physical activity commonly conduct epidemiological research. Dishman, Heath, and Washburn (in press) in their book, *Physical Activity Epidemiology,* address the topic. Neutens and Rubinson (1997) have a chapter on analytical epidemiological studies. Epidemiological research can be descriptive, with the intent to identify patterns, trends, and so on, in disease, injury, or death. However, epidemiological research can be more than descriptive, with the intent to determine *causation* of disease, injury, or death. This is what Neutens and Rubinson (1997) call analytic epidemiology. They state that epidemiology may be thought of as the study of health. There is a body of knowledge and methodology which is common to epidemiological research, but there may be slight variations in terms and methods, depending on the area in which the research is being conducted. Dishman, Heath, and Washburn (in press) discuss epidemiology in terms of physical activity. Other authors approach the topic in terms of factors other than physical activity as these effect health.

Research Designs

Dishman, Heath, and Washburn (in press) state that a research design is the way research participants are grouped according to some variable like physical activity or fitness, or other factors that might explain the occurrence of health-related events like injury, disease, or death. The intent of the research design is to allow the researcher to conclude that the independent variable (e.g., physical activity or fitness) explains changes in the dependent variables (e.g., disease, injury, or death). Thus, there needs to be a period of time between the change in the independent variable and the change in the dependent variable. When change in the independent variable is influenced by the researcher, the design is experimental. However, if the change occurs as a result of everyday life, the design is observational (descriptive). If the independent and dependent variables are manipulated or observed over time, the design is longitudinal or prospective. If, in the study, the researcher looks back in time after the dependent variable (disease, injury, or death) occurred to see the influence of the independent variable, the design is retrospective.

Neutens and Rubinson (1997) present basically the same information as Dishman, Heath, and Washburn (in press) but in a slightly different manner. Neutens and Rubinson state that there are two commonly used methods in analytic epidemiological research. The purpose of each is to determine if there is a cause-and-effect relationship between a risk factor (e.g., smoking, obesity) and a disease, injury, or social condition (e.g., welfare classification). **Cohort studies,** also called **prospective studies,** begin with a group of people (a cohort) who are observed over a period of time. The members of the group will differ in exposure to a risk factor being observed (e.g., smoking). They are observed to determine if there is a relation between degree of exposure to a risk factor and rate at which a characteristic (disease, injury, or death) occurs. Neutens and Rubinson list advantages and disadvantages of the cohort study. **Case control studies,** also called **retrospective studies,** have a group who already have the characteristic (health problem) and a group who do not have the characteristic. The groups are compared in terms of a risk factor (e.g., smoking) to determine if there is a relationship between the risk factor and the characteristic. The group who have the characteristic are called the **case group** while the group who do not have the characteristic are called the **control group.**

Dishman, Heath, and Washburn (in press) state that clinical trials are used to determine if a relationship between an independent and dependent variable is a cause-and-effect relationship. This requires a study (clinical trials) with a treatment group and a control group selected from a population. Many times the treatment (e.g., exercise) would have to be administered for years before any effect might be seen on the dependent variable (e.g., heart attack). Thus, a study of this type is prohibitively expensive. An alternative to a study of this type might be to study survivors of heart attacks to determine if the amount of exercise after the heart attack had any effect on the recurrence of heart attacks, or on the seriousness of recurring heart atttacks, if any recurred. Studies of this type have been done on a small scale on a few occasions.

Dishman, Heath, and Washburn (in press) indicate that there are a variety of other research designs which could be used to investigate a cause-and-effect relationship between physical activity, or fitness, and disease, injury, or death. The limitations of each design are dependent on how well the design satisfies the ten cardinal principles of causal inference presented by Paffenbarger (1988). These ten principles are listed in table 11.1 of this text. The ten principles are not ones we have considered in other research approaches. Further, the ten principles are essentially criteria for judging whether a research design is a good one. Dishman, Heath, and Washburn (in press) discuss each of the ten principles in detail. Such a discussion is beyond the scope of this chapter, but a few comments about each principle should help you understand them. For principle one, strength of association, Dishman, Heath, and Washburn (in press) indicate that studies must show a statistically meaningful association between physical activity, or fitness, and health (disease, injury, or death). The most common statistics used to measure the size of an association are relative risk, odds-ratio, and attributable risk. These statistics are not presented in all statistics books and not presented in chapters 12 and 13 of this book. They are commonly presented in research and statistics books in health and epidemiology. In addition to Dishman, Heath, and Washburn (in press), Kuzma (1998), *Basic Statistics for the Health Sciences,* and Neutens and Rubinson (1997), *Research Techniques for the Health Sciences,* present the formulas for these statistics. So, we find some statistics in the epidemiological approach to research which are not used in some other approaches. An overview of these three measures of association is presented below.

Data in an epidemiological study are typically organized and analyzed in a two rows and two columns table (2x2 table). The rows correspond to the levels of the independent variable (risk factor) and the columns correspond to the levels of the dependent variable (health characteristic). In a 2x2 table, the value in each of the four cells (squares) is the number of people with the row and column classification. For example, in table 11.2 the rows are inactivity (no exercise) and the columns are a health problem (a disease). In table 11.2, 200 people were inactive and 60 of them had health problems. **Relative risk** (RR) is the percent of incidence (health problem) rate for inactive people divided by the percent of incidence rate for active people:

TABLE 11.1 The Ten Cardinal Principles of Causal Inference

1. Strength of Association
2. Dose-Response Relationship
3. Independence
4. Temporal Sequence
5. Persistence
6. Alterability
7. Agreement
8. Consistency
9. Biologic Plausibility
10. Experimental Confirmation

Table adopted from Paffenbarger, R. (1988). Contributions of epidemiology to exercise science and cardiovascular health. *Medicine and Science in Sports and Exercise, 20* (5), 426–438.

TABLE 11.2 Example of a Two-by-Two (2 x 2) Table				
		HEALTH PROBLEM		
		Yes	**No**	**Total**
INACTIVITY	**Yes**	60	140	200
	No	40	360	400
	Total	100	500	600

Inactive percent rate = 60/200 = 30,   Active percent rate = 40/400 = 10

$$RR = 30/10 = 3.0$$

RR is interpreted as the health problem is three times more likely to occur in the inactive group than in the active group.

Odds ratio (OR) is the most common measure of association in case-control or retrospective studies. It is an estimate of relative risk. It is the ratio or odds of health problems in inactive people relative to the odds of health problems in active people. In table 11.2 , OR = (60)(360)/(140)(40) = 3.8. The interpretation of the odds ratio is similar to relative risk. Inactive people have 3.8 times the odds of having health problems as compared to active people. Neutens and Rubinson (1997) state that relative risk and attributable risk are used in cohort studies while odds ratio is used in case-control studies.

Attributable risk (AR) is an index of the percent of cases in the total group that occur in the inactive group, so it is calculated as the difference in the percent of cases for the total group and the inactive group divided by the percent of cases for the total group. In table 11.2,

Total group percent = 100/600 = 16.7   Inactive group percent = 60/200 = 30.0

$$AR = (30 - 16.7)/16.7 = 80\%$$

Principle two from Dishman, Heath, and Washburn (in press), dose-response relationship, means that there is a pattern of relationship between change in the independent variable (e.g., physical activity) and change in the dependent variable (e.g., disease, injury, or death). If every time the independent variable changes by one, the dependent variable changes by a constant amount, this would be the dose-response relationship. Principle three, independence, means that the dose-response pattern is unrelated to or independent of other factors which are related to the independent and dependent variables. Thus, changes in the independent variable caused the dependent variable to change. Temporal sequence, principle 4, deals with groups starting out equal in an experiment. For example, active and inactive participants started the research study equally healthy, so if at a later date the physically active group are more healthy than the inactive group, it may be due to the amount of exercise. Also, temporal sequence means the measurement of activity must precede the measurement of health (disease, injury, or death) and the time lag between the measurement of activity and the measurement of health is long enough to permit the change in the health measure to occur. Persistence, principle 5, is considered once a temporal sequence has been established. The researcher should determine whether the association between physical activity and health (disease, injury, or death) holds (persists) over time. If it doesn't hold, the beginning determination that physical activity and health are associated is a chance occurrence. Alterability, principle 6, deals with showing that changing or altering people's fitness level changes their health (disease, injury, or death) level. Changing fitness levels may be accomplished by a treatment in an experiment or observing change in fitness level over time. Agreement, principle 7, deals with the findings of many studies showing the same results. When studies do not agree, it must be determined why they differ and whether it is a design problem. Consistency, principle 8, is determining that findings of a research study are similar for different types of people, different parts of the country, etc.

Biologic plausibility, principle 9, is considered if all the preceding principles have been met. The researcher still must show that the association found between physical activity and health is due to physical activity causing biological changes in the research participants which are in agreement with present-day knowledge about the injury, disease, or death. Finally, experimental confirmation, principle 10, is needed. Experimental confirmation is conducting an experimental research study on a large number of people and confirming that increased physical activity caused a reduction in the rate of injury, death, or disease. So, we see ten things to consider in epidemiological research which we have not considered in other research approaches. Neutens and Rubinson (1997) discuss establishing causation and list seven possible ways which are similar to or the same as the ten cardinal principles presented by Dishman, Heath, and Washburn (in press).

Dishman, Heath, and Washburn (in press) discuss several research designs based on how well these satisfy the ten cardinal principles of causal inference. Discussed are the cross-sectional design, retrospective case-control design, and prospective cohort design. The authors indicate that the cross-sectional design is not a strong design. The retrospective case-control design is a common design used to discover the cause of health-related events (disease, injury, or death) after these have occurred. The prospective cohort design is a common design which permits observation of the characteristics and behaviors of a group or cohort of people across time. It is better than a retrospective design for showing cause and effect. Neutens and Rubinson (1997) also present an informative discussion of epidemiological designs, including advantages and disadvantages of the cohort method and the case-control method.

Epidemiological Research

There is an epidemiological section in the journal *Research Quarterly for Exercise and Sport.* There is not an epidemiological article in each issue, but many articles can be found. The December 1995 special issue is devoted to epidemiological related research. The journal *Medicine and Science in Sport and Exercise* has an epidemiology section with at least one article in each issue. The references for any epidemiological study found in a research journal can lead you to many more articles. The *American Journal of Public Health* and the *International Journal of Epidemiology* are two other sources for epidemiological research articles.

SINGLE PARTICIPANT APPROACH

Participants in a research study used to be called "subjects," so this approach used to be called "single subject research." Since researchers are now encouraged to use a term other than *subject,* we use the term *participant,* and discuss the single participant approach or **single participant research.** Single participant research is quite common in some areas and seldom used in other areas. It is conducted on the individual level with the performance of each research participant analyzed, rather than on the group level with the performance of the group analyzed. When the group of research participants is small and/or when each research participant responds to a treatment in a different manner, analyzing the performance of each research participant is often the best research approach. Single participant research is not a new approach. Books are published on single participant research (Johnson and Pennypacker 1993; Poling and Fuqua 1986; Kratochwill and Levin 1992), and college courses are taught on the topic. Basically with the single participant approach, for each research participant in a group the initial status or **baseline** for the participant is determined, a treatment is administered to the participant, the participant is measured again, and the treatment score is compared to the baseline score of the participant. In cases where the treatment does not cause a permanent change in the ability of a participant (e.g., a drug is administered and the effect of the drug wears off in time), the participant may be measured a third time to see if he/she has returned to baseline. In fact, the procedure of collecting a baseline measure, measuring the effect of a treatment, and measuring to determine if a research participant has returned to baseline can be expanded to multiple trials of the same treatment or more than one treatment. What has just been described is found in exercise physiology, biomechanics, pharmaceutical, teaching/learning, adapted physical education, and adult fitness studies.

Background

Recognition must be given where credit is due. At the 1998 National Convention of the American Alliance for Health, Physical Education, Recreation and Dance, Dr. Hans van der Mars from Oregon State University presented a half-day workshop on single participant research. Also, at the 8th Measurement and Evaluation Symposium in 1996 at Oregon State University, Drs. Roger James and Barry Bates presented a paper on single participant designs. Much of the material presented in this section of the chapter comes from these two sources.

Some people believe that number of research participants equals one is new, that research using single participant designs is not as rigorous as, research using group designs, that maybe single participant designs are not even research, and, finally, that research using one or several research participants is always single participant research. None of these are true. Single participant research was conducted in the 1960s and in areas like chemistry and physics. There are defined procedures in single participant research; thus, a case study with one person is not necessarily single participant research. Single participant research is often conducted with more than one research participant.

Van der Mars (1998) discussed single participant designs with reference to Applied Behavior Analysis (ABA). ABA is "applied" because the focus is on important behavior which is important to an individual or to society, "behavior" because the focus is on behavior to be changed, and "analytic" because the intent is to show enough experimental control to establish a functional relationship. Additional features of ABA are "technology," which is describing the experimental procedures so well that others can replicate them; "generality," which relates to behavior change which continues after the treatment is terminated and may spread to other behaviors, persons, and/or situations; "effective," which relates to how much behavior change is required for it to be considered important; and "conceptually systematic," in that the procedures should be tied to principles of behavior. So, ABA can occur in many different settings. A common question in exercise and sport science is what environmental variables are basic to having a particular behavior occur. This question can be addressed using ABA.

With ABA the data collected are often of frequency (how often something occurs) or duration (how long did a response last). Since the focus is on the individual, the analysis is on the individual. If the analysis had been on the group level, often no pattern of response would have been found, but with the analysis at the individual level, some patterns were identified. For example, if each person followed a different pattern of response across multiple treatments or measurements, the average (mean) score for the group might not change across treatments but each individual changed considerably across treatments.

James and Bates (1997) discussed single participant research as used in biomechanics, in a variety of other areas of exercise science, and in related areas. There is a great deal of similarity between what they and van der Mars (1998) presented. James and Bates (1997) have a good discussion of "individual analysis techniques" as compared to "group analysis techniques." Individual analysis techniques were the practice, but based on the work of statisticians in agriculture, group analysis techniques are the practice today. The question for the researcher is whether the interest is in the performance of a group or the performance of the individual.

Biomechanically, the many differences among individuals result in a huge number of different ways to perform a physical task. The Caster and Bates study

(1995) is a good example. Landing force before and after adding weight to a participant's ankles was measured. The difference in the landing force measures of a participant was negative, zero, or positive, depending on the participant. The authors explained that this was because the participants used a variety of different landing strategies. Bates (1996) suggested that a wide variety of movement options exist among different individuals and at different times for the same individual. Numerous other authors have shown the existence of strategies affecting performance scores.

Bates (1996) stated that individuals should be the unit of analysis in a research design when the goal is to understand or affect behavior in areas like high level performance, learning, injury, and so forth. James and Bates (1997) defined a single participant design as one where one individual serves as the unit of study. This is consistent with what van der Mars (1998) presented. The behavior or performance of each participant is evaluated across time and under different treatment conditions with the participant serving as his own control (Kazdin 1982). Single participant designs are used when studying the behavior of individuals and when large groups are not available (Bouffard 1993). Bates (1996) presented an excellent discussion of the rationale for and use of single participant designs as well as did James and Bates (1997). When the amount of variability among research participants suggests that they are heterogeneous rather than homogeneous in their response to a treatment, the use of a single participant design rather than a group design seems in order. If research participants respond in a variety of ways to a treatment so that positive, negative, and no change occur, a group design will probably lead the researcher to conclude that the treatment was not effective, whereas an appropriate single participant design will identify the fact that there were three different types of response to the treatment. A criticism of single participant designs is that it seems to be impossible to generalize results from the sample in the research study to a population. However, considering possible problems in analyzing the data of a heterogeneous group, the same criticism might be made of group designs.

James and Bates (1997) summarized the arguments for using single participant designs and recommended the following: (1) use single participant designs to examine an individual's performance, (2) use a series of similarly conducted single participant experiments to support generality of conclusions, and (3) use both single participant and group data analysis to better interpret the data. For the reader with a real interest in single participant designs, following the James and Bates (1997) paper is Zhu's (1997) response to that paper.

Data Collection and Analysis

The starting point is collecting baseline data. Before any behavior change treatment is applied, baseline data is collected on each research participant. Van der Mars (1998) used the terms "independent variable" and "intervention" where "treatment" may be used more in this chapter. All terms are intended to indicate an effort to change the "dependent variable" which in the broadest terms is some behavior. This baseline data is seldom based on one occasion (trial, session, day). Baseline data is collected until stability in the data of a research participant is established. Usually this is established by graphing the data for each research participant and seeing that the data path is reasonably flat. A graph is presented in figure 11.1 with "A" the baseline data and "B" the treatment data. Graphing is nice because you can see the data path developing as you collect data rather than at the end of the study as in a group analysis. A stable baseline enables the researcher to "predict" or expect that the data path would continue in the same manner if more data were collected. Also, a stable baseline allows the researcher to "verify" that the data path changed when a behavior modification treatment was applied and that the data path returned to baseline when the treatment was removed. Finally, a stable baseline allows the researcher to "replicate" the response to the behavior modification treatment by repeatedly applying the treatment and observing that it caused a response. This reduces the likelihood that other variables may have caused the response to the behavioral change treatment.

In terms of data analysis issues in single participant research designs, James and Bates (1997) suggested that the interested reader consult Barlow and Hersen (1984) and Edgington (1987). James and Bates (1997) and Bates (1996), among others, encourage researchers to consider the use of nonparametric rather than the more commonly used parametric statistical tests. In chapter 13 of this book, many common parametric statistical tests and a few common nonparametric statistical tests are presented.

As with all research approaches, there are many methodological and technical issues that must be addressed. Some formal training, background reading, careful planning of the research, experience with the research approach, and so forth, are essential to successful conduct of a research study using a single participant design. Addressing the methodological and technique issues in a study conducted with a single participant is beyond the scope of this book. Consulting books on the topic and reading research articles where the single participant approach was used is vital for students who want to use the single participant approach. Representative articles other than those cited elsewhere are DeLuca and Holborn (1992), Grant, Ballard, and Glen (1990), Houston-Wilson, Dunn, van der Mars, and McCubbin (1997), and Rushall and Pettinger (1969).

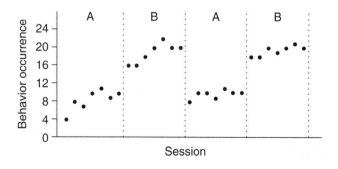

FIGURE 11.1
Graph of the data for a single participant study (A = baseline data; B = treatment data).

Designs

Remember, designs are just ways of organizing and conducting a research study. A number of designs are commonly used in the single participant approach. The simplest design is an A-B design where A represents collecting baseline data and B represents collecting treatment data. The design is seldom used any more. A more common design is an A-B-A-B design. In this design the baseline and treatment scores are replicated. A variation of this basic design is an A-B-A-B-A-B-A-B design. Notice replications seem to be in multiples of two (2, 4, 8). Another variation is utilizing two treatments in an A-B-A-BC-A-C-A-BC design. This design has limitations. On occasion you may see a B-A-B design. In all these designs the treatment (B) must be such that it wears off and research participants have the potential to return to baseline. If the treatment was an exercise program which would cause a permanent change, an A-B-A design would be impossible to use.

Single participant designs do not have to be simple. Multiple baseline designs are available. Sharpe, Lounsbery, and Bahls (1997) used one. There are changing criterion designs where each phase serves as the baseline for the next phase. A group design (3x3x2x2 Analysis of Variance Design with 30 scores per cell) could be duplicated with a single participant design. However, with all designs there are some concerns about the interpretation of data from single participant designs (Schutz and Goodman 1982; Bates, Defek, and Davis 1992).

CREATIVE ACTIVITIES

Introduction

If a person develops or produces something new, unique, or beautiful, some people call it **creative research;** others call it **creative activity.** Creative research, or creative activity, is presented in this text because it is important to be aware of the possible alternatives in situations where research is a job requirement. In the first edition of their introduction to research text, Thomas and Nelson (1985) included a chapter titled "Creative Research." At many colleges and universities, promotion is based partially on research productivity in the form of research publications. However, at many of these institutions the promotion guidelines list the requirement as "research or creative activity." That reference has allowed faculty members in fine arts departments to substitute creative activities for research productivity. Generally, faculty members outside fine arts departments have not been allowed to make this substitution.

So, what is creative research or creative activity in a fine arts department? For an artist, it is producing a beautiful picture; for the sculptor or potter, it is producing a beautiful object. Creative activity for the musician is playing beautiful music or writing beautiful music. The individual in dance or drama who performs at a very high level or produces outstanding dances or plays is engaging in that particular form of creative activity.

Creative research or creative activities are not restricted to a fine arts department. The writer who produces a best-seller or the poet who produces an outstanding poem or book of poetry would seem to qualify as having been creative. There are numerous examples of creativity, some of which will be discussed later in the chapter.

At the University of Georgia the graduate faculty in the School of Health and Human Performance met to discuss what constitutes research. They decided that creative involvement should be considered a creative activity and not referred to as creative research. Further, the group recognized that creative activities, as an alternative to research productivity, may be appropriate in the department of dance. So, for the rest of the chapter the term used will be "creative activity."

People in health and human performance who publish in research journals about their creative activities are credited with doing research, although it may not be called creative research. Thus, it seems that writing for publication about a creative activity conducted in a manner that resembles research seems to be an important criteria for determining whether a creative venture is considered creative activity or research. Within the historical-descriptive-experimental system of classifying research, most creative activities leading to publication are descriptive. Most of the creative activities typical of fine arts departments (creating a beautiful object or performance) probably could not or would not be described in a journal article, and thus would not qualify as research. Thus, creative activities are accepted as an alternative to traditional research productivity in certain situations.

Examples in HHP

Earlier in the chapter it was suggested that creative activities take place in the health and human performance discipline. Many faculty members in dance, as members of dance departments or physical education departments housed within schools or colleges of HHP, engage in the same type of creative activities as dance faculty members in fine arts departments. They may be very skillful performers or be skilled at choreographing dance movements. The development of large and complex computer programs for computer-assisted instruction or for some application could be considered a creative activity. Developing, perfecting, or performing a new gymnastic move or routine could be classified as a creative activity. Finally, developing a new piece of equipment or a new procedure is certainly creative. Usually, a description of the procedures followed and the results obtained in developing the new equipment or procedure is published, so it qualifies as research.

Procedures and Evaluation

Procedures for executing a creative activity and evaluating that activity vary considerably depending on the type of activity and the context within which it takes place. We will discuss how procedures and evaluation take place in fine arts departments because they have been doing it for a long time and may serve as a model.

In fine arts departments the artist, sculptor, and potter produce their art object. Their art objects are displayed at shows or exhibits where one or more well-qualified judges or critics evaluate the art object. The quality of the art object is established based on these evaluations. The more art objects a person produces and the higher the evaluations of these art objects, the more highly a person is judged in terms of their creativity or capability. One problem in this procedure occurs when the art object is very heavy or large in size; a two-ton statue or mural is difficult to transport to a show or exhibit.

The music, dance, and drama person in fine arts may face a slightly different situation. These people may either perform themselves or produce the music, dance, or play that others perform. If they themselves perform, their situation is the same as that of the artist, sculptor, and potter. If on the other hand, they produce an artistic work that others perform, how the artistic work is evaluated is dependent on the skill of the performers. Highly skilled performers can make an average artistic work look great, and average skilled performers can make an excellent artistic work look average. In addition, problems and great expense arise with transporting instruments, costumes, props, and backdrops (not to mention large groups of people) great distances to regional and national competitions for judges to evaluate the artistic work. More will be said about some of these problems when discussing procedures for developing a dance and having it evaluated.

Dancers choreograph a dance. This involves selecting the music for the dance and developing the dance by recording each step and movement every dancer will execute. This takes a vast amount of time and energy. Once this stage has been accomplished, the dancers are taught the dance and are rehearsed until they are ready to perform. Some time prior to performance, the costumes for the dancers must be selected and obtained, the lighting of the dance must be established, and props and scenery or backdrops for the dance must be built or bought. Ultimately, the dance must be performed and evaluated if the choreographer is to receive credit for creative activities.

As indicated earlier, the skill of the dancers affects how well the dance is executed. Also, the budget for the dance costumes, scenery, music, and lighting influence how the dance looks. Ideally, a well-qualified and recognized dance critic would be readily available to evaluate the dance on its merits alone, allowing for the ability of the dancers and any budget restraints affecting the appearance of the dance and dancers. However, such resources are uncommon on many university campuses, so less-qualified and less-recognized dance critics are used. Or, dance critics are used who have outstanding credentials but apply the same standards they use to evaluate professional dance company performances. Budget restraints usually make it difficult to take the dance to regional or national competition. Asking another member of the dance faculty to evaluate the dance choreographed usually causes problems because the person is not a recognized authority, others suspect the evaluation is overly high, the choreographer thinks the evaluation was too critical and faculty personal relations may suffer. Some choreographers choose to have the dance professionally taped and then mail it to a recognized authority for evaluation. Not only is this a tremendous expense for the choreographer, but much of the quality of the dance is lost on a tape.

Standards and Documentation

What follows are excerpts from The University of Georgia Guidelines for Appointment, Promotion, and Tenure (1995) in regard to creative activities. Notice that "the standard" is for creative activities in the fine arts, architecture and landscape design, and the performing arts. Notice that research or creative activities are expected of all faculty, and high quality is more important than quantity.

The Standard

Creative activities include innovative work in the fine arts, for example, the production of original paintings, sculptures, ceramics, musical compositions, novels, plays, poetry, and films; the development of plans for projects in architecture and landscape design; and fresh interpretations in the performing arts of music, drama, and dance.

Inquiry and originality are central functions of the University. Faculty are to discover new ideas, to fashion new interpretations of enduring ideas, and to participate in the application of these ideas. Consequently, faculty should conduct research or engage in other creative activities appropriate to their disciplines and to the missions of their promotion/tenure units, and they should disseminate the results of their work through media appropriate to their disciplines.

Faculty whose work assignments include research or other creative activities should clearly demonstrate high quality in these endeavors. The University distinguishes between the routine and the outstanding as judged by the candidates' peers at The University of Georgia and elsewhere. The principal standard should always be quality, rather than quantity.

Documentation

Evidence of creative activities includes, but is not limited to, the sources listed below. In joint endeavors, the evidence should specify the extent of each person's contribution.

1. Honors and awards for creative activities.
2. Generation of creative products and values.
3. Acknowledgment of creative activities.
4. Obtaining grants related to creative activities.
5. Election to offices, committee activities, and important service to professional associations and learned societies, including editorial work and peer reviewing as related to creative activities.

6. Departmental and institutional governance and academic policy and procedure development as related to creative activities.

Evidence of the creative activities listed is not all-inclusive but is excellent in that it clearly indicates there are many ways to document productivity.

Creative Activities for Graduate Students

Since research or creative activities are accepted for college professors it would seem that, in some situations, creative activities should be acceptable for graduate students. Creative activities for graduate students can be developed using the same guidelines set for faculty and using the Master of Fine Arts (MFA) requirements. Most MFA programs require a creative project and a paper explaining the project. The creative project must be evaluated. The paper must explain how the final outcome of the creative activity (e.g., dance, art piece) was developed and provide background on why the final outcome was developed in the manner it was. Every aspect of the development of the final outcome of the creative project is defended based on literature review, experience, trying several alternatives, and so forth. Depending on the situation, it would seem that an evaluation of the creative activity of a college professor could require an assessment of the outcome and a document explaining the creative activity, just as is required of a graduate student.

Summary

Three other research approaches have been discussed. Each of them allows the researcher to investigate research questions that may have been difficult or impossible to investigate with research approaches discussed in earlier chapters. Certainly, many of the techniques utilized in the three research approaches discussed in this chapter are unique to the research approach. You should be able to discuss each of the research approaches in terms of what are the basic techniques, and what research questions can be investigated.

Creative activities as an alternative to research have been discussed. You need to be aware of why creative activities are an acceptable alternative to research and what are some common creative activities.

Formative Evaluation of Objectives

Objective 1   Understand what each of the three research approaches are and how they are conducted.

1. What are the major techniques used with each of the three research approaches?

2. What are two research questions which could be answered with each of the research approaches?

Objective 2   Understand the issues involved with creative activities and why they are an alternative to research.

1. What are five creative activities commonly conducted by college/university personnel?

2. What are four problems in getting creative activities evaluated in terms of their quality?

Part Three

Data Analysis

Data are the measures, scores, and other information collected in a research study. Usually, the term *data* is used to refer to the scores of the participants for a variable, although it is not uncommon to have multiple data sets because information was collected on multiple variables. Researchers draw their conclusions based on the data. Presented in chapters 12 and 13 of Part III are a variety of commonly used data analysis techniques. It will be useful to be aware of what techniques are available in selecting the most appropriate one for use in your research. Knowledge of these techniques will also make the research literature easier to understand. These techniques typically require some mathematical calculation.

There are three distinct steps in data analysis: (1) select the technique appropriate for the data and the research questions; (2) apply the technique or calculate using the technique; and (3) interpret the result of the technique. Step 2 is often quite difficult when a large amount of data is involved or the analysis technique is complex. Thus, step 2 is best accomplished with the aid of the computer. A computer package will be frequently referenced in chapters 12 and 13, and no calculational formulas or computational examples will be presented in these chapters unless they help the reader understand the data analysis technique. Using the computer for step 2 takes nothing away from the researcher in terms of decision making but is of great benefit in terms of the time saved and the accuracy of the result. An excellent reference on interpreting statistics is Huck and Cormier (1996).

In most research studies, a population is identified, a sample is drawn from the population, the research study is conducted on the sample, and the results for the sample are inferred to the population. Thus, sample information (**statistics**) are used to estimate population information (**parameters).** For example, the mean, or arithmetic average, for a sample is a statistic used as an estimate of the mean for a population, which is a parameter. All calculated values in chapters 12 and 13 will be called statistics. Statistics can be classified in a number of ways. One classification is the **descriptive** versus **inferential statistic.** A descriptive statistic is used to describe characteristics of a group, while an inferential statistic is used in the process of making an inference from a sample to a population. Some statistics (the mean is one) can be used in either a descriptive or inferential manner. Another classification is the **parametric** versus **nonparametric statistic.** Most of the statistics presented in Part III are parametric. Parametric statistics usually require interval data and a normal distribution (see chapter 12). Nonparametric statistics have neither of these requirements. A third classification is the **univariate** versus **multivariate statistic.** Most of the statistics presented in Part III are univariate. With univariate statistics each subject contributes one score on one variable to the analysis, while with multivariate statistics each subject contributes multiple scores on multiple variables to the analysis. Any statistics book can be consulted on calculating statistics, but Ferguson and Takane (1989) is excellent.

12 *Descriptive Data Analysis*

KEY WORDS

Central tendency
Coefficient of determination
Continuous scores
Correlation
Correlation coefficient
Curvilinear relationship
Descriptive statistics
Discrete scores
Frequency polygon
Histogram
Inferential statistics
Interval scores

Leptokurtic
Linear relationship
Line of best fit,
    regression line
Mean
Median
Mode
Multivariate statistic
Negatively skewed curve
Nominal scores
Nonparametric statistic

Normal curve,
    bell-shaped curve
Ordinal scores
Outlier
Parameters
Parametric statistic
Percentile, percentile rank
Platykurtic
Positively skewed curve
Range
Ratio scores

Rho, Spearman's rho,
    rank order correlation
    coefficient
Scattergram
Simple frequency distribution
Standard deviation
Standard scores
Statistics
Univariate statistic
Variability
Variance
z score

OBJECTIVES

This chapter presents statistical techniques that can be applied to evaluate a set of scores. You should be familiar with them in order to select the appropriate one for a given situation and to understand the research literature.

After reading chapter 12, you should be able to

1. Select the appropriate statistic(s) for each research situation.
2. Interpret correctly each of the statistics commonly used by researchers.
3. Use the computer to statistically analyze a set of scores.

This chapter covers techniques and statistics commonly used to describe the characteristics and performance of a group and to interpret the scores of individuals within a group. There are many reasons why we analyze data. For a large group, a simple listing of the scores has no meaning to the researcher or the person reading the research report. Only by applying some analysis to the data can it be condensed to a point where it can be meaningful to all interested people in terms of overall performance or characteristics of the group. Also, to make comparisons between groups there must be a single score for each group representing the typical score of the group.

Sometimes it is necessary to describe the performance of an individual within a group. Some data analysis is necessary before the performance of an individual can be compared to the performance of others in the group or to the overall group performance. Before presenting various descriptive data analysis techniques, types of scores, common units of measure, and computer analysis must be discussed, since these elements influence the data analysis.

Types of Scores

Scores can be classified as either continuous or discrete. **Continuous scores,** as most are in HHP, have a potentially infinite number of values allowing variables to be measured with varying degrees of accuracy. Between any two values of a continuous score are countless other values that may be expressed as fractions. For example, 100-yard dash scores are usually recorded to the nearest tenth of a second, but they could be recorded in hundredths or thousandths of a second if timing equipment accurate to that level of precision was available. Body weight accurate to the closest five-pound interval, to the whole pound, or to the half-pound might be recorded depending on how exact the measurement needs to be. **Discrete scores** are limited to a specific number of values and usually are not expressed as fractions. Scores on a throw or shot at a target numbered 5-4-3-2-1-0 are discrete because whole number scores of 5, 4, 3, 2, 1, or 0 are the only ones possible. A score of 4.5 or 1.67 is impossible.

Most continuous scores are rounded off to the nearest unit of measurement when they are recorded. For example, the score of a student who runs the 100-yard dash in 10.57 seconds is recorded as 10.6 because 10.57 is closer to 10.6 than to 10.5. Usually when a number is rounded off to the nearest unit of measurement, it is increased only when the number being dropped is 5 or more. Thus 11.45 is rounded off to 11.5, while 11.44 is recorded as 11.4. A less common method is to round off to the last unit of measure, awarding the next higher score only when that score is actually accomplished. For example, an individual who does eight sit-ups but cannot complete the ninth receives a score of 8.

We can also classify scores as ratio, interval, ordinal, or nominal (Ferguson and Takane 1989). How scores are classified influences what calculations may be performed on the data. **Ratio scores** have a common unit of measurement between each score and a true zero point so that statements about equality of ratios can be made. Length and weight are examples, since one measurement may be expressed as two or three times that of another. **Interval scores** have a common unit of measurement between each score but do not have a true zero point. (A score of 0 as a measure of distance is a true zero, indicating no distance. However, a score of 0 on a knowledge test is not a true zero because it does not indicate a total lack of knowledge; it simply means that the respondent answered none of the questions correctly). Most physical performance scores are either ratio or interval. **Ordinal scores** do not have a common unit of measurement between each score but are ordered in a way that makes it possible to characterize one score as higher than another. Class ranks, for example, are ordinal: If three students receive sit-up scores of 16, 10, and 8, respectively, the first is ranked 1; the next, 2; and the last, 3. Notice that the number of sit-ups necessary to change the class ranks of the second and third students differs. Thus there is not a common unit of measurement between consecutive scores. **Nominal scores** cannot be hierarchically ordered and are mutually exclusive. For example, individuals can be classified by church preference, but we cannot say that one religion is better than another. Gender is another example.

Common Units of Measure

Many scores are recorded in feet and inches or in minutes and seconds. To analyze scores, they must be recorded in a single unit of measurement, usually the smaller one. Thus distances and heights are recorded in inches rather than feet and inches, and times are recorded in seconds rather than minutes and seconds. Recording scores in the smaller unit of measure as they are collected is less time consuming than translating them into that form later.

Computer Analysis

Score analysis should be accurate and quick. Particularly when a set of scores is large, say fifty or more, computers should be used to ensure both accuracy and speed. Computers are increasingly available in school districts and universities, agencies, and businesses. Each statistical example in this chapter is accompanied by an example of the desktop computer application. Sometimes the output from the desktop computer program will include more information than will have been discussed in the chapter. Do not be concerned if this information is unfamiliar or you do not understand what it means.

Many computer program packages for statistical computations have been developed. Some nationally distributed packages of statistical programs such as SAS and SPSS run on both mainframe and desktop computers. These packages are available on many college campuses. Other packages of statistical programs run on only one type of desktop computer (IBM or MacIntosh). Most computer programs provide similar information for any particular statistical technique. The computer examples in chapters 12 and 13 were generated using a package of statistical programs for a desktop computer because most students, both at present and once they have a job, will have access to desktop computers.

Chapters 12 and 13 will reference computer programs from the SPSS (1999) version 10.0 package. If you don't have access to and/or familiarity with any other package of computer programs, you may decide to use this one. SPSS version 10.0 was selected because there is a Windows version of the package and SPSS is commonly used in schools, agencies, labs, and organizations across the country. Also, SPSS is quite complete in meeting the needs of the researcher. There is a small version of SPSS version 10.0 which is called SPSS Student Version 10.0 (2000). It can be bought in a box containing the program disk and a manual for approximately $65. One nice feature is that the SPSS and SPSS Student Version operate basically the same, so learning how to use one of them prepares a person to use the other one. Another desirable feature is that data entered with another computer program package can be used by SPSS and data entered using SPSS can be used with another computer program package. A third nice feature of SPSS is that it has graphic capacities. The manuals available with SPSS and SPSS Student Version programs are quite good. Some of these manuals are listed at the back of the SPSS 10.0 for Windows Basics part of appendix A.

For a small additional cost (around $20), a copy of the SPSS Student Version 10.0 program disk can be purchased with this book. Check with the publisher or your book representative for details. Directions for using SPSS version 10.0 and SPSS Student Version 10.0 are presented in appendix A. Pavkov and Pierce (2001) is a short and inexpensive guide to using SPSS version 10.0.

There is not a Macintosh version of SPSS version 10.0. However, there are some excellent packages of computer programs for Macintosh. One of these is Statview version 5 (SAS 1998) with both a Macintosh and a Windows version. Most packages of computer programs are quite similar in terms of what they can do and how they do it. So, there is not much difference among packages of computer programs. Once you learn one package of computer programs, you can easily use another package. Larose and Jin (1998) is a short and inexpensive guide to using SAS for Windows.

The SPSS package of programs requires that the data be entered and then an analysis program selected. Normally after the data are entered they will be saved to disk before any analysis is undertaken. If the data are not saved to disk, when the computer is turned off the data are lost. If the data ever need to be reanalyzed because of a mistake in the original analysis, or if a different analysis becomes necessary, the data must be entered again. Doing additional analysis on the data happens quite often. If there are large amounts of data, reentering the data represents a considerable inconvenience. Thus, when using SPSS or some other computer program package, it is a good idea to enter and save the data to disk prior to analyzing the data.

All instructions in chapters 12 and 13 and appendix A concerning how to use the computer assume that the Windows version of SPSS version 10.0 is being used. The instructions for other versions of SPSS and for Student SPSS 10.0 are quite similar. The example computer printouts in the book are based on SPSS output.

The steps to follow in getting into SPSS, entering the data, saving the data, and editing the data are presented in sections 1 through 4 of the SPSS 10.0 for Windows Basics part of appendix A. The steps used to analyze the data and print the output of the analysis are presented in sections 5 and 6 of the document. Sections 7 through 9 of this part of appendix A have additional useful information. Note that in the SPSS 10.0 for Windows Statistical Procedures part of appendix A there are directions for using the analysis procedure selected in section 5 of the SPSS 10.0 for Windows Basics part of appendix A.

Organizing and Graphing Test Scores

Simple Frequency Distributions

The fifty scores in table 12.1 are not very useful in their present form. They become more meaningful if we order the scores to find out how many participants received each score. To do this, we first find the lowest and highest scores in the table. Now we find the number of participants who received each score between the lowest (46) and the highest (90).

Once the scores are ordered, it is easy to make up a simple frequency distribution of the results (see columns 1 and 2 of table 12.2). We used to make the simple frequency distribution by hand listing the scores in descending order with the best score first. Now we use the computer and the SPSS Frequencies program by default (automatic setting) lists scores in ascending order with the smallest score first. This assumes that the smallest score is the worst score. We might as well start following what is done by SPSS if we make a simple frequency distribution by hand. In most cases, the higher scores are better scores, but this is not true when, for example, distance running event

TABLE 12.1 Knowledge Test Scores for Fifty Participants

66*	67	54	63	90
56	56	65	71	82
68	68	76	55	78
47	58	68	78	76
46	68	68	90	62
58	49	62	84	75
75	65	66	72	73
71	75	83	83	64
60	76	65	79	56
68	70	48	77	59

*Number correct

times, number of accidents, or number of errors are being measured. A **simple frequency distribution** of times from a distance running event should list the higher scores first. We always want to list the scores from worst to best with the worst score first. In SPSS, if the smallest score is the worst score, nothing has to be done. However,

TABLE 12.2 Simple Frequency Distribution of Knowledge Test Scores of Fifty Participants in Table 12.1

SCORE	FREQUENCY	PERCENT	VALID PERCENT	CUMULATIVE PERCENT
46.00	1	2.0	2.0	2.0
47.00	1	2.0	2.0	4.0
48.00	1	2.0	2.0	6.0
49.00	1	2.0	2.0	8.0
54.00	1	2.0	2.0	10.0
55.00	1	2.0	2.0	12.0
56.00	3	6.0	6.0	18.0
58.00	2	4.0	4.0	22.0
59.00	1	2.0	2.0	24.0
60.00	1	2.0	2.0	26.0
62.00	2	4.0	4.0	30.0
63.00	1	2.0	2.0	32.0
64.00	1	2.0	2.0	34.0
65.00	3	6.0	6.0	40.0
66.00	2	4.0	4.0	44.0
67.00	1	2.0	2.0	46.0
68.00	6	12.0	12.0	58.0
70.00	1	2.0	2.0	60.0
71.00	2	4.0	4.0	64.0
72.00	1	2.0	2.0	66.0
73.00	1	2.0	2.0	68.0
75.00	3	6.0	6.0	74.0
76.00	3	6.0	6.0	80.0
77.00	1	2.0	2.0	82.0
78.00	2	4.0	4.0	86.0
79.00	1	2.0	2.0	88.0
82.00	1	2.0	2.0	90.0
83.00	2	4.0	4.0	94.0
84.00	1	2.0	2.0	96.0
90.00	2	4.0	4.0	100.0
Total	50	100.0	100.0	

if the smallest score is the *best* score, the SPSS program must be told to list the scores in descending order (largest score first and best score last). The Frequencies program directions explain how to do this.

From a simple frequency distribution we can determine the range of scores at a glance, as well as the most frequently received score and the number of participants who received each score. For example, from table 12.2 we can see that the scores ranged from 46 down to 90, that the most frequently received score was 68, and that scores had a frequency of 3 or less in all cases but one.

Where the number of scores is large, forming a simple frequency distribution is time consuming without a computer. Using a computer, scores can be entered and analyzed with any one of a number of programs. Most statistical packages for mainframe and desktop computers include a frequency count program.

The Frequencies program in SPSS is one such program. The directions for using the Frequencies program are presented in section 1 of the SPSS 10.0 for Windows Statistical Procedures part of appendix A.

The output from SPSS for the data in table 12.1 is presented in table 12.2. From table 12.2 it can be seen that test scores ranged from 46 to 90, and six participants scored 68.

Some researchers use a frequency count program to screen their data for extreme scores or incorrect scores before conducting any more complex analysis. It is a wise thing to do because scores do get incorrectly recorded and entered into the computer.

Grouping Scores for Graphing

The scores and their frequencies in table 12.2 could be presented in the form of a graph that shows the general shape of a score distribution. Based on the shape of a score distribution, decisions are made about how to interpret the performance of the group measured. If there are many different scores, the graph is usually formed by grouping like scores together. In grouping a set of scores, we try to form about fifteen (10-20) groupings by dividing the difference between the largest and smallest scores by 15, and rounding off the result to the nearest whole number if necessary.

$$\text{interval size} = (\text{largest score} - \text{smallest score}) \div 15.$$

The interval size tells us how many scores to group together. Design the first grouping to contain the worst score. Table 12.3 is a grouping of the data in table 12.2 using an interval size of three.

Figure 12.1 is a graph of the data in table 12.1 using SPSS. SPSS used different intervals from those in table 12.3. Test scores (sometimes midpoints of intervals) are listed along the horizontal axis with low scores on the left to high scores on the right. The frequency is listed on the vertical axis starting with 0 and increasing upward. Going up from a score until the graph line is hit and then going to the left

TABLE 12.3 Grouping of the Knowledge Test Scores in Table 12.2

GROUPING	FREQUENCY
44–46	1
47–49	3
50–52	0
53–55	2
56–58	5
59–61	2
62–64	4
65–67	6
68–70	7
71–73	4
74–76	6
77–79	4
80–82	1
83–85	3
86–88	0
89–91	2

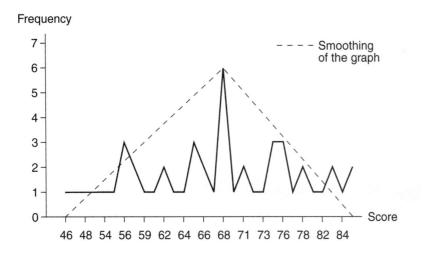

FIGURE 12.1
Graph of the knowledge test scores in table 12.1.

until the vertical axis is hit, the frequency for a score can be obtained. For example, the frequency for the score 56 is 3. This graph was formed by connecting the plotted frequencies for the scores. The graph is called a **frequency polygon.**

Smoothing out the frequency polygon creates a curve that, by its shape, tells us the nature of the distribution. In figure 12.1, the smoothing out is indicated by the broken line. If that line resembles the curve in figure 12.2, the graph is called a **normal curve** or **bell-shaped curve.** The normal curve is often used as a model. If the graph of the data resembles the normal curve (data are normally distributed) one decision is made, but if the graph does not resemble the normal curve a different decision is made.

When a smoothed graph has a long, low tail on the left, indicating that few participants received low scores, it is called a **negatively skewed curve.** When the tail of the curve is on the right, the curve is called **positively skewed.** A curve is called **leptokurtic** when it is more sharply peaked than a normal curve and **platykurtic** when it is less sharply peaked (fig. 12.3). Leptokurtic curves are characteristic of extremely homogeneous groups. Platykurtic curves are characteristic of heterogeneous groups.

A computer can be utilized to form a graph. An option of most computer programs is any number of groupings and several different types of graphs. Another type of graph that is quite common is a **histogram.** Again, the frequencies for the scores (sometimes midpoints of intervals) are plotted and bars are constructed at the height of the frequency running the full length of the interval. A histogram for the data in table 12.1 is presented in figure 12.4. Several types of graphs can be obtained with SPSS by clicking on Graphs and then clicking on the type of graph desired. The Histogram program forms a histogram with about 10 scores (interval midpoints) by default and the Line Chart program forms a frequency polygon with about 15 to 20 scores (interval midpoints) by default. An option with the Histogram program is to have a normal curve superimposed on the histogram as was done in figure 12.4. Directions for these programs are in sections 17 and 18 of the Statistical Procedures part of appendix A. Other types of graphs and how to construct graphs are presented in most basic statistics books, such as Ferguson and Takane (1989).

FIGURE 12.2
A normal curve.

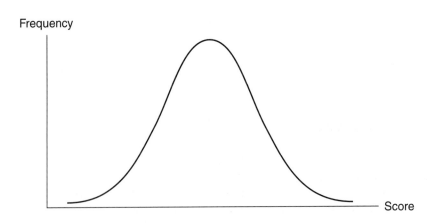

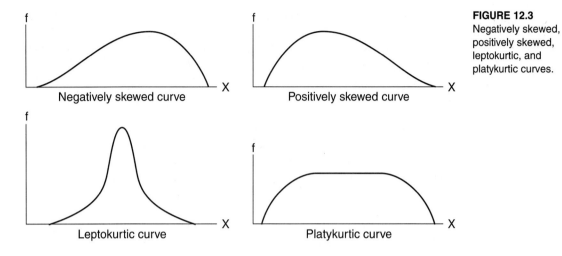

FIGURE 12.3
Negatively skewed, positively skewed, leptokurtic, and platykurtic curves.

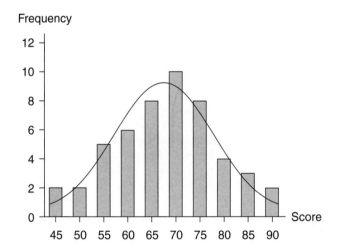

FIGURE 12.4
Histogram for table 12.1 data.

Descriptive Values

Once a large set of scores has been collected, certain descriptive values can be calculated; these values will summarize or condense the set of scores and give it meaning. Descriptive values are used by researchers primarily to describe the performance of a group or compare its performance with that of another group.

Measures of Central Tendency

One type of descriptive value is the measure of **central tendency,** which indicates those points at which scores tend to be concentrated. There are three measures of central tendency: the mode, the median, and the mean.

Mode.   The **mode** is the score most frequently received, and it is used with nominal data. In table 12.2 the mode is 68: More participants received a score of 68 than any other one score in the set. It is possible to have several modes if a number of scores tie for most frequent. The mode is not a stable measure because the addition or deletion of a single score can change its value considerably. Unless the data are nominal or the most frequent score is desired, other measures of central tendency are more appropriate.

Median.   The **median** is the middle score; half the scores fall above the median and half below. It requires data that are at least ordinal. It cannot be calculated unless the scores are listed in order from best to worst. For example, the median score for the nine numbers 4, 3, 1, 4, 10, 7, 7, 8, and 6 is 6 since it is the middle score.

$$10, 8, 7, 7, 6, 4, 4, 3, 1$$

$$\uparrow \text{ Median}$$

Notice that the value of the median is affected only by the position, not the value, of each score. If, in the example above, the scores were 10, 8, 7, 7, 6, 3, 2, 1, and 0, the median would still be 6. This characteristic of the median is sometimes a limitation.

When scores are listed in a simple frequency distribution, we can obtain a value of the median by a computational formula. This value of the median is usually a fractional number.

Mean.   The **mean** is ordinarily the most appropriate measure of central tendency for interval or ratio data. It is affected by both the value and the position of each score. The mean ($\bar{x}$) is the sum of the scores divided by the number of scores. Notice that the scores need not be ordered hierarchically to calculate the mean. For example, the mean for the scores in table 12.1 is 67.78, the sum of the randomly ordered scores divided by 50.

When the graph of the scores is a normal curve, the mode, median, and mean are equal. When the graph is positively skewed, the mean is larger than the median; when it is negatively skewed, the mean is less than the median. For example, the graph for the scores 2, 3, 1, 4, 1, 8, and 10 is positively skewed with a mean of 4.14 and a median of 3.

The mean is the most common measure of central tendency. But when scores are quite skewed or lack a common interval between consecutive scores (e.g., with ordinal scores), the median is the best measure of central tendency. The mode is used only when the mean and median cannot be calculated (e.g., with nominal scores) or when the only information wanted is the most frequent score (e.g., most common uniform size, most frequent error).

Measures of Variability

A second type of descriptive value is the measure of **variability,** which describes the data in terms of their spread or heterogeneity. For example, consider these scores for two groups:

Group 1	Group 2
9	5
1	6
5	4

For both groups, the mean and median are 5. If you simply report that the mean and median for both groups are identical without showing the data, another person could conclude that the two groups have equal or similar ability. This is not true: Group 2 is more homogeneous in performance than is group 1. A measure of variability is the descriptive term that indicates this difference in the spread, or heterogeneity, of the data. There are two such measures: the range and the standard deviation.

Range.   The **range** is the easiest measure of variability to obtain and is the one used when the measure of central tendency is the mode or median. The range is the difference between the highest and lowest score. For example, the range for the data in table 12.2 is 44 (90-46). The range is neither a precise nor stable measure because it depends on only two scores and is affected by a change in either of them. For example, the range for the data in table 12.2 would have been 38 (84-46) if the subjects who scored 90 had instead scored 84 or less.

Standard Deviation.   The **standard deviation** is the measure of variability used with the mean. It indicates the amount that all the scores differ from the mean. The more the scores differ from the mean, the larger the standard deviation. The minimum value of the standard deviation is 0, indicating that all scores were the same value. Presented below is a formula illustrating how the standard deviation is defined.

$$s = \sqrt{\frac{\sum (x - \bar{x})^2}{n - 1}}$$

In the formula, s is the standard deviation, x is a score, $\bar{x}$ is the mean, n is the number of scores, and Σ is a summation sign. There is a much easier formula than this one for calculating s.

If the data are normally distributed, few if any scores will be more than three standard deviations away from the mean. For example, if the mean is 60 and the standard deviation 10, the lowest score might be around 30 ($\bar{x} - 3s = 60 - 30$) and the highest score might be around 90. Often, when a score is more than three standard deviations from the mean, it is called an **outlier** and may be removed from the data. The researcher is concerned that the outlier score is not correct or the participant did not belong in the group.

The mean, standard deviation, and other useful statistics can be obtained with SPSS using either the Descriptives program or the statistics option in the Frequencies program. Because the median is provided with the Frequencies program but not with the Descriptives program, many researchers use the Frequencies program. Directions for these programs are presented in sections 1 and 2 of the Statistical Procedures part of appendix A. Read the directions for both programs before selecting one. If the Frequencies program is selected, pay attention in the directions to selecting and turning off options in the program. The output from the Frequencies program for the data in table 12.1 is presented in table 12.4.

Variance.   A third measure of variability is the **variance.** It is not a descriptive statistic like the range or standard deviation, but rather, a useful statistic in certain

---

TABLE 12.4 All the Statistics Output from SPSS for the Data in Table 12.1

N	Valid	50
	Missing	0
Mean		67.7800
Std. Error of Mean		1.5184
Median		68.0000
Mode		68.00
Std. Deviation		10.7367
Variance		115.2771
Skewness		−.058
Std. Error of Skewness		.337
Kurtosis		−.392
Std. Error of Kurtosis		.662
Range		44.00
Minimum		46.00
Maximum		90.00
Sum		3389.00

other statistical procedures and interpretations of statistics that will be discussed later. The variance is the square of the standard deviation. If, for example, the standard deviation is 4, the variance is 16.

Measuring Group Position

Percentile Ranks and Percentiles

Sometimes a researcher needs to indicate the position or rank of participants within a group based on their test scores. This can be accomplished by the use of **percentile ranks** and **percentiles.** Although their calculations differ, their interpretations are basically the same, so the two terms are used interchangeably in the literature. Both statistics indicate the percentage of participants below a particular score. Thus, if a researcher reports that the percentile rank (PR) for a score of 28 is 60, this indicates that 60 percent of the participants scored below the score of 28. However, the researcher might report that a participant with a score of 28 scored at the 60th percentile (P). Percentile ranks and percentiles are often calculated when developing norms.

One disadvantage of percentile ranks is that they are ordinal scores. There is no common unit of measure between consecutive percentile rank values because they are position measures. Thus, it is inappropriate to add, subtract, multiply, or divide percentile rank values. Another disadvantage of percentile ranks is that small changes in score values near the mean result in large changes in percentile ranks. Baumgartner and Jackson (1999) present a detailed coverage of percentile ranks and percentiles.

Percentiles and percentile ranks computer programs are available but they are not common in packages of statistical programs like SPSS. Some researchers use the CUM. % values presented in table 12.2 as an estimate of percentile ranks. Computer programs usually assume that a large score is good. When this is not true (score is number of auto accidents), subtract the percentile rank of each participant from 100 to get the correct value. How to obtain percentiles and percentile ranks using SPSS are presented in sections 13 and 14 of the Statistical Procedures part of appendix A. Percentiles for the data in table 12.1 are presented in table 12.5.

Standard Scores

Researchers use **standard scores** when they have data on participants from several different tests, and they want all the data in the same unit of measurement. An example of this is the sit-up, mile-run, skin-fold, and sit-and-reach tests common to many fitness batteries. Test scores for a test are converted to standard scores by the formula

$$z = (x - \bar{x})/s$$

TABLE 12.5 Percentiles for the Data in Table 12.1	
PERCENTILE	**SCORE**
5	47.5500
10	54.1000
15	56.0000
20	58.0000
25	59.7500
30	62.3000
35	64.8500
40	65.4000
45	66.9500
50	68.0000
55	68.0000
60	70.6000
65	72.1500
70	75.0000
75	76.0000
80	76.8000
85	78.3500
90	82.9000
95	86.7000
100	90.0000

where z is a standard score, x is a test score, $\bar{x}$ is the mean for the test, and s is the standard deviation for the test. Thus, for each test, test scores are converted to z **scores** by using the formula. Once all test scores are converted to z scores, the researcher can obtain the sum of the z scores for each participant or determine on which test the participant scored best.

A z score indicates how many standard deviations a test score is from the mean. Thus, a z score of 1.5 indicates the test score was 1.5 standard deviations above the mean. Typically z scores are between -3.0 and 3.0 and are fractional. The mean z score is 0, and the standard deviation for a distribution of z scores is 1.0.

Computer programs to obtain z scores are usually available. Most packages of statistical programs have a transformation feature that could be used to calculate new scores (like z scores) using scores already entered into the computer. To accomplish this, first enter the scores into the computer, then obtain the mean and standard deviation for the scores using the computer, and finally, using the transformation feature, calculate z scores. With SPSS, z scores can be obtained using an option in the Descriptives program. In sections 15 and 16 of the Statistical Procedures part of appendix A, there is a description of how to get z scores and the sum of z scores. The z scores for the data in table 12.1 are presented in table 12.6.

TABLE 12.6 *z* Scores for the Data in Table 12.1

CASE	SCORE	z SCORE	CASE	SCORE	z SCORE
1	66	−0.166	26	62	−0.538
2	56	−1.097	27	66	−0.166
3	68	0.020	28	83	1.418
4	47	−1.935	29	65	−0.259
5	46	−2.029	30	48	−1.842
6	58	−0.911	31	63	−0.445
7	75	0.672	32	71	0.300
8	71	0.300	33	55	−1.190
9	60	−0.725	34	78	0.952
10	68	0.020	35	90	2.070
11	67	−0.073	36	84	1.511
12	56	−1.097	37	72	0.393
13	68	0.020	38	83	1.418
14	58	−0.911	39	79	1.045
15	68	0.020	40	77	0.859
16	49	−1.749	41	90	2.070
17	65	−0.259	42	82	1.324
18	75	0.672	43	78	0.952
19	76	0.766	44	76	0.766
20	70	0.207	45	62	−0.538
21	54	−1.283	46	75	0.672
22	65	−0.259	47	73	0.486
23	76	0.766	48	64	−0.352
24	68	0.020	49	56	−1.097
25	68	0.020	50	59	−0.818

Mean   = 67.78
Std Dev = 10.74

There is another standard score called a *T* score, which physical education teachers often use in preference to *z* scores. Baumgartner and Jackson (1999) discuss *T* scores in detail.

Determining Relationships between Scores

There are many situations in which researchers would like to know the relationship between scores on two different tests (e.g., the relationship between beliefs about the importance of leisure time pursuits and leisure time practices). Sometimes the major objective of the research is to determine relationships, but in other studies it may be a minor objective. To determine if there is a relationship between two variables, every participant must be measured on each variable. There are two different techniques to determine score relationships: a graphing technique and a mathematical technique called correlation.

The graphing technique is not as precise as the mathematical technique, but prior to computers it was easier and quicker. Many of the terms used in the mathematical technique come from the graphing technique. Presently, with the availability of computers, many researchers are using the graphing technique initially to check some of the assumptions underlying the mathematical technique and as a way to graphically show the relationship. They then use the mathematical technique to obtain a value that precisely indicates the amount of relationship between the two variables.

The Graphing Technique

To graph a relationship, the computer develops a coordinate system with values of one variable listed along the horizontal axis and values of the other variable listed along the vertical axis. It plots a point for each participant above his/her score on the horizontal axis and opposite his/her score on the vertical axis, as shown in figure 12.5. The graph that results is called a **scattergram.**

The point plotted for participant A is at the intersection of sit-up score 15 and push-up score 10, the scores the participant received on the two tests. The straight line—the **line of best fit** or the **regression line**—represents the trend in the data, in this case that participants with large sit-up scores have large push-up scores, and vice versa. When large scores on one measure are associated with large scores on the other measure, the relationship is positive. When large scores on one measure are associated with small scores on the other measure, the relationship is negative (fig. 12.6).

FIGURE 12.5
Graph of a positive relationship between scores.

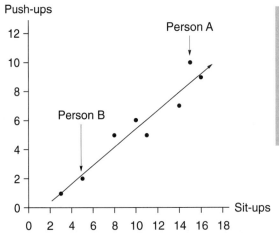

Person	Sit-ups	Push-ups
A	15	10
B	5	2
C	11	5
D	10	6
E	14	7
F	3	1
G	16	9
H	8	5

The closer the plotted points to the trend line, the higher or larger the relationship. The maximum relationship occurs when all plotted points are on the trend line. When the plotted points resemble a circle, making it impossible to draw a trend line, no linear relationship exists between the two measures being graphed (fig. 12.7).

Computer programs contain scattergram graphic programs that facilitate plotting data. An example of a computer-generated graph using SPSS and the data in figure 12.5 is presented in figure 12.8. To obtain a scattergram using SPSS, follow the directions in section 19 of the Statistical Procedures part of appendix A.

The Correlation Technique

Correlation is a mathematical technique for determining the relationship between two sets of scores. The formula was developed by Karl Pearson to determine the degree of relationship between two sets of measures (called X measures and Y measures).

A **correlation coefficient** (r) has two characteristics, direction and strength. Direction of the relationship is indicated by whether the correlation coefficient is positive or negative, as indicated under the graphing technique. Strength of the

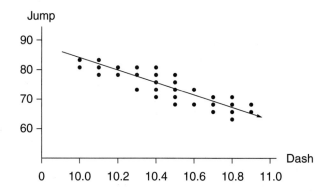

FIGURE 12.6
Graph of a negative relationship between scores.

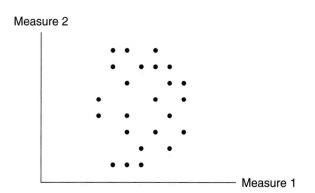

FIGURE 12.7
Graph of no relationship between scores.

FIGURE 12.8
Computer-generated
scattergram of the data
in figure 12.5.

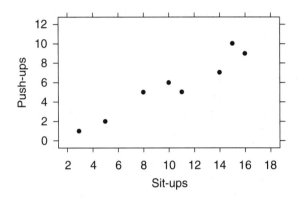

relationship is indicated by how close the *r* is to 1, the maximum value possible. A correlation of 1 (*r* = 1) shows a perfect positive relationship, indicating that an increase in scores on one measure is accompanied by an increase in scores on the second measure. A perfect negative relationship (*r* = −1) indicates that an increase in scores on one measure is accompanied by a decrease in scores on the second. (Notice that a correlation of −1 is just as strong as a correlation of 1). Perfect relationships are rare, but if one exists, it is exactly described by a mathematical formula. An example of a perfect positive and a perfect negative relationship is shown in table 12.7. When the correlation coefficient is 0 (*r* = 0), there is no linear relationship between the two sets of scores.

Because the relationship between two sets of scores is seldom perfect, the majority of correlation coefficients are fractions (e.g., .93, −.85). The closer the correlation coefficient is to 1 or −1, the stronger the relationship. When the relationship is not perfect, the scores on one measure only tend to change with a change in the scores on the other measure. Look, for example, at table 12.8. The correlation between height and weight is not perfect: Participant C, whose height is 75 inches, is not heavier than Participant E, whose height is only 70 inches.

When the scores for the two sets of scores are ranks, a correlation coefficient called **rho** or **Spearman's rho** or the **rank order correlation coefficient** may be calculated. The formula is just a simplification of the Pearson correlation formula and will produce the same result when applied to the two sets of ranks, provided that no tied ranks exist. Rho is commonly included in computer statistical programs.

Interpreting the Correlation Coefficient. A high correlation between two measures does not usually indicate a cause-and-effect-relationship. The perfect height and weight relationship in table 12.7, for example, does not indicate that an increase in weight *causes* an increase in height. Also, the degree of relationship between two sets of measures does not increase at the same rate as does the correlation coefficient. The true indicator of the degree of relationship is the **coefficient of**

TABLE 12.7 Examples of Perfect Relationships

PARTICIPANT	HEIGHT	WEIGHT	PARTICIPANT	100-YARD DASH	PULL-UPS
A	60	130	A	10.6	14
B	52	122	B	10.6	14
C	75	145	C	11.2	8
D	66	136	D	11.7	3
E	70	140	E	10.5	15
	$r = 1$			$r = -1$	
Exact formula: weight = height + 70			Exact formula: dash = 12 − .1 (pull-ups)		

TABLE 12.8 Example of an Imperfect Correlation

PARTICIPANT	HEIGHT	WEIGHT
A	60	130
B	52	125
C	75	145
D	66	136
E	70	150
	$r = .91$	

determination—the amount of variability (variance) in one measure that is explained by the other measure. The coefficient of determination is the square of the correlation coefficient (r^2). For example, the square of the correlation coefficient in table 12.8 is .83 ($.91^2$), meaning that 83 percent of the variability in height scores is due to the individuals having different weight scores.

Thus, when one correlation coefficient is twice as large as another, the larger coefficient really explains four times the amount of variation that the smaller coefficient explains. For example, when the r between height and weight is .80 and the r between strength and athletic ability is .40, the r^2 for height and weight is $.80^2$, or 64 percent, and the r^2 for strength and athletic ability is $.40^2$, or 16 percent.

Remember: When you interpret a correlation coefficient, there are no absolute standards for labeling a given r as "good" or "poor"; only the relationship you want or expect determines the quality of a given r. For example, a correlation coefficient of .67 between leg strength and distance run scores for males might lead you to expect a similar correlation coefficient in comparing leg strength and distance run scores for females. If the relationship between the females' scores were only .45, you might label that correlation coefficient "poor" because you expected it to be as high as that of the males.

There are two reasons why correlation coefficients can be negative: (1) opposite scoring scales and (2) true negative relationships. When a measure on which a small score is a better score is correlated with a measure on which a larger score is a better score, the correlation coefficient probably will be negative. Consider, for example, the relationship between scores on a speed event like the 50-yard dash and a nonspeed event like the high jump. Usually, the best jumpers are the best runners, but the correlation is negative because the scoring scales are reversed. Two measures can be negatively related as well. We would expect, for example, a negative correlation between body weight and measures involving support or motion of the body (e.g., pull-ups).

The Question of Accuracy. In calculating r we assume that the relationship between the two sets of scores is basically linear. A **linear relationship** is best shown graphically by a straight line, as is the trend line in figure 12.5. However, a relationship between two sets of scores may be best represented by a curved line, indicating a **curvilinear relationship.** If a relationship is truly curvilinear, the correlation coefficient will underestimate the relationship. For example, r could equal 0 even when a definite curvilinear relationship exists. Learning curves and fatigue curves are typically curvilinear. The correlation between age and most physical performance measures (e.g., strength) is curvilinear. An example of a curvilinear relationship is presented in figure 12.9.

FIGURE 12.9
Example of a curvilinear relationship between group performance and practice trials within a day when learning a new skill.

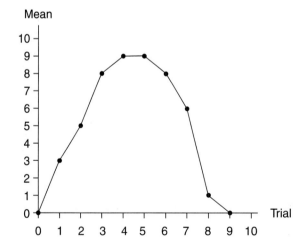

Practice trial	Group mean
1	3
2	5
3	8
4	9
5	9
6	8
7	6
8	1

Although we need not assume when calculating r that the graph of each of the two sets of scores is a normal curve, we do assume that the two graphs resemble each other. If they are dissimilar, the correlation coefficient will underestimate the relationship between the scores. Considerable differences in the two graphs are occasionally found, usually when the number of people tested is small. For this reason, the correlation coefficient ideally should be calculated using the scores of several hundred people.

Other factors also affect the correlation coefficient. One is the reliability of the scores; low reliability reduces the correlation coefficient. Another factor is the range in the scores; the correlation coefficient will be smaller for a homogeneous group than for a heterogeneous group. Ferguson and Takane (1989) suggest that, generally, the range in scores increases as the size of the group tested increases. Certainly, the measurements or test scores for small groups exhibit a greater tendency than those of large groups to be either more homogeneous or more heterogeneous than is typical for the group measured and the test administered. This is another reason to calculate the correlation coefficient for only large groups. Ferguson and Takane (1989) cover this subject in greater detail.

When the group tested is large or when the researcher wants the correlation between all possible pairings of more than two variables (sex, age, height, weight, etc.), a computer is the most efficient way to generate the correlation coefficients. Programs for calculating correlation coefficients are commonly found in statistical packages for computers. In SPSS, correlations are obtained by following the directions presented in section 10 of the Statistical Procedures part of appendix A. Before clicking on Ok to do the analysis, click on Listwise deletion (Listwise deletion is not using the scores of a subject who has any missing scores. Pairwise deletion is not using the scores of a subject who has missing scores on the two variables being correlated.).

The correlations for the data in table 12.9 are presented in table 12.10 using SPSS. The correlations between any two variables are found by finding the value listed in the cell formed by the row and column of the two variables. For example, the correlation between height and weight is .91.

Summary

The importance of selecting the appropriate statistic for the situation and interpreting it correctly has been stressed in this chapter. This ability to choose and interpret statistical measures is of consequence for both a researcher and a person reading research journals. A variety of descriptive statistics were presented and the student will need a thorough understanding of these statistical techniques in order to fully grasp the material in chapter 13.

Finally, the student should have some ability to use the computer and have practiced using some package of statistical programs by the time this chapter has been covered. This skill is assumed in the next chapter and should prove valuable in the future as well.

TABLE 12.9 Individual Physical Characteristic Data of 40 Participants

PARTICIPANT	SEX	AGE	HEIGHT	WEIGHT	PARTICIPANT	SEX	AGE	HEIGHT	WEIGHT
1	0	6	123.0	22.5	21	1	7	122.7	23.8
2	0	6	115.0	24.9	22	1	7	132.9	33.9
3	0	6	115.0	22.7	23	1	7	128.8	28.3
4	0	6	121.5	24.3	24	1	7	133.6	30.2
5	0	6	116.5	19.7	25	0	8	136.0	31.8
6	1	6	119.6	21.9	26	0	8	129.0	26.8
7	0	7	124.6	24.5	27	1	8	128.2	27.6
8	0	7	111.8	19.3	28	1	8	131.1	28.8
9	0	7	120.3	19.8	29	1	8	139.1	31.1
10	0	7	119.0	21.3	30	1	8	124.1	25.4
11	0	7	119.5	21.3	31	1	9	137.1	34.8
12	0	7	132.0	26.9	32	1	9	134.6	31.9
13	0	7	122.5	22.7	33	1	9	137.6	29.8
14	0	7	128.5	31.6	34	1	9	140.1	34.4
15	0	7	119.5	21.3	35	1	9	140.2	32.3
16	1	7	126.0	24.3	36	1	9	149.9	36.6
17	1	7	132.2	29.3	37	0	10	140.5	29.0
18	1	7	136.8	28.9	38	0	10	131.5	29.6
19	1	7	125.8	25.5	39	0	10	146.4	35.5
20	1	7	116.9	22.6	40	0	10	136.5	28.1

Sex: 0 = Female, 1 = Male
Age: In years
Height: In centimeters
Weight: In kilograms

TABLE 12.10 Correlations Among All Variables for the Data in Table 12.9

	SEX	AGE	HEIGHT	WEIGHT
SEX	1.00			
AGE	0.13	1.00		
HEIGHT	0.36	0.77	1.00	
WEIGHT	0.41	0.67	0.91	1.00

Formative Evaluation of Objectives

Objective 1   Select the appropriate statistic(s) for each research situation.

1. In each situation below, what statistic(s) are needed?

   a) Describe the characteristics or scores of a group.
   b) Determine if the scores of a group are normally distributed.
   c) Allow scores from tests differing in unit of measurement to be combined into a total score.
   d) Determine how much the performance of a group changed from the pretest to the posttest.
   e) Identify the degree of relationship between the scores of a group on two different tests.

Objective 2   Interpret correctly each of the statistics commonly used by researchers.

1. In each situation below, how is the statistic reported correctly interpreted?

   a) The median score for the group is 11.6.
   b) The mean score for the group is 7.5.
   c) The standard deviation for the scores of the group is 6.6.
   d) Participant 17 has a percentile rank of 53 based on her score of 16.
   e) The correlation between IQ scores and knowledge test scores is .77.
   f) Number of mistakes on a job proficiency test correlated $-.35$ with scores on a job knowledge test.

Objective 3   Use the computer to statistically analyze a set of scores.

1. In terms of the statistical package of computer programs available to you, answer the following questions.

   a) What is the procedure followed in analyzing the data no matter what program in the statistical package is used?
   b) What program in the statistical package provides descriptive statistics (e.g., mean, standard deviation)?
   c) What program in the statistical package provides all possible correlations between the variables when scores on three or more variables are collected on each participant?

13 *Inferential Data Analysis*

KEY WORDS

Alpha level
Analysis of covariance
  (ANCOVA)
Analysis of variance
  (ANOVA)
Beta (ß)
Cell
Correlation
Covariate
Critical region
Critical value
Cross validation
Degrees of freedom
Expected frequency
Experiment-wise error rate
Factorial design

Matched pairs
Mean square (MS)
Multiple prediction
Multivariate tests
Nonparametric
Nonsignificant
Null hypothesis
Observed frequency
One-group *t* test
One-way ANOVA
One-way (goodness of fit)
  chi-square test
Parametric
Per-comparison error rate
Polynomial regression
Prediction

Random blocks ANOVA
Real difference
Regression
Repeated measures
Repeated measures ANOVA
Research hypothesis
Sampling error
Significant
Simple effects tests
Simple prediction
Slope
Standard error of prediction
Statistical hypothesis
Statistical power
Sums of squares (SS)

Two dependent groups *t* test
Two-dimensional ANOVA
Two group comparisons,
  multiple comparisons, *a*
  posteriori comparisons
Two independent groups
  t test
Two-way ANOVA
Two-way (contingency table)
  chi-square test
Type I error
Type II error
Univariate tests
Variate
Y-intercept

OBJECTIVES

This chapter presents statistical tests that researchers commonly use in analyzing their data. You should be familiar with them in order to select the appropriate one(s) in your research and to understand the research of others as reported in research journals.

After reading chapter 13, you should be able to

1. Identify the different research designs and statistical tests commonly used.
2. Understand the five-step hypothesis-testing procedure and how it is reported in research journals.
3. Understand and evaluate common statistical tests when they are used in the research literature.

The data analysis techniques discussed in this chapter are those most commonly used by researchers to analyze their data. These are the techniques you are most likely to use as a researcher and to see in the research literature as a consumer of research. Not all data analysis techniques available can be discussed in this context. On occasion you will need to use techniques or will see techniques in the literature that have not been discussed in this chapter. It is hoped that, what you learn here will provide you with the foundation you will need to put these additional techniques to work.

No statistical training is assumed in order to understand the material in this chapter. The material presented should prepare you to understand the statistical information presented in the research literature. This chapter is not a comprehensive coverage of each statistical technique as would be found in a statistics book, so some of you may want to consult a statistics book. Others may want to skip some of the more advanced topics (e.g., two-way ANOVA). Ferguson and Takane (1989) is an excellent statistics book covering most of the statistical techniques presented. Selected statistics books are referenced throughout the chapter.

Inference

A researcher typically identifies or defines a population to which the findings of the research are to apply; states a research hypothesis about the population; selects a sample(s) from the population, using random sampling procedures conducts the research study on the sample(s); and, finally, infers the results of the study to the population (see steps in research, chapters 2 and 7).

Example: The researcher wants to determine which of three teaching methods (A, B, or C) is the best way to teach rope skipping to third-grade boys. The researcher defines the population as third-grade boys in Georgia. The research hypothesis is that teaching method A is superior to the other two methods. Using random sampling procedures, the researcher selects three samples of fifty participants each from the population. The study is conducted by teaching a different method of skipping rope to each sample and administering a rope-skipping test to all participants. After analyzing the rope-skipping data, the researcher finds that method B is the superior teaching method. The researcher infers this finding to the population by stating that the research hypothesis is false and method B is the superior method for teaching third-grade boys in Georgia.

Let us examine this example further. The rope-skipping test has 20 points possible. The mean rope-skipping test scores for groups A, B, and C are 10.5, 15.9, and 12.1, respectively. In regard to the differences in the means, one position the researcher could take is that any difference indicates that the teaching methods are not equally effective and that teaching method B is the superior method. This position however, ignores the possibility of **sampling error** which may have partially or totally caused the differences among the groups in mean score. Sampling error occurs when a sample is not 100 percent representative of the population. Blommers and Forsyth (1983) define sampling error as the difference between the value of a population parameter and that of the corresponding sample statistic. Therefore, the differences among groups A, B, and C in mean score could be due to sampling error. Essentially, all samples should have started the experiment with the same mean, but due to sampling error the sample means differed. This could be what caused the differences at the end of the experiment, rather than any differences in the effectiveness of the three treatments. As a result, the differences among the sample means may be a **real difference** due to the treatments not being equally effective, or the differences may be due to sampling error.

If the differences among the means in the rope-skipping example are large, it is reasonable to conclude the differences are real and the treatments are not equally effective. However, if the differences among the means are small, they may well be due to sampling error. The question becomes, Are the differences among the sample means (10.5, 15.9, 12.1) large enough to indicate a real difference? Posing this question to a group of people, some would say yes and some would say no, but many would say they could not tell. The researcher needs a standard procedure to follow in reaching such a decision. Standardization increases the likelihood that researchers following the procedure will reach the same conclusion. Agreement among researchers in this situation is desirable.

Hypothesis-Testing Procedure

Hypothesis testing involves a five-step procedure that researchers use to decide whether to accept or reject the research hypothesis based on the information collected on the sample(s) in the research studies. Though they may execute these steps, researchers may not report all five in their written report or journal article. This five-step procedure, which can be used in a variety of situations, is explained below. Following this explanation, a number of different research designs are presented showing how the hypothesis-testing procedure is used.

Step 1: State the Hypotheses

A researcher starts out with a statement concerning what may be the situation at the population level. If the research involves multiple groups, the statement is that the groups are equal in terms of the measure of interest in the research. Since this is a statement of no or null difference, this statement is called the **null hypothesis** and is indicated using the symbol H_0. This is the **statistical hypothesis,** and it does not have to agree with the **research hypothesis.** In the rope-skipping example, the research hypothesis is that method A is superior, but the null hypothesis is that all three methods are equally good. At least one, and often two, alternate hypotheses symbolized by H_1 and H_2 must be stated to provide a hypothesis to accept if H_0 is rejected.

Step 2: Select the Probability Level

The difference between the population statement in the null hypothesis and what is found in the sample(s) in the research studies is due either to the null hypothesis being false or to sampling error. To make an objective decision, the researcher will conduct a statistical test at the fourth step of the five-step hypothesis-testing procedure. The results of the statistical test provide the probability of the sample finding occurring if the null hypothesis is true. If the probability is small, the null hypothesis is rejected and the difference is considered to be real. Otherwise, the null hypothesis is accepted and the difference is considered to be due to sampling error. In step 2 the researcher selects some probability level that warrants rejection of the null hypothesis. This probability level is called the **alpha level** (a) and is usually specified as .05 or .01.

Step 3: Consult the Statistical Table

Most researchers examine the appropriate statistical table to find the value that the statistical test of the sample would need to equal or exceed in order to reject the null hypothesis at the chosen alpha level. Many computer programs provide a probability value (p) for the value of the statistical test selected in step 4. In this case, the researcher rejects the null hypothesis if the p value is less than or equal to the alpha level.

Step 4: Conduct the Statistical Test

In this step the statistical test is calculated. The statistical test may be calculated by hand or by using a computer.

Step 5: Accept or Reject the Null Hypothesis

In the final step, the decision is made either to accept or to reject the null hypothesis. If the value of the statistical test is greater than the table value or if the p value for the value of the statistical test is less than the alpha level, the null hypothesis is rejected. If the opposite is true, the null hypothesis is accepted.

Accepting the null hypothesis does not prove it is true, only that it is plausible. The null hypothesis could be false by such a small amount that the statistical test did not detect it (e.g., H_0: $\mu = 10$ when really $\mu = 10.03$). So, some researchers use the terms *fail to reject* and *reject* rather than *accept* and *reject*. A statement in the research literature that the statistical test was **significant** indicates that the value of the statistical test warranted rejection of the null hypothesis. More specifically, it indicates that the difference between the null hypothesis population statement and what was found in the sample(s) in the research seems to be a real difference and not due to sampling error. Therefore, a statement that the statistical test was **nonsignificant** indicates that the null hypothesis was retained, and any differences were attributed to sampling error.

The five-step hypothesis-testing procedure is applied in the examples that follow. Each uses a different research design and statistical test. Some additional explanation of the steps in the research process is provided along with the examples. The most extensive explanation of the steps occurs in the first example. The presentation of the five-step hypothesis-testing procedure in subsequent examples is abbreviated to save space. Since the same five-step procedure is followed in each example, make sure you understand the one-group t test example well before venturing on to other examples. The t test and analysis of variance (ANOVA) examples generally apply to situations in experimental research (chapter 7) while the chi-square test examples usually apply to situations in descriptive research (chapter 8).

One-Group t Test

A researcher believes the mean percentage of body fat for a population of male workers is 18 percent. To test this hypothesis, the researcher randomly selects a sample of forty-one men from the population and measures their percentage of body fat.

Step 1: The researcher's hypothesis is that the mean percentage of body fat is 18, so the null hypothesis is that the population mean (μ) is 18 (H_0: $\mu = 18$). As alternatives to this hypothesis, the researcher thought it possible that the mean could be less than 18 (H_1: $\mu < 18$) or greater than 18 (H_2: $\mu > 18$).

Step 2: An alpha level of .05 is selected.

Step 3: A **one-group t test** will be the statistical test, and the sample size is 41. The researcher uses the t tables to find that in order to reject the null hypothesis at an alpha level of .05, the value of the t test has to be at least ± 2.021. Step 3 is not needed if a microcomputer program is used because a p value is calculated and can be compared to the selected alpha level in step 2 (.05 in this case).

Step 4: The researcher calculates the mean for the body fat measurements and calculates the t test.

$\bar{x} = 16.50$, $s = 2.50$

$$t = \frac{\bar{x} - \mu}{SE} = \frac{16.50 - 18}{SE} = -3.85,$$ where SE is the standard error (calculated by using a formula presented in a statistics book or by the computer program). In this case because the formula is simple, $SE = s/\sqrt{n} = 2.50/\sqrt{41}$.

Step 5: Since the calculated value of t (-3.85) at step 4 is less than the tabled value of t (-2.021) at step 3, the researcher concludes that the difference between the null hypothesis value (18 percent) at step 1 and the sample value (16.50 percent) at step 4 is real and not due to sampling error. The researcher rejects the null hypothesis and accepts the most likely alternate hypothesis, which in this case is H_1. The population mean is less than 18 percent, since the sample mean is less than 18 percent.

Summary of Example

At step 3 when the researcher used the t tables (see appendix B) to identify the t value needed for rejecting the null hypothesis, the **degrees of freedom** and the alpha level had to be lined up to find the t value. The degrees of freedom for this t test was (n-1) where n is the sample size. Because there are two alternate hypotheses, the researcher uses the alpha level under a two-tailed test. For a two-tailed test this value is always interpreted as both plus and minus. If there is only the one alternate hypothesis, the alpha level under the one-tailed test is used; the value read from the table is interpreted as plus if the alternate hypothesis is greater than (H_1: $\mu >$) and minus if the alternate hypothesis is less than (H_1: $\mu <$). The tabled value is sometimes called the **critical value.** All values at or beyond the critical value are in the **critical region.** If the value of the statistical test used at step 4 is equal to or greater than the tabled value found at step 3 (in the critical region), the difference and the statistical test are called significant (the difference is considered to be real), and the null hypothesis is rejected at step 5. If the value of the statistical test is not equal to or greater than the table value, the difference and statistical test are called nonsignificant (the difference is considered to be due to sampling error), and the null hypothesis is accepted.

At step 4, the larger the difference between the hypothesized population mean (18) and the sample mean (16.50), the larger the value of t. Also, the standard error (SE) is an indication of the amount of sampling error.

This one-group t test just studied is one of three t tests available. Fortunately, most computer packages of statistical programs contain all three t tests. In SPSS, the t test for one group is called One-Sample T Test. Directions for its use are presented in section 3 of the Statistical Procedures part of appendix A.

The scores of three groups on a first aid test are presented in table 13.1. The scores of group A are analyzed using SPSS to test the null hypothesis that the population mean equals 10 (H_0: $\mu = 10$). The t test output is presented in table 13.2. Notice that the computer provides a probability value (p value—.025, in our example) so that it is not necessary to look up the table value.

Two Independent Groups t Test

The **two independent groups t test** is used either when two samples are drawn from the same population and each is administered a different treatment or when a sample is drawn from each of two populations. In the first case, two samples of seventy-five each are drawn from a population of female college freshmen and each sample is

TABLE 13.1 Scores for Three Groups on a First Aid Test

GROUP A	GROUP B	GROUP C
12	7	13
15	10	14
10	11	10
11	8	9
9	9	12
14	10	11
12	12	11
13	9	15

TABLE 13.2 Output for the One-Group t Test of Group A in Table 13.1

N	8
Mean	12.00
Std. Deviation	2.00
Mean Difference	2.00
t	2.83
df	7
Sig. (2-tailed)	.025

taught by a different method. After the treatments (methods) are administered, each sample represents a different population: a population of freshmen who have received or will in the future receive the particular treatment. In the second case, two samples of forty are drawn, one from a population of athletes and one from a population of nonathletes. Both samples represent different populations; the question is whether there is a difference between the two samples in mean performance as an indication of a difference at the population level.

The t test for two independent groups can be obtained with SPSS. The data of groups A and B in table 13.1 are used to demonstrate this analysis and the five-step hypothesis-testing procedure. When entering the data into the computer each participant must have two scores: one identifying group membership and the other being the score of the participant. An example of this for the first two scores in group A and then group B in table 13.1 is shown below.

Case	ID	Score	
1	1	12	ID was the name the researcher used to identify
2	1	15	group membership (1 =A group, 2 =B group)
3	2	7	and SCORE was the name the researcher used
4	2	10	for the score of a subject.

To conduct the t test using SPSS, refer to section 4 of the Statistical Procedures part of appendix A.

Step 1: H_0: $\mu_A - \mu_B = 0$ (hypothesis that population means are equal)

H_1: $\mu_A - \mu_B > 0$ (hypothesis that A population mean is greater)

H_2: $\mu_A - \mu_B < 0$ (hypothesis that B population mean is greater)

Step 2: Alpha = .05

Step 3: The t test table critical value is based on degrees of freedom equal to $(n_1 + n_2 - 2)$ where n_1 is the sample size for group A and n_2 is for group B. The degrees of freedom is 14 (or $8 + 8 - 2$). The table value for an alpha of .05 under a two-tailed test and degrees of freedom 14 is ± 2.145.

Step 4: The scores of each group are analyzed and the t test calculated.

$$t = \frac{\bar{x}_A - \bar{x}_B}{SE}$$, where SE is based on the two sample variances and is an estimate of the amount of sampling error.

The results of the computer analysis are presented in table 13.3.

Step 5: The calculated t value from step 4 is compared with the table t value at step 3 or the computer p value with the alpha level at step 2.

The computer provided a p value of .015. No matter whether the calculated t value of 2.76 is compared with the table t value of ± 2.145, or the p value of .015 is compared with the alpha level (.05) in step 2, the difference between the means for A and B groups is significant and the null hypothesis (H_0) is rejected in favor of H_1 because the t value is positive and group A has the larger mean.

Two Dependent Groups t Test

One example of the **two dependent groups t test** is a **repeated measures** design, and the other example is a **matched pairs** design. In either case there are two columns of scores and some degree of correlation or dependency between them.

TABLE 13.3 Output for the Two Independent Groups *t* Test for Groups A and B in Table 13.1

ITEM	GROUP A	GROUP B
N	8	8
Mean	12.00	9.50
Std. Deviation	2.00	1.60
t	2.76	
df	14	
Sig. (2-tailed)	.015	

With the repeated measures design, a population is defined from which a sample is drawn using random sampling procedures. Participants are tested initially, an experimental treatment is administered, and the participants finally retested. Usually, the same test is administered both before and after the treatment so the research situation is called a test-retest design or pretest-posttest design. With paper-and-pencil tests, one form of the test (form A) could be administered at pretest and form B of the test could be administered at posttest. The purpose of this research design is to determine if an experimental treatment is effective.

The research question could also be investigated using two independent groups, with one group receiving the experimental treatment (experimental group) and the other receiving no treatment (control group). The repeated measures design is more efficient and precise than the two independent groups design because all participants receive the treatment and act as their own control. The experimental research chapter describes the repeated measures design as having numerous internal and external validity problems; however, this design is commonly used.

With the matched pairs design, a population is defined and some measure(s) is collected on each member of the population that the researcher feels must be controlled in the research study. The researcher wants the two groups involved in this design to start the experiment basically equal in terms of the measure(s) collected. Participants are paired on this measure(s), with one participant from each pair randomly assigned to each of the two groups. Each group receives a different treatment, so there may be one experimental group and one control group, or there may be two experimental groups. After the groups receive the treatments, they are measured and the data are analyzed to determine if the groups seem equal in mean performance.

Example: The population is college freshmen at a large university. Two different methods of teaching a large lecture class are going to be compared. A gender score and IQ score are obtained for each of the 600 members of the population. For two students to be paired, they have to be of the same gender and have IQ scores that differ by no more than 5. One hundred pairs are formed. One participant from each pair is randomly assigned to each teaching method. Participants are taught by their assigned teaching method for fifteen weeks. After that, all participants take a knowledge test. The data are analyzed to determine if the two teaching methods seem to be equally effective.

The matched pairs design is an alternative to the two independent groups design but is more precise in that the two groups start the experiment equal on at least the measure(s) used for forming pairs. Loss of participants can be a problem with the matched pairs design because some members of the population cannot be paired, and during the experiment, if one member of a pair is lost from the experiment, the other member of the pair must be removed from the study.

The t test is the same for the repeated measures design and matched pairs design.

$$t = \frac{\bar{x}_I - \bar{x}_F}{SE}$$ for repeated measures where $\bar{x}_F$ is the mean for the final scores

or

$$t = \frac{\bar{x}_1 - \bar{x}_2}{SE}$$ for matched pairs where $\bar{x}_2$ is the mean for group 2,

with degrees of freedom equal to $n - 1$, where n is the number of participants for a repeated measures design or the number of pairs for a matched pairs design. An example of the five-step hypothesis-testing procedure with a repeated measures design is presented below.

Suppose eight participants are selected and initially (I) measured for number of mistakes made when juggling a ball. The participants are then taught to juggle and finally (F) measured. Let us say that, in table 13.1, the group A scores are the initial scores and the group B scores are the final scores. To determine if the participants improved in juggling ability as a result of the juggling instruction, a t test for dependent groups is conducted.

Step 1: H_0: $\mu_I - \mu_F = 0$ (hypothesis that final and initial means are equal
            H_1: $\mu_I - \mu_F < 0$ at the population level)

Step 2: Alpha = .05

Step 3: Find the t test table value with degrees of freedom equal to $n - 1$, where n is the number of participants. In this example, the degrees of freedom is 7 (8 − 1) and the tabled t value is −1.895 for an alpha of .05 in a one-tailed test.

Step 4: Analyze the initial and final data, and calculate the t test.

$$t = \frac{\bar{x}_I - \bar{x}_F}{SE}$$

The repeated measures t test can be obtained with SPSS. The data are entered in pairs by participant with the initial and final score for participant 1 (12, 7) entered first, followed by the initial and final score for participant 2 (15, 10), and each of the remaining participants. To conduct the t test using SPSS, follow the procedures presented in section 5 of the Statistical Procedures part of appendix A. The printout of this analysis is presented in table 13.4.

Step 5: Because the p value in table 13.4 is less than the .05 alpha level selected at step 2, the difference between the initial and final means is significant and the null hypothesis is rejected. Notice that the calculated t exceeds the tabled t, and the same conclusion is drawn. Also notice that because the measured variable is number of mistakes, the final mean of 9.50 is superior to the initial mean of 12.00. Therefore, the researcher concludes that the treatment is effective.

Decision on Alternate Hypotheses and Alpha Level

Before considering other research designs and statistical tests, selection of alternate hypotheses and the alpha level must be explained in greater detail. With the five-step hypothesis-testing procedure at least one, and often two, alternate hypotheses are stated. Usually two alternate hypotheses are stated because the null hypothesis and the two alternate hypotheses cover all possibilities. The researcher believes that if the null hypothesis is false it could be in either direction, and the researcher is interested in both alternatives. For example, all possibilities are covered in the situation where H_0: mean IQ is 100; H_1: mean IQ is less than 100; and H_2: mean IQ is greater than 100. The researcher may have decided that the teaching method to be used will

TABLE 13.4 Output for the Repeated Measures t Test Treating the A and B Group Data in Table 13.1 as Repeated Measures

ITEM	SCORE 1	SCORE 2
N	8	8
Mean	12.00	9.50
Std. Deviation	2.00	1.60
Mean Difference	2.50	
t	2.89	
df	7	
Sig. (2-tailed)	.023	

depend on which hypothesis is accepted. However, in situations where the researcher knows there is only one alternative to the null hypothesis or only one alternative is of interest to the researcher, only one alternative hypothesis is stated. For example, in a repeated measures design the researcher usually knows that the treatment will either have no effect or a positive effect; the treatment will not make the participants worse. Another example is situations where a traditional method is being compared with a new method. Only if the new method is superior to the traditional method will the researcher recommend a change in method.

It is important to remember that the number of alternate hypotheses determines whether the statistical test is one-tailed or two-tailed. If there are two alternate hypotheses, the statistical test is two-tailed. Notice in the *t* tables that for any degrees of freedom and alpha level, the value for a one-tailed test is smaller than for a two-tailed test. The smaller the table value, the easier it is to reject the null hypothesis. Thus, acceptance or rejection of the null hypothesis may be dependent on the number of alternate hypotheses.

While examining the *t* table, notice that for any degrees of freedom, the smaller the alpha level, the larger the table value. Selection of the alpha level also influences the acceptance or rejection of the null hypothesis. Traditionally researchers have used an alpha level of .05 unless there were reasons for selecting a different value. The second most commonly used alpha level is .01. Using an alpha level of .01 rather than .05 makes it more difficult to reject the null hypothesis, meaning the smaller the alpha level, the larger the difference must be between what is hypothesized at the population level and what is found at the sample level. In situations where rejecting the null hypothesis has major implications, researchers tend to use alpha levels of .01 or even .001. For example, if rejecting the null hypothesis means that an effective traditional drug is going to be replaced by a new drug, the researcher might use an alpha level of .01 or .001 because the researcher wants to be particularly confident that the new drug is superior to the effective traditional drug.

A diagram of the four possible outcomes of a research study is presented in figure 13.1. In any research study, the null hypothesis is either true or false, but the researcher never knows for sure which is correct. Based on the statistical test, the researcher either accepts or rejects the null hypothesis. If the null hypothesis really

	Decision	
	Accept	**Reject**
H_0 **True**	Good decision	Type I error
False	Type II error	Good decision

FIGURE 13.1
Four possible outcomes in a research study.

is true, and based on the statistical test the researcher accepts it, this is a good decision. However, if the researcher rejects a null hypothesis that is really true this is called a **type I error.** A type I error is defined as rejecting a true null hypothesis. The probability of making a type I error is equal to the alpha level. Therefore, the researcher usually selects the alpha level based on the seriousness of a type I error. Researchers always use small alpha levels as a way of protecting themselves against making a type I error.

If the null hypothesis really is false, and based on the statistical test the researcher rejects it, this is also a good decision. But if the researcher did not reject a false null hypothesis, this is called a **type II error** and is symbolized by **beta (β).** A type II error is defined either as accepting a false null hypothesis or not rejecting a false null hypothesis. Many things can influence the probability of making a type II error. The larger the alpha level, the smaller the probability of making a type II error. Since the alpha level also affects the probability of a type I error, most researchers do not try to influence the probability of a type II error with the alpha selection. The larger the sample size, the smaller the probability of a type II error, and sample size is often something the researcher can control. The more false the null hypothesis, the less likely a type II error will occur. This is not something the researcher controls, but it should be kept in mind when small differences are found in a research study.

The term **statistical power** is commonly found in the research literature. Statistical power is the probability of not making a type II error, so power is the probability of rejecting a false null hypothesis. Power equals one minus beta ($1 - \beta$). One-tailed tests have more statistical power than two-tailed tests, and a two dependent groups design has more statistical power than a two independent groups design. Everything that decreases the probability of making a type II error, increases statistical power.

Analysis of Variance

Many research problems or questions involve more than two treatment groups. In these situations, **analysis of variance (ANOVA)** is used to analyze the data. Actually, ANOVA can also be used when there are just two treatment groups, so in this situation it could be used rather than a *t* test. There are many different ANOVA designs. An overview of the technique should help in understanding each design.

Using the ANOVA technique, the total variability in a set of scores is divided into two or more components. These variability values are called **sums of squares (SS).** A degrees of freedom value (df) is obtained for both the total variability value and each of the component values. The sum of squares value for each component is divided by its degrees of freedom value to obtain a **mean square (MS) value.** The ratio of two mean square values is an *F* statistic, which is used to test the null hypothesis. The *F* test is conducted at step 4 of the five-step hypothesis-testing procedure.

One-Way ANOVA

One-way ANOVA is an extension of the two independent groups design already discussed, but typically involves statistical analysis of three or more independent groups. Ferguson and Takane (1989) refer to this test as a one-way ANOVA because each score only has one classification (group membership). The placement of the score in the group has no effect on the data analysis. Actually, a one-way ANOVA can be used with two or more independent groups, so it could be used in place of the *t* test for two independent groups. The null hypothesis being tested is that the populations represented by the groups (samples) are equal in mean performance. The one alternate hypothesis is that the population means are not equal.

Some explanation of the one-way ANOVA is necessary to understand how the technique is used and how to interpret the output from the computer analysis. Also, a few symbols are necessary in order to develop formulas for determining degrees of freedom.

Two or more independent groups each receive a different treatment. The number of groups will be represented symbolically by K, and the total number of scores by N. For the data in table 13.1, $K = 3$ and $N = 24$. All the scores in all the groups are combined into one set of scores and the mean is calculated. The variability of the scores from this mean is the total variability for the set of scores and is called the sum of squares total (SS_T). The sum of squares total is divided into sum of squares among groups (SS_A) and sum of squares within groups (SS_W).

$$SS_T = SS_A + SS_W$$

Group means are calculated; if these group means are not equal, the sum of squares among groups is greater than zero. Thus, SS_A is an indication of differences among the groups. The sum of squares within groups is an indication of how much the scores in the groups differ from their group mean. Thus, if in any groups all scores are not the same value, SS_W will be greater than zero.

Each sum of squares has a degrees of freedom value. The degrees of freedom for total (df_T) is divided into a degrees of freedom among (df_A) and within (df_W) groups.

$$df_T = df_A + df_W,$$
$$\text{where } df_T = N - 1, df_A = K - 1, df_W = N - K.$$

Applied to the data in table 13.1.

$$df_T = 24 - 1 = 23$$
$$df_A = 3 - 1 = 2$$
$$df_W = 24 - 3 = 21$$

The sums of squares values for among and within groups are divided by their degrees of freedom to provide mean square (MS) values and an F statistic is calculated from the two mean square values:

$$MS_A = \frac{SS_A}{df_A}, \; MS_W = \frac{SS_W}{df_W}, \; F = \frac{MS_A}{MS_W}$$

Any F statistic is represented by two degrees of freedom values in the F table. The first degrees of freedom value is for the numerator and the second degrees of freedom value is for the denominator of the F statistic. The numerator degrees of freedom is df_A and the denominator degrees of freedom is df_W. So,

$$F = \frac{MS_A}{MS_W} \text{ has degrees of freedom equal to } (K - 1) \text{ and } (N - K).$$

The F table is presented in appendix C. The first degrees of freedom value is read across the top of the table, and the second degrees of freedom value is read down the left side of the table. Two table values appear where the line down from the first degrees of freedom value and across from the second degrees of freedom value intersect. The larger value is the F value needed for significance at the .01 alpha level, and the other level is for the .05 alpha level. If the degrees of freedom is 2 and 21, the table values are 3.47 for alpha equals .05 and 5.78 for alpha equals .01.

An example of the five-step hypothesis-testing procedure using the data in table 13.1 follows:

Step 1: H_0: $\mu_A = \mu_B = \mu_C$ (the three population means are equal)
H_1: $\mu_A \neq \mu_B \neq \mu_C$ (the three population means are not equal)

Step 2: Alpha = .05

TABLE 13.5 Output for the One-Way ANOVA for the Data in Table 13.1

SOURCE	SS	DF	MS	F	SIG.
Among	31.75	2	15.88	4.45	.024
Within	74.88	21	3.57		
Total	106.63	23			

GROUP	N	MEAN
A	8	12.00
B	8	9.50
C	8	11.88

Step 3: Find the critical value in the F test table with degrees of freedom ($K - 1$) and ($N - K$) at the alpha level selected. In this example, the degrees of freedom are 2 and 21 so the table value is 3.47 for alpha equals .05.

Step 4: Analyze the data using a one-way ANOVA. In SPSS, one-way ANOVA is conducted by following the directions in section 6 of the Statistical Procedures part of appendix A. As in the t test for two independent groups, when the data are entered, there must be a variable identifying group membership and a score for each participant. In SPSS, the Dependent variable is the data variable and the Factor variable is the variable identifying group membership. Applied to the data from table 13.1, the one-way ANOVA output is presented in table 13.5. The statistical test is the F ratio, and it can be seen that the F ratio is 4.45 and the p value of the F ratio is .024.

Step 5: Since the p value of .024 is less than the alpha level of .05, a researcher concludes that there is a significant difference among the group means and accepts the alternate hypothesis. The same decision is made if the F ratio of 4.45 is compared with the table value of 3.47 in step 3.

Repeated Measures ANOVA

The **repeated measures ANOVA** design is an extension of the t test for two dependent groups design, using repeated measurement of participants. Each participant is measured on two or more occasions. If there are only two measures for each participant, the repeated measures ANOVA design is an alternative to the t test for dependent groups design. However, if there are more than two measures for each participant, the repeated measures ANOVA design must be used. The repeated measures ANOVA design is also referred to as a one-way ANOVA with repeated measures. The null hypothesis being tested is that, at the population level, the means for the repeated measures are equal. The alternate hypothesis is that the means are not equal.

Suppose a group of participants is drawn from a population using random sampling procedures. Before the experimental treatment is administered the participants are initially tested. The experimental treatment is then administered for nine weeks, and every three weeks the participants are tested. The data layout for this study is presented in table 13.6.

The data layout is two-dimensional since each score has two classifiers—a row designation (participant) and a column designation (repeated measure). The score of 10 for participant A must be placed in the Initial Test column of the row for participant A (each row-column intersection is called a **cell**) or it is in the wrong cell. Notice in the one-way ANOVA previously discussed, that each score had only the single classification of group membership.

Again, some symbolism is needed to develop degrees of freedom formulas. The total number of scores is N, the number of repeated measures is K, and the number of participants is n. In table 13.6, $N = 32$, $K = 4$, and $n = 8$. In this ANOVA design, sum of squares total (SS_T) is partitioned into the following components: sum of squares participants (SS_P); sum of squares repeated measures (SS_M); and sum of squares interaction (SS_I).

$$SS_T = SS_P + SS_M + SS_I$$

The minimum value for each of the sum of squares values is zero. The SS_T is greater than zero if all N scores are not the same. The SS_P is greater than zero if participants differ in mean score across repeated measures. The SS_M is greater than zero if the means for repeated measures are not equal. The SS_I is greater than zero if all participants did not follow the same scoring pattern across the repeated measures. In table 13.6, SS_I is greater than zero because the scores for participant A increased by three, then by two, then by one from test to test, but the other participants demonstrated different patterns. Each of these terms has a degrees of freedom (df) value.

$$df_T = df_P + df_M + df_I$$

The formulas for the degrees of freedom are as follows:

$$df_T = N - 1 \qquad df_P = n - 1 \qquad df_M = K - 1 \qquad df_I = (n - 1)(K - 1)$$

In table 13.6, $df_T = 32 - 1 = 31$, $df_P = 8 - 1 = 7$, $df_M = 4 - 1 = 3$, and $df_I = (8 - 1)(4 - 1) = 21$.

Mean square values are obtained for participants, for repeated measures, and for interaction components. The statistical hypothesis being tested is that the means for the repeated measures are equal. To form the F statistic the mean square value

TABLE 13.6 Repeated Measures ANOVA Example Data

PARTICIPANTS	INITIAL TEST	3-WEEK TEST	6-WEEK TEST	9-WEEK TEST
A	10	13	15	16
B	5	9	10	13
C	11	12	12	13
D	6	9	12	14
E	6	8	10	12
F	5	6	10	13
G	8	10	11	13
H	9	11	13	14

indicating the differences among the means for the repeated measures (MS_M) becomes the numerator, and the mean square value indicating sampling error (MS_I) becomes the denominator. The F test takes this form:

$$F = \frac{MS_M}{MS_I}, \quad \text{with } K - 1 \text{ degrees of freedom and} \\ (n - 1)(K - 1) \text{ degrees of freedom}$$

An example of the five-step hypothesis-testing procedure is presented using the data in table 13.6.

Step 1: H_0: $\mu_{initial} = \mu_3 = \mu_6 = \mu_9$
H_1: $\mu_{initial} \neq \mu_3 \neq \mu_6 \neq \mu_9$

Step 2: Alpha $= .05$

Step 3: Find the table value of F with degrees of freedom $K - 1$ and $(n - 1)$ $(K - 1)$ at the .05 alpha level. The value of F with degrees of freedom 3 and 21 at the .05 alpha level is 3.07.

Step 4: This repeated measures ANOVA design is not possible on Student SPSS. The easiest way to conduct a repeated measures ANOVA with SPSS is to use the Reliability program. In this program the columns are called items, so for the repeated measures ANOVA the repeated measures are the items. To get the column (repeated measure) means and the ANOVA summary table, the Statistics option in the Reliability program must be selected as described in the directions for the Reliability program (see section 12 of the Statistical Procedures part of appendix A). The Reliability program was used to analyze the data in table 13.6. The output from the computer is presented in table 13.7. The repeated measures F

TABLE 13.7 Output for the Repeated Measures ANOVA for the Data in Table 13.6

SOURCE	SS	DF	MS	F	SIG.
Between People	82.47	7	11.78		
Between Measures	158.34	3	52.78	48.39	.000
Residual	22.91	21	1.09		
Total	263.72	31	8.51		

	Measure	Mean	Std. Deviation
	Initial	7.50	2.33
	3-week	9.75	2.25
	6-week	11.63	1.77
	9-week	13.50	1.20

value is 48.39, which is greater than the table value of F at step 3. The p value of .000 for repeated measures is less than the alpha level at step 2. Using either indicator, the calculated F value for repeated measures is significant. The F value for participants is not of interest in this analysis.

Labels for the sources or components in the ANOVA vary among statistics books and computer programs. Knowing what to expect in the ANOVA summary table helps the reader interpret the labels. In table 13.7 the residual source is the interaction source. Other computer programs may label the interaction source as error, or as PT to suggest a participant (P) by treatment (T) interaction.

Step 5:   Based on step 4, conclude that H_0 is false; accept H_1 that the treatment means are not equal.

Random Blocks ANOVA

Earlier in this chapter, a matched pairs t test design was presented. In this design pairs are formed by pairing two participants. Then, using random procedures, one participant from each pair is assigned to one group, and the other participant is assigned to a second group. The **random blocks ANOVA** design is an extension of the matched pairs t test when there are three or more groups, and is the same as the matched pairs t test when there are two groups. In the random blocks design, participants similar in terms of a variable(s) are placed together in what is called a *block,* rather than a *pair* as in the t test. The number of participants in each block is equal to the number of treatment groups in the research study. The procedures used in the matched pairs t test might serve as a helpful reference for this design.

After participants are assigned to groups, each group receives a different treatment, and at the end of the study the data are collected. The random block design has all the advantages and disadvantages of the matched pairs t test.

Table 13.8 is an example data layout for a random blocks design. Notice that the same notation is used in this design as is used for the repeated measures ANOVA design. In fact, blocks are like participants, treatment groups are like repeated measures, and the hypothesis tested is that the group means are equal. Thus, the analysis for the random blocks design is the same as the analysis for the repeated measures ANOVA design.

Two-Way ANOVA, Multiple Scores per Cell

Two-way ANOVA is a term used by Ferguson and Takane (1989) and some other authors of statistics books and computer programs. A variety of other terms referring to the same design are commonly found in statistics books and the research literature as well. In a two-way ANOVA design, each score has a row and a column classifier.

TABLE 13.8 Example Data Layout for a Random Blocks ANOVA Design

BLOCK	GROUP 1	GROUP 2	GROUP 3	• • •	GROUP K
1	X	X	X	• • •	X
2	X	X	X	• • •	X
3	X	X	X	• • •	X
•	•	•	•		•
•	•	•	•		•
•	•	•	•		•
n	X	X	X	• • •	X

The two ANOVA designs previously discussed involved just one score per cell. Three examples of two-way ANOVA designs with multiple scores in each cell are presented next. The data analysis is the same in all three examples. In each example, it is possible to test several statistical hypotheses that require different F tests. An explanation of the data analysis follows each example.

The first example is a random blocks design with more than one score per cell. This is the same as the previous random blocks design except that enough participants are placed in each block to have multiple scores per cell. For example, if there are five treatment groups, the number of participants in each block has to be ten, fifteen, or some other multiple of five. The statistical hypothesis is always that the treatment groups are equal in mean score; additional statistical hypotheses of interest are tested in certain situations.

The second example is referred to as **factorial design.** In this two-way data layout, the rows represent some classification of the participants (e.g., gender, age, school grade), the columns identify the treatment group, and there are multiple participants in each cell. In table 13.9, participants are classified by gender with five females and five males randomly assigned to each treatment group. Data are collected at the end of the research study after the groups experienced the treatments. The analysis for this example design could be referred to as a **two-dimensional ANOVA** or a 2 × 3 (Gender × Treatment) ANOVA. Gender has two levels and treatment has three levels because there are two classifications of gender and three treatment groups.

In this example, the researcher is interested in testing the statistical hypothesis that the treatment group (column) means are equal. The row variable may be a dimension if the researcher wants to test a second statistical hypothesis that the row means are equal. Or, it is possible that this hypothesis is not of interest to the researcher, so the row variable is a dimension used to gain experimental control as discussed in the experimental research chapter. In the table 13.9 example, gender as a dimension will be a source in the ANOVA summary table. If gender is not a dimension, the design is a one-way ANOVA with three treatment groups, gender is not a source in the ANOVA summary table, and any differences between the genders in

TABLE 13.9 Example Data Layout for a Factorial ANOVA (Gender × Treatment)			
	TREATMENT GROUP		
GENDER	**A**	**B**	**C**
Female	2, 1, 3, 2, 3	6, 3, 4, 5, 6	5, 4, 7, 6, 8
Male	4, 3, 2, 3, 1	4, 5, 7, 6, 8	10, 9, 10, 8, 11

mean score are put into the "within" component of the one-way ANOVA. Since in the one-way ANOVA, $F = \text{MS}_{among}/\text{MS}_{within}$, putting the gender difference into the within component will decrease the value of the F test and increase the chances of making a type II error.

A third statistical hypothesis can be tested in this example: no interaction between the row variable and the column variable. In terms of table 13.9, this hypothesis states that any differences in the effectiveness of the treatments are the same for both genders. The no interaction hypothesis will be discussed later in the chapter.

The third example is also a factorial design, but rows are levels of one treatment, columns are levels of a second treatment, and there are multiple participants in each cell. It is commonly used because it is a combination of two treatments. For example, in table 13.10 treatment A, is the number of days per week people participated in an adult fitness program (A1 = 1 day, A2 = 3 days); treatment B, is how many minutes per participation day people participated (B1 = 15 minutes, B2 = 30 minutes, B3 = 45 minutes). Five participants are randomly assigned to receive each treatment combination. For example, the A1B1 group participated 1 day a week, 15 minutes a day. The experimental period is six months. At the end of that period, all participants are tested on a fitness test where a low score reflects high fitness.

Three null hypotheses are usually tested in this ANOVA design. The first hypothesis is that there is no interaction between the row and column variables. If there is no interaction, the difference between any two column means is the same for each row, and vice versa. If there is no interaction effect, the difference between the A1B1 and A1B2 cell means is the same as the difference between the A2B1 and A2B2 cell means. The second hypothesis is that the row means are equal. If the hypothesis is true, the A1 and A2 row means are equal. The third hypothesis is that the column means are equal. If the hypothesis is true, the B1, B2, and B3 column means are equal.

The particular symbols used to represent two-way ANOVA designs with multiple scores per cell apply to all three of the example designs that have been presented. The symbol C represents the number of columns in the design; the number of rows in the design is R. The number of scores in each cell is represented by n; the total number of scores in the whole design is represented by N, which is equal to CRn (columns × rows × cell size). In table 13.10, $C = 3$, $R = 2$, $n = 5$, and $N = 30$.

In the two-way ANOVA design with multiple scores per cell, the sum of squares total (SS_T) is partitioned into a sum of squares columns (SS_C), a sum of squares rows (SS_R), a sum of squares interaction (SS_I), and a sum of squares within (SS_W):

TABLE 13.10 Example Data Layout for a Factorial ANOVA (Days × Minutes)			
TREATMENT	B1	B2	B3
A1	12, 10, 9, 11, 10	10, 11, 9, 10, 11	10, 9, 8, 7, 8
A2	14, 12, 13, 15, 12	8, 9, 10, 9, 11	6, 7, 5, 6, 4

Note: A1 = 1 day/week; A2 = 3 days/week; B1 = 15 minutes/day; B2 = 30 minutes/day;
B3 = 45 minutes/day.

$$SS_T = SS_C + SS_R + SS_I + SS_W$$

The minimum value for each of these sum of squares is zero. The SS_T is greater than zero if all N scores are not equal. The SS_C is greater than zero if the means for the columns are unequal. The greater the inequality among the columns, the larger SS_C. Likewise, the more the row means differ, the larger is SS_R. There will be no interaction ($SS_I = 0$) if the pattern of differences among column means is the same for each row, and vice versa. Finally, SS_W will equal zero if for each cell all scores in the cell are the same value.

Each of these sum of squares values has an associated degrees of freedom value. So,

$$df_T = df_C + df_R + df_I + df_W, \text{ where}$$
$$df_T = N - 1,$$
$$df_C = C - 1,$$
$$df_R = R - 1,$$
$$df_I = (C - 1)(R - 1),$$
$$df_W = (C)(R)(n - 1).$$

As always, each of the parts of SS_T is divided by its degrees of freedom (df) to produce a mean square (MS) value. So,

$$MS_C = SS_C/df_C,$$
$$MS_R = SS_R/df_R,$$
$$MS_I = SS_I/df_I,$$
$$MS_W = SS_W/df_W.$$

These mean square values are used to form the F tests for the various statistical hypotheses. All three potential hypotheses are presented below; although a researcher might not test a hypothesis if it is not of interest.

Typically the first hypothesis tested is one of no interaction. The alternate hypothesis (H_1) is one of interaction. The hypothesis is tested with $F = MS_I/MS_W$ with degrees of freedom $(C - 1)(R - 1)$ and $(C)(R)(n - 1)$. A significant F value could affect how subsequent F tests are calculated and/or how the overall data analysis is conducted. Discussion of this issue is left to books such as Winer, Brown, and Michels (1991), Maxwell and Delaney (1990), Keppel (1991), and other experimental design books.

A second hypothesis tested is that the column means are equal. The alternate hypothesis is that the column means are not equal. This test is usually with $F = MS_C/MS_W$ and degrees of freedom $(C - 1)$ and $(C)(R)(n - 1)$. Occasionally, the denominator is not MS_W; this will alter the second degrees of freedom value. Remember, for any F test the first degrees of freedom value is for the numerator and the second degrees of freedom value is for the denominator. In the F test just presented, the numerator will always be MS_C. Notice that the numerator of any F test corresponds to the hypothesis being tested. The hypothesis in the last example dealt with the column means, so the numerator of the F test was MS_C.

A third hypothesis tested is that the row means are equal. The alternate hypothesis is the row means are not equal. This hypothesis is seldom tested in a random blocks design. The F test is normally $F = MS_R/MS_W$ with degrees of freedom $(R - 1)$ and $(C)(R)(n - 1)$.

The following is an example of the data analysis for a factorial design using the data in table 13.10. Remember, this data are fitness test scores, so small scores are better than large scores.

Step 1: A. First hypothesis tested is that there is no interaction between rows and columns.

H_0: $\mu_I = 0$ (mean interaction $[\mu_I] = 0$)
H_1: $\mu_I \neq 0$ (mean interaction > 0)

B. Second hypothesis tested is that the row means are equal.

H_0: $\mu_1 = \mu_2$ (row means are equal)
H_1: $\mu_1 \neq \mu_2$

C. Third hypothesis tested is that the column means are equal.

H_0: $\mu_1 = \mu_2 = \mu_3$ (column means are equal)
H_1: $\mu_1 \neq \mu_2 \neq \mu_3$

Step 2: Alpha $= .05$

Step 3: Find the table value for each of the three hypotheses stated in step 1 for the alpha level stated in step 2.

A. $F(2,24) = 3.40$ (for testing interaction) (F with 2 and 24 degrees of freedom $= 3.40$)

B. $F(1,24) = 4.26$ (for testing row means)

C. $F(2,24) = 3.40$ (for testing column means)

Step 4: A factorial ANOVA is conducted on the data in table 13.10 using SPSS. In entering the data there is a variable for treatment A, treatment B, and the score of a participant. The directions for using SPSS to conduct a factorial ANOVA are presented in section 7 of the Statistical Procedures part of appendix A. The Dependent variable is the data variable and the Factors variable is the variable used to form the rows and columns in the factorial ANOVA. Select the Means option. The output of the data analysis is presented in table 13.11. Notice that a summary of the ANOVA, row means, column means, and cell means are provided in this output.

Based on table 13.11, there is a significant interaction effect. This is determined either by noting that the F ratio for the interaction effect from the computer (15.89) exceeds the tabled F (3.40) or noting that the significance value (p value) for the interaction effect from the computer (.000) is less than the alpha level (.05) specified in step 2. Figure 13.2 is a plot of the means that illustrates the significant interaction. The significant interaction can be easily seen in the graph because the lines formed by the cell

TABLE 13.11 Output for the Two-Way ANOVA for the Data in Table 13.10

SOURCE	SS	DF	MS	F	SIG.
Rows	0.53	1	0.53	0.42	.523
Columns	116.27	2	58.13	45.89	.000
Rows × Columns	40.27	2	20.13	15.89	.000
Error	30.40	24	1.27		
Total	187.47	29	6.46		

Row	N	Mean
1:	15	9.67
2:	15	9.40

Column	N	Mean
1:	10	11.80
2:	10	9.80
3:	10	7.00

Row/Column	N	Mean
1 and 1	5	10.40
1 and 2	5	10.20
1 and 3	5	8.40
2 and 1	5	13.20
2 and 2	5	9.40
2 and 3	5	5.60

FIGURE 13.2
A plot of the cell means for
the data in table 13.10.

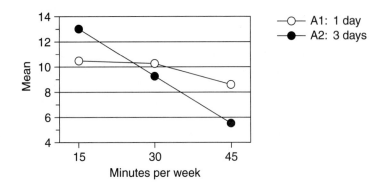

means are not parallel. For those who exercised only one day per week (A1), 45 minutes of exercise per week is better than 15 or 30 minutes; however, the group that exercised three days per week (A2) improved their fitness by exercising more minutes per day.

Significant interactions are reacted to in many different ways depending on the research situation and the type of interaction that the graph of the means appears to show. A discussion of how to interpret significant interactions is beyond the scope of this book. However, in the factorial design example discussed, the significant interaction might invalidate the F tests on row means and on column means. In this case, **simple effects tests** are conducted. Simple effects tests could be comparing the column means for each row or the row means for each column. For example, the test could check for differences among the three column means for row 1 and then for row 2.

As presented in table 13.11, there is not a significant difference between the row means ($F = .42$, $p = .523$). For the difference to be significant, the F value would have to be at least 4.26, or the p value would have to be .05 or smaller.

There is, however, a significant difference among the column means. In table 13.11 the F value for columns is 45.89, which exceeds the table value of 3.40; the p value is .000, which is less than the alpha level of .05. An inspection of the column means shows that the means get progressively smaller as the participants exercise longer per day.

Step 5: The researcher concludes, based on the findings at step 4, that there is an interaction between number of days per week of exercise (rows) and length of each exercise session (columns). Also, the researcher concludes that the three lengths of an exercise session (columns) are not equally effective. However, the researcher concludes that the number of days per week of exercise (rows) are equally effective.

Other ANOVA Designs

The ANOVA designs presented are those most often found in the research literature. Many more ANOVA designs are possible and can be found in the research literature. Whole statistics courses are taught on ANOVA designs from texts like Dayton (1970), Keppel (1991), Kirk (1982), Maxwell and Delaney (1990), and Winer, Brown, and Michels (1991). One- and two-way ANOVA designs have been discussed, but three- and four-way ANOVA designs are not uncommon in the research literature. Many computer programs will analyze up to an eight-way ANOVA. However, researchers should be cautious when designing studies that require an ANOVA design larger than a three-way because they are usually complex and the many interaction terms are difficult to interpret.

Assumptions Underlying Statistical Tests

The statisticians who developed the t and F statistical tests based these tests on certain assumptions. Researchers should be aware of these assumptions and try to satisfy them. Failure to at least partially satisfy the assumptions underlying a statistical test invalidates the test. The assumptions underlying statistical tests sometimes vary from test to test. Assumptions underlying each of the statistical tests discussed up to this point are presented in most statistics books. Presented below is a discussion of assumptions common to most of these statistical tests.

First, it is assumed scores are at least interval (see chapter 12). In some situations, and with some data, it may be acceptable to use the statistical tests with ordinal scores.

Random sampling of participants is assumed when using the statistical tests. In theory, the researcher has access to all members of the population, and from this population one or more samples is randomly selected. Sample size should be a small percentage of population size. However, in many studies the researcher does not have access to all members of the population, and almost all of the accessible members of the population are included in the sample. If random sampling is used for sample selection in such cases, most researchers accept that the random sampling assumption is met.

With the t test for two independent groups, one-way ANOVA, and factorial ANOVA, it is assumed that the groups are independent of each other. Groups are independent if the selection and placement of any individual into a particular group has no bearing on what other participants are selected or placed into that group. The assumption of independence is not totally met in some studies where volunteer participants are used. For example, a researcher wants to have an experimental group and a control group. If potential participants are volunteers, ideally some are randomly selected and assigned to the experimental group, some are randomly selected and assigned to the control group, and some are not selected as participants. However, only sixty people volunteer and five people say they will not participate in the study unless they are in the experimental group. So, the researcher puts the five people in the experimental group, randomly selects twenty-five other people for the experimental group, and places the remaining thirty volunteers in the control group. Basically, the assumption of independence is met.

It is also assumed that scores are normally distributed at the population level (i.e., the graph resembles a normal curve; see chapter 12). The best evidence that this assumption is true is that sample scores are normally distributed. With small sample sizes, scores are often not normally distributed even if scores at the population level are normally distributed. For this reason, a group size of thirty is considered the minimum sample size, and larger sample sizes are recommended. Often researchers have fewer than thirty available participants for each group, so the groups are smaller. Fortunately, as long as the assumption of normal distribution is basically met, the statistical tests are justified.

In studies using multiple samples, the populations they represent are assumed to be equally variable. The assumption is checked by comparing the samples. If the variance (see chapter 12) for any group equals the variance for the other groups, the assumption is met. As long as the assumption of equal variability is basically met, the application of the statistical test is appropriate.

A researcher can do several things to improve the probability that the assumptions underlying a statistical test are basically met. Be sure that the members of the population available for selection as participants are truly representative of the population; in most studies this means having a large number of people from which to sample. Large sample sizes are definitely advantageous. With multiple groups, it is recommended that approximately the same number of participants be included in each group.

Statistical Design Sensitivity

Statistical design refers to the way the data are analyzed. The statistical design influences the probability of type I and type II errors which were discussed earlier. The interpretation of the statistical test results relate to this issue. It is hoped that you will find the discussion which follows sufficient and not too technical and/or lengthy.

An example is used to discuss statistical design sensitivity. Suppose there were three groups (A, B, and C) with 15 male and 15 female undergraduate college students in each group. Each group received a different experimental treatment. A one-way ANOVA could be applied to the data to test the null hypothesis that the populations the groups represent are equal in mean score. The ANOVA summary table and F test are as follows:

Source	SS	DF	MS	F
Among	—	2	—	—
Within	—	87	—	
Total	—	89	—	

F = (MS Among)/(MS Within).

As noted in the discussion of one-way ANOVA, the MS Among is an indication of difference among the groups in mean score and the MS Within is an indication of difference (variability) among the scores within groups. In this example, if there is a large difference in scores between males and females, the MS Within will be inflated (much larger than if should be or would be if all participants were the same gender). Since the inflated MS Within is in the denominator of the F test, the value of the F test is decreased. This decreases the likelihood of rejecting the null hypothesis and increases the chances of a type II error if the null hypothesis really is false.

In this example, one way to reduce or eliminate the problem of the inflated denominator for the F test is to change the design of the statistical analysis. In this case the conduct of the research study is not changed. There are still three groups with 15 males and 15 females in each group, and each group receives a different experimental treatment. The statistical analysis design is a two-way ANOVA.

		TREATMENT		
		A	B	C
GENDER	Male	n=15	n=15	n=15
	Female	n=15	n=15	n=15

The ANOVA summary table is as follows:

Source	SS	DF	MS	F
Gender	—	1	—	—
Treatment	—	2	—	—
Gender x Treatment	—	2	—	—
Error	—	84	—	
Total	—	89		

Note: the Treatment source in this two-way ANOVA is the same as the Among source in the one-way ANOVA. The Total source is the same in both designs since the same data are being used. Thus, the Within source in the one-way ANOVA is partitioned into the Gender, Gender x Treatment, and Error sources in the two-way ANOVA. The F test for difference among the treatments in mean score is F = (MS Treatment)/(MS Error) in the two-way ANOVA and F = (MS Among)/(MS Within) in the one-way ANOVA. The numerators are the same value in both F tests but the denominator for the F test in the two-way ANOVA should be smaller than the denominator for the F test in the one-way ANOVA since the Error source is just a part of the Within source. Thus, the F test value in the two-way ANOVA should be larger than that in the one-way ANOVA. The larger the F test value, the less likely a type II error will occur. In summary, the two-way ANOVA is a more sensitive design than the one-way ANOVA in this example.

In this example situation, another way to reduce or eliminate the problem of the inflated denominator for the F test is to have all of the participants be the same gender. In this case a one-way ANOVA would be used. However, this one-way ANOVA is more sensitive (more statistical power) than the original one-way ANOVA.

Effect Size

Statistically significant differences among groups in mean score are not necessarily practically significant differences. For example, if there was a statistically significant difference between two groups in mean IQ with the means 101.55 and 102.49, this is really not enough difference to have any practical significance in that both groups are basically average in mean IQ. Although not very obvious from what has been presented concerning t tests and F tests in ANOVA, the larger the sample size, the larger the statistical power to reject the null hypothesis—even when it is false by a very small and practically unimportant amount. Thus, in the IQ example above, since the sample size was very large, the difference between 101.55 and 102.49 was statistically significant. If the sample size had been smaller, probably the difference would not have been significant. You can see an example of the influence of sample size (n) on the statistical test by looking at the formula for a single group t test which was presented earlier in this chapter: $t = (\overline{x} - \mu)/(s / \sqrt{n})$. Notice as n gets larger, the denominator gets smaller and the t test value gets larger. If the t test value is large enough, the null hypothesis can be rejected.

A way to decide whether the statistically significant difference is a practically significant difference is to calculate an **effect size** (ES). We studied effect size in chapter 10, Meta-analysis.

ES = [mean score of Group A—mean score of Group B] / [standard deviation for one group or the standard deviation for the combined (pooled) groups].

Cohen (1988) states that an effect size less then .20 is small, around .50 is medium, and greater than .80 is large. In most cases, if the effect size is large, the difference between the two means has practical implications, whereas a small-effect size is less likely to have practical significance. Statistics books like Winer, Brown, and Michels (1991) have an excellent discussion of statistical power and effect size. Lipsey (1990) is totally devoted to the topic.

Overview of Two-Group Comparisons

Two-group comparisons are sometimes referred to as **multiple comparisons** or *a posteriori* **comparisons.** These techniques are used to compare groups two at a time following a significant F test in ANOVA. Having rejected H_0 that the group means are equal and accepted H_1 that the group means are not equal, the researcher wants to compare pairs of means to determine if they differ significantly. For example, if there are three groups (A, B, and C), this involves comparing A to B, A to C, and B to C.

There are several techniques developed specially for two-group comparisons. It is important for beginning researchers to know something of these techniques in case there is need to use them and in order to have some understanding of their application in the research literature. Some of the techniques commonly used are by Scheffe, Tukey, Duncan, Newman-Keuls, and Bonferroni. Discussion of the techniques can be found in statistics books like Ferguson and Takane (1989), and Winer, Brown, and Michels (1991). Which technique to use is influenced partly by personal preference and partly by the research situation.

Two-group comparison techniques may differ in terms of three important attributes: per-comparison error rate, experiment-wise error rate, and statistical power. Each of these attributes should be considered when selecting a technique for a particular research situation. **Per-comparison error rate** is the probability of making a type I error in a single two-group comparison. **Experiment-wise error rate** is the probability of making a type I error somewhere in all of the two-group comparisons conducted. Statistical power is the probability of not making a type II error in a two-group comparison.

Scheffe's technique, for example, controls type I errors very well, but is lacking in statistical power unless sample sizes are large. Tukey's technique does not control type I errors as well, but has better statistical power than Scheffe.

Two-group comparisons are conducted after a significant F test in any ANOVA design, provided there are three or more levels or groups associated with the F test. For example, if for the data in table 13.10 there is a significant F test for columns, then two-group comparisons are conducted; but a significant F test for rows indicates that the two row means are not equal, making two-group comparison unnecessary.

In statistics books, two-group comparisons are very often discussed after one-way ANOVA, and in packages of statistical computer programs two-group comparisons are often part of the one-way ANOVA program. Further, computer programs may not contain all of the two-group comparison techniques. Thus, using a particular two-group comparison with ANOVA designs other than a one-way may require hand calculation of the two-group comparison. A hand calculation is not difficult with the information provided in the computer printout for the ANOVA conducted to justify the two-group comparisons. SPSS provides many two-group comparison techniques with both the one-way and two-way programs. Within these programs, click on Post Hoc Tests to select the desired two-group comparison. With a two-way ANOVA, you must specify if two-group comparisons are for rows or columns or both.

Overview of Analysis of Covariance

Analysis of covariance (ANCOVA) was discussed briefly in the experimental research chapter; it would be helpful to review that material before proceeding. ANCOVA is an alternative to most ANOVA designs, and it is commonly found in the research literature. Basically, ANCOVA statistically adjusts the difference among the group means on the criterion (data) variable to allow for the fact that the groups differ in mean score on some other variable(s) and then applies ANOVA to the adjusted criterion variable. A variable used for adjusting the data is called the **covariate,** and the data variable is called the **variate.** If there is no adjustment in the variate, ANOVA and ANCOVA yield the same results.

One reason for using ANCOVA is to reduce error variance (reflected in the denominator of the F test) in a design. Another reason is to adjust for the inequality of groups at the start of the research study in terms of one or more variables that need to be controlled in the research study.

ANCOVA is more complex than ANOVA in terms of the assumptions underlying its use, data collection, and analysis. Prior to using ANCOVA the researcher should become familiar with the technique by consulting statistics books like Huck and Cormier (1996), Keppel (1991), and Winer, Brown, and Michels (1991). Manuals for packages of statistical computer programs often include good explanations of statistical techniques. In SPSS, ANCOVA is in the two-way ANOVA program referenced earlier.

Overview of Nonparametric Tests

All of the statistical tests discussed so far have been **parametric** tests in that interval data and normal distribution of the scores for each population are assumed. This section discusses statistical tests that do not require that these two assumptions be met. **Nonparametric** statistical tests are used when the data are not interval or the data are interval but not normally distributed. For example, small sample sizes per group ($n < 10$) seldom yield data that are normally distributed. An overview of nonparametric statistical tests is presented and then one commonly used test, chi-square, is discussed in detail.

Books devoted entirely to nonparametric statistical tests include Siegel (1956), which is a classic but is out of print; Siegel and Castellan (1988), which is a revision of Siegel; Hollander and Wolfe (1973); and Marascuilo and McSweeney (1977). Nonparametric statistics courses are available at most universities. Many statistics books (e.g., Ferguson and Takane [1989]) have a chapter devoted to the common nonparametric statistical tests. For each of the common parametric statistical tests discussed in this chapter, there is an alternative nonparametric statistical test. Where parametric statistical tests deal with the mean, nonparametric statistical tests deal with the median, ranks, and frequencies. Note that the second-best measure of central tendency is the median, and the mode is based on frequencies. Often, nonparametric statistical tests do not have as much statistical power as parametric statistical tests. However, random sampling is still assumed with nonparametric statistical tests.

The Kruskal-Wallis one-way ANOVA by ranks and the Friedman two-way ANOVA by ranks are two nonparametric statistical tests commonly found in the research literature. Both of these statistical tests can be found in statistical packages for the computer. SPSS has a Nonparametric Tests program.

The chi-square (χ^2) statistical test is a nonparametric test often used by researchers conducting descriptive research. Most general statistics books discuss the chi-square test. The **one-way (goodness of fit)** and **two-way (contingency table) chi-square tests** are discussed in detail in subsequent paragraphs because of their many uses in research studies.

One-Way Chi-Square

In a research study where a one-way or goodness of fit chi-square test is used to analyze the data, the researcher hypothesizes some distribution for the data of a population. Based on the distribution of sample data, the researcher either accepts or rejects the hypothesis. Again, the five-step hypothesis-testing procedure is used. An example will help to clarify this test.

Suppose a researcher is interested in determining whether freshmen at a university are satisfied with living in a dorm. The population of university freshmen is 6,000. A sample of 1,000 students is selected using random procedures. A four-item questionnaire with five possible answers (strongly agree, agree, neutral, disagree, strongly disagree) per item is sent to the sample. Eight hundred students return the questionnaire. Prior to mailing the questionnaires to the sample, the researcher hypothesizes that the population distribution on items is 10 percent strongly agree, 10 percent strongly disagree, 20 percent agree, 20 percent disagree, and 40 percent neutral. These hypothesized percentages generate the **expected frequency** for each answer, whereas the number of participants in the sample selecting each answer generates the **observed frequency** for each answer. Presented in table 13.12 are the frequencies of response (observed frequencies) for the sample to each item of the questionnaire. Presented in table 13.13 are the expected frequencies for each answer to the questionnaire in table 13.12. Are the observed frequencies and expected frequencies for a questionnaire item in close enough agreement to accept the hypothesized distribution of responses?

TABLE 13.12 Frequency of Responses of a Sample ($n = 800$) to a Four-Item Questionnaire about Dorm Conditions

ITEM	STRONGLY AGREE	AGREE	NEUTRAL	DISAGREE	STRONGLY DISAGREE	N
1. Food is great.	50	135	400	200	15	800
2. Roommate is terrible.	70	150	350	170	60	800
3. Public dorm area is a mess.	100	200	325	145	30	800
4. Own room is nice.	20	100	200	300	180	800

TABLE 13.13 Expected Frequencies for Questionnaire Items in Table 13.12 ($n = 800$)

ANSWER	HYPOTHESIZED %	EXPECTED FREQUENCY
Strongly Agree	10	80
Agree	20	160
Neutral	40	320
Disagree	20	160
Strongly Disagree	10	80
Total	100	800

The one-way or goodness of fit chi-square test is used with the five-step hypothesis-testing procedure to determine whether the observed and expected frequencies are in agreement with each other. This chi-square test is called *one-way* because the response of each subject to an item has only one classification—which answer was selected. The *goodness of fit* name comes from the chi-square test as a test of the extent to which the expected and observed frequencies were in agreement. The less the agreement between the expected and observed frequencies for the answers to an item, the larger the chi-square value. If there were perfect agreement, the chi-square value would be zero. The one-way chi-square test has degrees of freedom equal to the number of different responses to an item or number of different observed values of a variable (K) minus one ($df = K - 1$). The tabled values of chi-square are provided in appendix D. Tabled values are positioned where the degrees of freedom row and alpha-level column intersect.

The five-step hypothesis-testing procedure is presented using the responses to item 1 in table 13.12.

Step 1: H_0: Model or distribution of responses is 10%–20%–40%–20%–10%
H_1: Model is not correct

TABLE 13.14	Output for the One-Way Chi-Square for Item 1 in Table 13.12 and the Expected Values in Table 13.13			
	N		800	
	Chi-Square		97.97	
	df		4	
	Sig.		.000	
Observed N				
50	135	400	200	15
Expected N				
80.00	160.00	320.00	160.00	80.00

Step 2: Alpha = .05

Step 3: Since there are five different answers to the item, the degrees of freedom is 4 (5 − 1). With df = 4 and alpha = .05, the tabled chi-square value is 9.49.

Step 4: Analyze the data item by item. The data for item 1 in table 13.12 is analyzed. Using the one-way Chi-Square program in SPSS the output presented in table 13.14 was obtained. Both the chi-square value and p value indicate significance. The directions for using this program are presented in section 8 of the Statistical Procedures part of appendix A.

Step 5: The researcher concludes that the hypothesized model is not correct.

Two-Way Chi-Square

In a research study where a two-way or contingency table chi-square test is used to analyze the data, the researcher has hypothesized that, for a population, two variables are independent of each other or uncorrelated. Based on the data of a sample from the population the researcher accepts or rejects the hypothesis. As always, the five-step hypothesis-testing procedure is followed. The following example is an easy way to present this chi-square test.

A questionnaire is sent to a sample of 100 former participants in an industrial fitness program and 30 of them return it. Participants are asked to indicate their gender, age, and response to each of three items about the fitness program. The data from the questionnaire is presented in table 13.15. The researcher hypothesizes that males and females respond in a similar manner to item 1. This is equivalent to believing that gender and response to item 1 are independent of each other.

The two-way or contingency chi-square test is applied to the data following the five-step hypothesis-testing procedure to determine whether the researcher's belief seems to be true. This chi-square test is called *two-way* because the response

TABLE 13.15 Data from a Questionnaire Completed by Former Participants in an Industrial Fitness Program

PARTICIPANT	GENDER	AGE	I-1	I-2	I-3
1	1	2	2	3	2
2	1	3	2	4	2
3	2	2	1	3	2
4	1	1	2	3	1
5	2	3	3	2	3
6	2	1	2	4	3
7	2	2	3	2	1
8	1	2	2	2	2
9	1	1	3	3	3
10	2	2	3	4	3
11	1	3	2	3	3
12	1	2	1	2	1
13	1	1	1	2	3
14	1	2	2	2	3
15	2	3	2	3	2
16	2	2	1	2	2
17	1	3	2	3	3
18	2	3	3	3	2
19	2	3	1	2	2
20	1	1	2	2	3
21	1	2	3	3	3
22	1	3	2	2	1
23	2	1	1	2	1
24	2	1	3	2	1
25	1	3	3	4	3
26	1	1	2	2	2
27	2	3	3	4	3
28	1	2	1	2	1
29	2	3	2	3	1
30	1	3	1	4	1

Gender: 1 = Female, 2 = Male
Age: 1 = 18–25, 2 = 26–39, 3 = 40–60
Item: 1 = Strongly Agree, 2 = Agree, 3 = Disagree, 4 = Strongly Disagree

of each participant to an item has two classifications on it. In this example, the two classifications are answer selected and gender. If the percent of males and females selecting an answer to an item is the same and this prevails for each answer choice within an item, the chi-square value of the item is zero (e.g., if 15 percent of the males and 15 percent of the females selected strongly disagree, 40 percent of each gender selected disagree, and so forth). In this example, response to the item is independent of gender since both genders responded in the same manner.

With a two-way chi-square test, a two-dimensional table is developed with the rows identifying the levels or values of one variable and the columns identifying the levels of the other variable. The number of participants in each cell of the two-dimensional table is then determined. The degrees of freedom for the two-way chi-square test is $(n - 1)(K - 1)$ where n = number of rows and K = number of columns in the two-dimensional table. Tabled values of chi-square are provided in appendix D.

The five-step hypothesis-testing procedure is presented using the gender and item 1 (I-1) data from table 13.15.

Step 1: H_0: Gender and I-1 are independent of each other
H_1: Gender and I-1 are dependent

Step 2: Alpha = .05

Step 3: Since gender has two levels or values (1 and 2) and I-1 has three levels (1, 2, and 3), the degrees of freedom is 2 [$(2 - 1)(3 - 1)$]. With df = 2 and alpha = .05, the tabled chi-square value is 5.99.

Step 4: Analyze the data item by item. The data for gender and I-1 in table 13.15 are analyzed using the Two-Way Chi Square program in SPSS. The directions for using this program are presented in section 9 of the Statistical Procedures part of appendix A. Note: In the directions a number of statistics and options should be selected to obtain a complete printout. Computer output for this analysis is presented in table 13.16.

First cell frequencies and total frequencies for each row and column are provided in table 13.16. Seventeen females (row code 1) and 13 males answered item 1. Eight participants strongly agreed (column code 1), 13 participants agreed, and 9 participants disagreed with item 1. Ten females agreed (row code 1 and column code 2) with item 1. Then percents of total, row percents, and column percents are provided for each cell. The females who strongly agreed (row code 1 and column code 1) are 13.33 percent of all 30 participants (percent of total), 23.53 percent of all 17 females (row percents), and 50 percent of all 8 participants who strongly agreed (column percents). Finally test statistics and coefficients (not introduced in this chapter) are provided. The Pearson Chi-Square is the statistic to use. Neither the chi-square value (4.313) nor p value (.116) indicate significance.

Step 5: Accept H_0 that males and females responded in a similar manner to I-1.

Overview of Multivariate Tests

The statistical tests discussed to this point have been **univariate tests** in that each participant contributed one score to the data analysis, or in the case of repeated measures contributed one score per cell. With **multivariate tests,** each participant contributes

---

TABLE 13.16 Output of the Two-Way Chi-Square for Gender and
I-1 in Table 13.15

GENDER * I1 CROSSTABULATION

				I1		
			1.00	**2.00**	**3.00**	**Total**
GENDER	1.00	Count	4	10	3	17
		Expected Count	4.5	7.4	5.1	17.0
		% within GENDER	23.5%	58.8%	17.6%	100.0%
		% within I1	50.0%	76.9%	33.3%	56.7%
		% of Total	13.3%	33.3%	10.0%	56.7%
	2.00	Count	4	3	6	13
		Expected Count	3.5	5.6	3.9	13.0
		% within GENDER	30.8%	23.1%	46.2%	100.0%
		% within I1	50.0%	23.1%	66.7%	43.3%
		% of Total	13.3%	10.0%	20.0%	43.3%
Total		Count	8	13	9	30
		Expected Count	8.0	13.0	9.0	30.0
		% within GENDER	26.7%	43.3%	30.0%	100.0%
		% within I1	100.0%	100.0%	100.0%	100.0%
		% of Total	26.7%	43.3%	30.0%	100.0%

CHI-SQUARE TESTS

	VALUE	**DF**	**ASYMP. SIG. (2-SIDED)**
Pearson Chi-Square	4.313[a]	2	.116
Likelihood Ratio	4.461	2	.107
Linear-by-Linear Association	.569	1	.450
N of Valid Cases	30		

---

multiple scores. So, for example, in the case of a multivariate one-way ANOVA, each participant contributes a knowledge test score, a physical performance score, and an attitude test score. The purpose of the data analysis is to determine if there is a difference among the groups in terms of a composite score composed of the three test scores.

Books devoted entirely to multivariate statistical tests are available, such as Tabachnick and Fidell (1989), Harris (1985), Stevens (1986), and Tatsuoka (1988). Multivariate statistics courses are offered at most universities. Usually these courses are the third to fourth course in a sequence of statistics courses. For each of the common univariate statistical tests discussed in this chapter there is usually a parallel multivariate statistical test. Multivariate statistical tests that parallel the *t* test and ANOVA procedures are common in the research literature. Other multivariate techniques often used by researchers are canonical correlation, discriminant analysis, and factor analysis. Discussion of these techniques is beyond the scope of this book.

Multivariate statistical tests can be found in statistical packages for the computer such as SPSS (1999). In SPSS multivariate tests are under General Linear Model. Use of multivariate statistical tests is common in the research literature.

As a word of caution, multivariate statistical tests are fairly complex, and so some formal training and experience is recommended before using them in a research study. The use and understanding of multivariate statistical tests is usually too much to expect of the typical master's student or doctoral student who have had only minimal statistical training. Just because a researcher collects some data and analyzes it by using a multivariate statistical test on the computer is no guarantee that the output from the computer is good or that the interpretation of the output is correct. There is a saying among computer users that applies here: Garbage in and garbage out. Bad data going into the computer results in bad information coming out of the computer.

Overview of Prediction-Regression Analysis

The terms *correlation, regression,* and *prediction* are so closely related in statistics that they are often used interchangeably. **Correlation** refers to the relationship between two variables. When two variables are correlated, it becomes possible to make a prediction. **Regression** is the statistical model used to predict performance on one variable from another. An example is the prediction of percent body fat from skinfold measurements.

Practitioners and researchers are interested in predicting scores that are either difficult or impossible to obtain at a given moment. **Prediction** is estimating a person's score on one measure based on the individual's score on one or more other measures. Although prediction is often imprecise, it is occasionally useful to develop a prediction formula.

Simple Prediction

Simple prediction involves predicting an unknown score (*Y*) for an individual by using that person's performance (*X*) on a known measure. To develop a simple prediction, or regression formula, a large number of participants must be measured, and a score on the independent or predictor variable *X* and the dependent or predicted variable *Y* must be obtained for each. Once the formula is developed for any given relationship, only the predictor variable *X* is needed to predict the performance of an individual on measure Y. An example of simple prediction is predicting college grade point average (Y) with high school grade point average (X). One index of the accuracy of a simple prediction equation is the correlation coefficient (r).

Prediction being a correlational technique, there is a line of best fit or regression line that can be generated (see graphing technique, p. 278). In the case of simple prediction, this is the regression line for the graph of the X variable on the horizontal axis and the Y variable on the vertical axis.

The general form of the simple prediction equation is

$$Y' = bX + c$$

where, Y' is a predicted Y score, b is a constant and represents the slope of the regression line. The **slope** is the rate at which Y changes with change on X. The constant c is called the **Y-intercept** and is the point at which the line crosses the vertical axis. It is the value of Y that corresponds to an X of 0. Sometimes computer programs report the simple prediction equation in terms of slope and Y-intercept.

An individual's predicted score Y' does not equal the actual score Y unless the correlation coefficient used in the formula is perfect—a rare event. Thus, for each individual there is an error of prediction. The standard deviation of this error is called the **standard error of prediction.** The standard error of prediction is another index of the accuracy of a simple prediction equation.

If the prediction formula and standard error seem acceptable, the researcher should check the accuracy of the prediction formula on a second group of individuals similar to the first. This process is called **cross-validation.** If the formula works satisfactorily for the second group, it can be used with confidence to predict score Y for any individual who resembles the individuals used to form and cross-validate the equation. If the formula does not work well for the second group, it is considered to be unique to the group used to form the equation and has little value in predicting performance in other groups.

Multiple Prediction

A prediction formula using a single measure X is usually not very accurate for predicting a person's score on measure Y. **Multiple prediction** (or regression) techniques allow Y scores to be predicted using several X scores (e.g., the prediction of college grade point average based on high school grade point average and SAT scores).

A multiple regression equation has one intercept and one b value for each independent variable. The general form of two- and three-predictor multiple regression equations are

$$Y' = b_1X_1 + b_2X_2 + c \text{ (two-predictor)}$$
$$Y' = b_1X_1 + b_2X_2 + b_3X_3 + c \text{ (three-predictor)}$$

The multiple correlation coefficient R is one index of the accuracy of a multiple prediction equation. The minimum and maximum values of R are 0 and 1, respectively. A second index, percentage of variance in the Y scores explained by the multiple prediction equation, is R^2. A third index of the accuracy of a multiple prediction equation is the standard error of prediction. Whole books have been written on multiple regression by Cohen and Cohen (1975) and Pedhazur (1982). Chapters on the topic can be found in Safrit and Wood (1989), and Ferguson and Takane (1989).

Simple prediction can be accomplished by using a multiple prediction computer program since, if only one X score is entered as data, it is simple prediction. In SPSS, Linear Regression is the program which does multiple prediction. The directions for using this program are presented in section 11 of the Statistical Procedures part of appendix A. There are many options in this program which are not discussed in this book.

Nonlinear Regression

The regression models discussed to this point assume a linear relationship, but this assumption is not the case for all data. For example, when relating age and strength, the relation is linear for the ages of 10 through 17 because the person is growing and gaining muscle mass; for ages 18 through 65, however, the relationship is nonlinear (or is curvilinear) because increasing age through this period is usually accompanied by a loss of strength. As explained earlier, if the relationship is curvilinear, the linear correlation will be lower than the true correlation. Computer programs have what is termed a **polynomial regression** program to compute the curvilinear correlation. Polynomial regression analysis is beyond the scope of this book.

Overview of Testing Correlation Coefficients

Correlation was introduced as a descriptive statistical technique in the previous chapter. As such, the correlation coefficient is usually viewed as an indication of the relationship between two variables for a group. However, it is not uncommon for a researcher to state a hypothesis about the correlation in a population, randomly select a sample from a population, calculate a correlation coefficient for the sample, and based on the sample correlation coefficient, accept or reject the hypothesis. It is common for a researcher to apply the five-step hypothesis-testing procedure to correlation coefficients. The commonly applied statistical tests on correlation coefficients are usually presented in general purpose statistics books like Ferguson and Takane (1989). Less commonly applied statistical tests on correlation coefficients and statistical tests involving multiple prediction or regression are presented in books like Pedhazur (1982). A brief overview of two statistical tests on correlation coefficients is presented because these tests are common in the research literature and will provide a basic understanding of their application.

Situation 1: H_0: The correlation coefficient at the population level is zero. H_1: The correlation coefficient is greater than zero. If the correlation coefficient for the sample is considerably larger than zero, H_0 is rejected. The researcher states that the correlation coefficient is significant, which indicates that the coefficient is significantly greater than zero and did not happen by chance.

Situation 2: H_0: The correlation between two variables is the same for each of two populations. H_1: The correlation coefficients are not equal. If the correlation coefficients for each of the two independent samples differ considerably in value, H_0 is rejected and the researcher concludes that there is a difference between the two correlation coefficients.

Selecting the Statistical Test

Selecting the appropriate statistical test for a given research situation is sometimes difficult for the inexperienced researcher. In terms of the statistical tests discussed in detail in this chapter, figure 13.3 may be helpful in selecting the appropriate statistical test. Starting at the top of the figure, move down the figure selecting options until a statistical test is selected at the bottom of a path of lines. For example, the null hypothesis concerns means (move to YES), there are three independent groups (move to 2 or more groups and then One-way ANOVA), and so the statistical test is a one-way ANOVA.

Summary

A number of different research designs and statistical tests have been presented in this chapter. As a result of studying this chapter, the student should understand the concept of inference from a sample to a population, the five-step hypothesis-testing procedure, and the related terminology. The first objective of this chapter is that the student be able to read the statistical analysis section of a research journal article with reasonably good understanding. The second objective is that a student researcher be able to select and execute a statistical analysis of some data with some guidance from a faculty member. If the student understands and is able to work with the research designs and statistical tests presented in this chapter, these two objectives have been met. However, mastery of this chapter certainly does not suggest that the student will understand the statistics presented in all research articles.

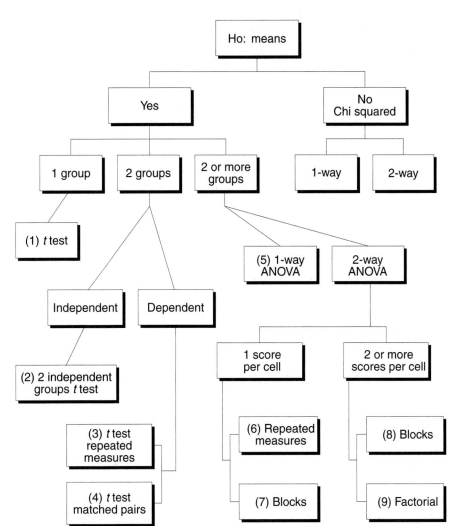

FIGURE 13.3
A chart for selecting the
appropriate statistical test.

Formative Evaluation of Objectives

Objective 1   Identify the different research designs and statistical tests commonly used.

1. F tests are commonly used in research studies. What other statistical tests are commonly used in research studies?

2. Research designs could be classified as independent groups or dependent groups. What are some other ways designs might be classified?

Objective 2   Understand the five-step hypothesis-testing procedure and how it is reported in research journals.

1. What are the five steps in the hypothesis-testing procedure and what occurs at each step?

2. In regard to the five-step hypothesis-testing procedure, what is a researcher indicating when he/she says

    a) the difference is significant?
    b) the difference is not significant?
    c) $F(2,57) = 3.17, p < .05$?
    d) the hypothesis is rejected at the .01 level?
    e) a type I error may have occurred?

3. What are the commomly used alpha levels and why would a researcher use them or other levels?

Objective 3   Understand and evaluate common statistical tests when they are used in the research literature.

1. In each situation below, what is the table value, the value needed for rejection?

    a) Two tailed t test, alpha $= .05$, df $= 8$.
    b) F test, alpha $= .01$, df $= 3,56$.
    c) Chi-square test, alpha $= .05$, df $= 8$.

2. In each situation below, what statistical test is appropriate?

    a) Each of the two groups received a different experimental treatment.
    b) Each of forty-two participants was measured at the beginning of the experiment and every two weeks after that for eight weeks.
    c) The gender and response (SA, A, D, SD) to a ten-item questionnaire was determined to see if gender influenced response to the questionnaire.

14

Measurement Issues in Research

KEY WORDS

Coefficient alpha	Intraclass correlation	Objectivity coefficient	Stability reliability
Concurrent validity	coefficient	Percent agreement	Standard error of
Construct	Kappa coefficient	Phi	measurement
Correlation coefficient	Kuder-Richardson	Rater reliability	Test
Cronbach's alpha	Logical validity	Reliability	Test is good
Good test	Modified kappa	Reliability coefficient	Validity
Internal consistency reliability			

OBJECTIVES

In this chapter, we present measurement concepts and techniques commonly used in research. You should be familiar with these concepts and techniques in order to select the appropriate techniques in your research and to understand the research reported in research journals.

After reading chapter 14, you should be able to

1. Discuss objectivity in terms of what it is, why it is important, and how it is estimated.
2. Discuss reliability in terms of what it is, why it is important, and how it is estimated.
3. Discuss validity in terms of what it is, why it is important, and how it is estimated.
4. Identify things to consider both when preparing to test participants in a research study and when testing them.

Measurement of the participants in a research study in regard to physical ability, physical characteristics, knowledge, attitudes, beliefs, practices, and so on, is part of conducting experimental research and most descriptive research studies. The data collected must have certain essential characteristics in order for them to be considered acceptable evidence upon which research conclusions are based. These essential characteristics are discussed and then a few other measurement considerations are presented. These measurement considerations contribute to the characteristics of acceptable data.

Essential Characteristics of Data

Data as used here means a set of scores. Data may be obtained by using a variety of techniques or instruments, such as knowledge tests, paper and pencil instruments, physical performance tests, testing equipment, and so on. From here on, a data-gathering technique will be called a **test** and the scores obtained by using a technique will be called *data* or *test scores*. Often people will say a good test must have objectivity, reliability, and validity, but it is actually the data that must be good because important decisions are made based on the data. From here on, the terms **good test** and **test is good** will be used as often as possible to mean a test for which acceptable objectivity, reliability, and validity of the data have been determined. That a test is good must be documented before data collection begins in the research study, no matter whether the test was developed by another person or by the researcher. Thus, documentation that a test is good almost always occurs in a pilot study with individuals who are similar to the participants in the research study. The age, sex, experience, and such characteristics, of the individuals used in the pilot study, as well as the test itself, may influence whether the test is good. So, a good test for one group may not be a good test for another group. Further, all tests do not have the same potential to yield data with objectivity, reliability, and validity. Some tests are better than others.

Objectivity, reliability, and validity were briefly discussed in chapter 3 as a step in the research process. Discussed in this chapter are methods used to document the objectivity, reliability, and validity of data and terms which are used in research articles to describe these methods. Thus, after studying this material, researchers will know what methods exist and readers of research will recognize the methods and terms. Usually, the computations involved with these methods are not shown, but if you are interested in the computations, consult measurement books like Baumgartner and Jackson (1999), Safrit and Wood (1989), Crocker and Algina (1986), and Nunnally and Bernstein (1994). In some situations, a formula must be presented for the reader to understand a method or see the difference between methods. In these cases, computations with these formulas may be presented in order for the reader to understand the formula. However, in these situations, computations are kept to a minimum and as simple as possible.

The three essential characteristics of data will be defined and briefly discussed in the order they should be determined. First is *objectivity*. If objectivity exists, two or more people could administer a test to a group and obtain the same or very similar data. If objectivity does not exist, the data of a group are unique to whomever administered and scored the test. Objectivity is important because the data obtained should not be dependent on who administered the test. If the data have objectivity, it is possible for them to have reliability. In fact, objectivity is sometimes called **rater reliability.**

Reliability is defined as consistency of test scores. If reliability exists, people's test scores are not changing over a short period of time. This could be from trial to trial if a test is administered multiple times within a day (like multiple trials one after another or multiple administrations with some short time elapsing between administrations). Or this could be from day to day if a test is administered on two different days. This could be from item to item of a knowledge test. Reliability is important because the researcher wants to be sure that the data collected are a true indication of the ability of the people tested. Without reliability, the data are unique to the testing session and would be entirely different if collected at some other time. If the data have reliability, it is possible for them to have validity.

If **validity** exists, the data measure what they are supposed to measure. In other words, the reason all people don't have the same test score is that they differ in terms of the attribute the test measures. To the extent that other things influence the data, the data are not perfectly valid. Validity is vital and the most important characteristic of data. It allows the researcher to make important decisions based on the data, with confidence that the decisions are based on correct information.

The essential characteristics of data (objectivity, reliability, and validity) must be established before collecting research data so the researcher is assured that conclusions are based on correct information. Occasionally, researchers estimate the objectivity, reliability, and validity of the data as part of the data collection procedure for the research study. This is taking a big risk—because if the data are not valid, they should be discarded. They are not good enough to use when drawing conclusions.

If it has been documented by another person that the test is good for the type of people to be tested in the research study, then it is quite acceptable for the researcher to use the test without documenting it himself/herself. However, it would be a good research practice if the researcher checked the objectivity and reliability himself/herself to get a better understanding of the test and the data the test provides. That another person has documented that the test is good indicates only that the test has the potential to be a good test. If the test is administered improperly, it will not be a good test.

If it has not been documented that the test is good for the type of people to be tested in the research study, then the researcher must take the time to develop this documentation. This could be necessary because the test is a new one the researcher developed, a major modification of a documented test, or documented for a different type of people than the researcher will be testing in the research study. The age, sex, experience, and such characteristics, of the people tested may influence the reliability and validity of the data. Documenting that the test is good does not have to be done with a large number of people, at least initially. If, for example, the test does not yield reliable data, this might as well be established using thirty rather than three hundred people. If the test yields reliable data for thirty people, it would be wise to check that this is true for a larger group. However, much of the documentation of tests found in the literature is based on the test scores of thirty to fifty people. Documenting that a test is good must be conducted in a systematic manner, starting with objectivity and ending with validity. If any of the three essential characteristics of data is not present, try to improve the test, and then check the characteristic again. There is no use in finding that a test does not yield valid data and not knowing whether that is due to lack of reliability or due to the test not measuring what it is supposed to measure.

Thus, when the researcher must document that a test is good, the documentation is done in a pilot study before conducting the actual research study. A small group, maybe thirty to fifty people, is used in the pilot study. After the test is found to yield good data, it is used with confidence in the research study. As will be found later in this chapter, usually more test scores per person must be collected in the pilot study than in the research study because it takes more test scores per person to determine objectivity, reliability, and validity of the data.

Many different techniques are used to document the objectivity, reliability, and validity of the data. The technique used may be dependent on what is to be documented. Whether the test is a paper-and-pencil test or a physical performance test may influence the technique used. The type of paper-and-pencil test or physical performance test may even influence the technique used. Finally, when several techniques are available, the technique used may be personal choice. Certainly one technique does not fit all situations, so the selection of a technique must be a knowledgeable one.

Before discussing techniques used to estimate objectivity, reliability, and validity, it must be recognized that the discussion is a brief overview of techniques which are available. The discussion should be enough that a researcher knows what techniques are available and can select the appropriate technique, or a reader of research articles can recognize and understand the techniques used. The techniques discussed are taught in measurement courses at the undergraduate and graduate level.

Objectivity, reliability, and validity are commonly determined by calculating a correlation coefficient. Correlation was discussed in chapter 12; you might review it before continuing. A **correlation coefficient** indicates the degree of relationship between two sets of scores collected on a group of people. Typically, correlation coefficients between zero and one (positive or negative) are obtained. The closer the correlation coefficient is to one, the higher the degree of relationship between the two sets of scores. There are a number of different types of correlation coefficients used to indicate the objectivity, reliability, and/or validity of the data. Most of the correlation coefficients can vary from -1.00 to $+1.00$, so the interpretation of the correlation coefficient is usually the same no matter the type of correlation coefficient.

Objectivity

To determine objectivity, at least two scorers, raters, or judges (usually two) must independently score a group of people on the test. With physical performance tests, this would be each scorer independently scoring each person as he/she performed the test. For example, two individuals independently time each person as he/she runs the mile for time. For paper-and-pencil tests or instruments like a questionnaire, this would be each scorer independently scoring the test or instrument. For example, two individuals independently grade a knowledge test. No matter what the situation, for each person tested there will be a score from each scorer. The score organization will be as presented in table 14.1.

The correlation coefficient indicating the relationship between the scores of the scorers is called the **objectivity coefficient.** The **intraclass correlation coefficient** (R) is the coefficient calculated as the objectivity coefficient. The R can vary from

TABLE 14.1 Data for Two Scorers to Determine Objectivity

PERSON	SCORER-1	SCORER-2
A	4*	4
B	4	3
C	3	3
D	2	3
E	3	2
F	3	3
G	5	4
H	4	3
I	1	2
J	3	2

*Scores are ratings on a 5-point scale with 5 = excellent and 1 = terrible.

0.00 to 1.00. It is calculated using values which come from a statistical technique called Analysis of Variance (ANOVA). The ANOVA technique was discussed in chapter 13. There are many different ANOVA designs; the design used is dependent on how the data are organized. We will always organize our data so the rows are people and the columns are a repeated measure, as in table 14.1. In table 14.1, scorers are the repeated measure because each person was scored by each scorer (each person has two scores on the measure). The ANOVA design we use to calculate R is called a two-way or repeated measures ANOVA with one score per cell. A cell in an ANOVA design is identified by a row and a column. For example, in table 14.1 the intersection of a row (Person A) and a column (Scorer 1) is a cell with the score four (4) in it. With the ANOVA technique a summary table is used to present the results of the ANOVA. The ANOVA is usually done using the computer, which provides the ANOVA summary table. Several different components are identified under a heading called "sources of variation" in the ANOVA summary table. For each of these sources, values called "sum of squares" (SS), "degrees of freedom" (DF), and "mean square" (MS) are presented in the ANOVA summary table. The data in table 14.1 were analyzed using a computer program called Reliability Analysis, in the SPSS package of statistical programs. The ANOVA summary table and other information for the analysis are presented in table 14.2. In terms of calculating an intraclass correlation coefficient (R), we are interested in the mean square (MS) value for the sources People and Interaction. The mean square for People is symbolized as MS People and the mean square for Interaction as MS Interaction in formulas presented for calculating R. In table 14.2, MS People = 1.49 and MS Interaction = .34. In other books, and using other computer programs, the sources of variation may be named differently than in table 14.2. For example, the sources of variation "Between People" might be called "Rows" and "Interaction" might be called "Residual" or "Error".

TABLE 14.2 Means and ANOVA Summary Table for the Data in Table 14.1			
	MEAN	STD. DEVIATION	CASES
Scorer 1	3.20	1.14	10
Scorer 2	2.90	.74	10

	ANALYSIS OF VARIANCE		
SOURCE OF VARIATION	SUM OF SQUARES	DF	MEAN SQUARE
Between People	13.45	9	1.49
Between Measures	.45	1	.45
Interaction	3.05	9	.34
Total	16.95	19	.89

In table 14.1, two scorers were used in the pilot study so that objectivity could be determined. Most likely in the research study, the researcher would like to have one person score the test with assurance that the data obtained are basically the same data any well-trained scorer would award. The intraclass correlation coefficient can be calculated using several different formulas. In this case the intraclass correlation coefficient (R) is calculated as

$$R = \frac{MS\ People - MS\ Interaction}{MS\ People + MS\ Interaction}, \tag{1}$$

where MS = mean square from a two-way Analysis of Variance (ANOVA) design; design is People X Scorers with two scorers; R = objectivity of a score for each participant which is from one scorer.

Applying formula (1) to the data in table 14.3, R = (1.49 − .34)/(1.49 + .34) = .63, which is not high objectivity since R can be as high as 1.0.

If you don't understand the ANOVA technique, don't worry; the ANOVA values needed to calculate R are obtained using the computer. If the R formula seems a little overwhelming at this time, don't be too concerned. Formulas are presented so you can see that techniques differ as to the formula used. The important thing to know is that an intraclass R should be used and the R formula is the one for this situation. Usually, objectivity is determined as presented in the example (data of two scorers in the pilot study; one scorer used in the research study). If this is the case, the researcher must indicate this when describing the procedures and findings for the research study. For example, since R = .63 using formula one, the researcher might state that, using an intraclass R, the objectivity of the data of a single scorer was .63.

TABLE 14.4 Means and ANOVA Summary Table for the Data in Table 14.3

	MEAN	STD. DEVIATION	CASE
Trial 1	7.85	2.06	20
Trial 2	8.10	2.31	20
Trial 3	8.50	2.50	20
Trial 4	8.65	2.32	20
Trial 5	9.30	2.43	20

ANALYSIS OF VARIANCE

SOURCE OF VARIATION	SUM OF SQUARES	DF	MEAN SQUARE
Between People	393.36	19	20.70
Between Measures	8.06	4	2.02
Interaction	122.74	76	1.62
Total	524.16	99	5.29

test, sex and age of the people tested, and so on, all influence the reliability of the data. Thus, a test which yields reliable data for one group may not yield reliable data for a group with different characteristics.

Multiple Days.   This is a typical situation with physical performance tests where the same test is administered to a group of people (thirty or more) on two different days, usually one to seven days apart. Thus, this testing procedure allows stability reliability to be determined. The data arrangement is as presented in table 14.5. Usually, in this situation, the reason the test was administered on two different days in the pilot study was to be able to determine reliability, but in the future the researcher would like to administer the test on one day with assurance that the data collected during the research study data collection have high stability reliability. An intraclass correlation coefficient is calculated to determine stability reliability using the formula

$$R = \frac{\text{MS People} - \text{MS Interaction}}{\text{MS People} + \text{MS Interaction}}. \qquad (4)$$

See formula (1) for definitions of MS values; design is People X Days with scores from two days; R = reliability of a score for each participant which is collected on one day.

The data for trials one and two in table 14.3 were analyzed treating the trials as if they were day-one and day-two scores, so that an example calculation of R using formula (4) is possible. Based on the analysis of the trial-one and trial-two data which are presented in table 14.6, $R = (7.97 - 1.63)/(7.97 + 1.63) = .66$. This is a low reliability coefficient.

The researcher stating that the objectivity was .63 is an inadequate description because neither the method of determining objectivity nor the score for which the objectivity is reported is indicated. If there are more than two scorers in the pilot study, and/or in the research study there are more than one scorer, the formula for R will change. There would be nothing wrong with having two scorers when determining objectivity in the pilot study and using two scorers during data collection in the research study. In this case the score for each participant in the research study would be the sum or mean of the participant's scores from the two scorers. In fact, as long as the number of scorers is the same in both the pilot study and the research study, the objectivity coefficient (R) would be calculated as

$$R = \frac{\text{MS People} - \text{MS Interaction}}{\text{MS People}}. \qquad (2)$$

See formula (1) for definitions of MS values; design is People X Scorers with two or more scorers; R = objectivity of a score for each participant which is the sum or mean of the participant's scores from the scorers.

Using the data in table 14.2 and formula (2), $R = (1.49 - 34)/(1.49) = .77$. Notice that formula (2) and formula (1) have the same numerator but different denominators. This is important since the formula for calculating R must be the correct one. The formula for R is dependent on the number of scorers used to determine objectivity in the pilot study and the number of scorers to be used when collecting the data in the research study. A common mistake is using a formula for R which is not consistent with the number of scorers used. Often researchers mistakenly use formula (2) with the pilot study data but have only one scorer in the research study. Again, when describing the procedures and findings for the research study, the researcher must indicate the method used to obtain R and the score for which R is reported. In fact, R can be calculated using information from a one-way ANOVA rather than the two-way ANOVA presented here, so the researcher should report that a two-way ANOVA was used. See Baumgartner and Jackson (1999) for additional information on calculating R.

You may read a research report in which the researcher used a Pearson correlation coefficient (r) to determine objectivity. This is an outdated technique. Sometimes the author of a research report will determine objectivity by calculating **Cronbach's alpha,** sometimes called **coefficient alpha.** The coefficient alpha is the same as the R using formula (2). Note this R is not the objectivity coefficient for a single score (one scorer) during the research study data collection. Thus, coefficient alpha is not the correct value to calculate and report as the objectivity coefficient for a single scorer, but it is the correct value if in the research study the number of scorers will be the same number as in the pilot study. Earlier, you were cautioned to use and make sure authors of research reports use a formula for R which is consistent with the number of scorers used. Usually, use of coefficient alpha as an objectivity coefficient is not appropriate because usually only one scorer is used in the research study.

Since the objectivity coefficient is influenced by the amount of agreement among scorers, characteristics of the group tested, like sex, age, experience, and such, usually have little influence on the objectivity coefficient. So a test documented as yielding data with objectivity for one group can be used with any group as long as the scorers are competent. The objectivity of data is dependent on the type of test. The more difficult the test to score accurately, the lower tends to be the objectivity coefficient. The minimal acceptable objectivity for a physical performance test is .70, but for knowledge tests and attitude scales the minimal value may be different. The minimal value is dependent on how much objectivity is needed, the objectivity obtained by other researchers, the objectivity obtained for similar tests, and so on.

The Reliability Analysis program in the SPSS package of statistical programs can be used to obtain an R as an estimate of objectivity. The program is quite versatile, calculating R for a score which is either a single scorer or the mean of several scorers and using either a one-way or two-way ANOVA model. The directions for this program are presented in section 12 of the Statistical Procedures part of appendix A.

Reliability (Relative)

To determine reliability each person must have at least two repeated measure scores. These scores might be (1) multiple trials (administrations) of a physical performance test within a day, (2) multiple administrations of a physical performance test with each administration on a different day, (3) multiple items on a knowledge test, (4) two different forms (A and B) of a knowledge test with both forms administered on different days or on the same day, or (5) other repeated measures. If the data are collected within a day, this allows a determination of **internal consistency reliability**, defined as consistency of the test scores within a day. If the data are collected on different days, this allows a determination of **stability reliability**, defined as consistency of the test scores across days. In all cases, some correlation coefficient is calculated to indicate the degree of relationship between the sets of scores. This correlation coefficient is called the **reliability coefficient**. Since it can vary from 0.00 to 1.00, 0.00 indicates no reliability and 1.00 indicates perfect reliability.

Multiple Trials within a Day. This is typically multiple trials of a physical performance test administered within a day (internal consistency). The physical performance test must be one in which multiple trials can be administered without fatigue or learning changing performance from trial to trial. Multiple trials of a maximum exertion test, such as a treadmill test, would not be administered within a day. Administering a test before participants had sufficient time to learn how to take the test by practicing it would cause learning to change performance from trial to trial. An example of a multiple trial physical performance test would be when each person in turn is scored on a flexibility test and the group continues to rotate taking turns until all people in the group of twenty people have been scored five times (five trials). Another example would be when each person is administered five trials of the flexibility test, then another person is administered five trials, and so on, until all twenty people have

five scores. So, the data arrangement is as shown in table 14.3. Usually, in this situation, the score of a participant is the sum or the mean of the participant's trial scores, and reliability is determined by using the intraclass correlation coefficient

$$R = \frac{\text{MS People} - \text{MS Interaction}}{\text{MS People}} . \tag{3}$$

See formula (1) for definitions of MS values; design is People X Trials with two or more trials; R = reliability of a score for each participant which is the sum or mean of the participant's trial scores.

The data in table 14.3 were analyzed using the Reliability Analysis program in the SPSS package of statistical programs and the results of this analysis are presented in table 14.4. Using this information and formula (3), $R = (20.70 - 1.62)/(20.70) = .92$. In this situation, the more trials, the higher tends to be the R. An R of .70 to .80 is usually the minimum accepted value. The R of .92 obtained is quite good. Type of

TABLE 14.3 Multiple Trial Data Arrangement

PERSON	TRIAL 1	TRIAL 2	TRIAL 3	TRIAL 4	TRIAL 5
1	8	7	9	7	9
2	10	9	9	12	12
3	7	7	7	8	9
4	7	10	12	9	9
5	10	7	11	11	8
6	10	6	8	10	11
7	6	6	6	6	6
8	9	11	12	8	8
9	9	9	8	10	8
10	6	6	6	7	5
11	8	10	10	9	11
12	7	9	6	7	6
13	5	8	6	7	6
14	5	5	5	5	5
15	6	5	6	7	6
16	5	6	5	5	5
17	10	10	12	12	12
18	10	10	10	12	8
19	12	14	11	12	11
20	7	7	11	9	11

TABLE 14.5 Multiple Day Data Arrangement

PERSON	DAY 1	DAY 2
1	X	X
2	X	X
3	X	X
•	•	•
•	•	•
•	•	•
n	X	X

n = number of people tested

TABLE 14.6 Means and ANOVA Summary Table for Trials One and Two in Table 14.3

	MEAN	STD. DEVIATION	CASES
Trial 1	7.85	2.06	20
Trial 2	8.10	2.31	20

ANALYSIS OF VARIANCE

SOURCE OF VARIATION	SUM OF SQUARES	DF	MEAN SQUARE
Between People	151.48	19	7.97
Between Measures	.63	1	.63
Interaction	30.88	19	1.63
Total	182.99	39	4.69

There are differences between formulas three and four in terms of how the data are collected (within a day or between days), the denominator of the formula, and the score for which R is reported [sum (mean) of scores or one score]. If formula (3) was used on the values in table 14.6, $R = (7.97 - 1.63)/(7.97) = .80$. This is an acceptable value for a reliability coefficient, but it requires that the score for each participant be based on scores for two trials or two days. Just reporting that the reliability is a value (like .66) is a totally inadequate description of the test reliability. The ANOVA model (one-way or two-way) (see Baumgartner and Jackson 1999 for more information), criterion score (one score or mean score), type of reliability (internal consistency or stability), and value of R must be reported to adequately describe the situation. Formula four is correct if in the pilot study the test was administered on two days to determine R and in the research study the test is administered on one day. Notice that formula (4) is the same as formula (1) for determining objectivity for a score of a single scorer. There would be nothing wrong with administering the test on each of two days during both the pilot study and the research study data collection and the score for each participant being the sum or mean of the participant's day-one and day-two scores. In fact, as long as the number of days the test is administered is the same in both the pilot study and the research study, the stability coefficient (R) is determined by the formula

$$R = \frac{\text{MS People} - \text{MS Interaction}}{\text{MS People}} . \tag{5}$$

See formula (1) for definitions of MS values; design is People X Days; R = reliability of a score for each participant which is the sum or mean of the participant's day scores.

General Case.   If the test was administered more than twice (three or more trials or days) to determine R, so each person has more than two scores, the formula changes, as presented by Baumgartner and Jackson (1999). This formula is:

$$R = \frac{\text{MS People} - \text{MS Interaction}}{\text{MS People} + (\text{K/K'} - 1)(\text{MS Interaction})} , \tag{6}$$

where K = the number of times the test was administered and K' = the number of scores used to form the score of a person. See formula (1) for definitions of MS values.

This formula is important because it is a general formula which can be used in any reliability or objectivity situation. If the test was administered on three days in the pilot study to determine R and the score of a participant in the research study will be from one day, K = 3 and K' = 1 in formula (6). If, for internal consistency reliability, five trials of a test were administered in the pilot study to determine R and the score of a participant in the research study will be the sum or mean of the best three of the five trials, K = 5 and K' = 3 in formula (6). Also, if the test was administered on more than two days in the pilot study to determine R and the score of each participant in the research study will be the sum or mean of the scores from more than one day, the formula for R changes, as presented by Baumgartner and Jackson (1999) and shown in formula (6).

The Reliability Analysis program in the SPSS package of programs can be used to obtain an R as an estimate of reliability. The program is quite versatile, calculating R for a score which is either a single score or the mean of several trials or days and using either a one-way or two-way ANOVA model.

Knowledge Test.   A knowledge test composed of many true-false and/or multiple choice items is administered to a group in a pilot study in order to determine internal consistency reliability. Each item measures some part of a total construct.

Notice that, for this type of test, each item is scored right (1 point) or wrong (0 point) and the total score of a person is the number of items correctly answered. The reliability of the total score is determined by calculating one of the **Kuder-Richardson** coefficients (#20 or #21) or the **Cronbach's Alpha** coefficient. These coefficients are correlation coefficients and they are easy to calculate, presented in most measurement books, and commonly found in packages of computer programs. Cronbach's alpha is the same as the R using formula (3) with items replacing trials in table 14.3. The type of test, sex and age of the people tested, and so on, influences the magnitude of the reliability coefficient. To decide whether the reliability coefficient for the data of a test is large enough, compare it to reliability coefficients obtained by other researchers and/or for similar tests. Probably a reliability coefficient of .70 or higher is required for sufficient reliability.

Stability reliability is seldom if ever determined for knowledge tests. If a knowledge test is administered on each of two different days, most participants score better on the second day because they remembered answers to items from the first-day administration and/or obtained answers to items between the first-day and second-day administrations.

Questionnaire.   A questionnaire may have a number of different forms. If the questionnaire has many items with potential answers provided, it is much like a knowledge test. For example, the questionnaire may be for measuring attitudes, with each item a statement to which the research participant responds *strongly agree, agree, disagree,* or *strongly disagree.* The responses are numerically coded with *strongly agree* = 4, *agree* = 3, *disagree* = 2, and *strongly disagree* = 1. Notice that these are just codes and not real scores. The codes could be any numbers (for example, 9,8,3,1), as long as each response has a different code. Further, note that there are no right answers to the items and for many questionnaires the items are unrelated to each other, not measuring a total construct as for a knowledge test. Thus, although a total score—which is the sum of the codes for the item responses—is possible, a total score is usually inappropriate and meaningless. This being the case, determining reliability with techniques used with knowledge tests is incorrect. It is not uncommon when reading a research article to find that a Kuder-Richardson coefficient or coefficient alpha has been used inappropriately to determine the reliability of the data from a questionnaire.

Internal consistency reliability of questionnaire data could be determined by using several pairs of items in the questionnaire. For example, items 11 and 32, 25 and 41 are paired. If participants respond in a similar manner to the two items in a pair and this is true for each pair, this is acceptable evidence that each item in the questionnaire provides reliable data. Reliability for each pairing of items is probably determined by using the coefficient alpha but an intraclass correlation coefficient (formula number 3) could be used. Again, characteristics of the questionnaire and the people tested influence the magnitude of the reliability coefficient. Reliability coefficients for questionnaire data are often not high; maybe .60 is an acceptable value. As with knowledge tests, stability reliability is seldom determined for questionnaires.

Dichotomously Scored Tests. Some tests are scored pass or fail, proficient or nonproficient, and so on. For these tests there is some score (standard) which, if obtained or exceeded, results in a person being classified as passing; otherwise, the person fails. For example, to pass a 100-point knowledge test, a score of at least 90 is required. To determine reliability of the data, the test must be administered twice (two trials within a day or two days), and each time the test is administered, each person is assigned a score of one (1) if the person passes, or zero (0) if the person fails. Thus, there is a data arrangement as shown in table 14.7.

Reliability for the data of this type may be determined by several different methods. One simple method is **percent agreement,** which indicates the percentage of the group classified the same on both administrations. This value can vary from zero to one. The formula is:

$$\text{Percent Agreement} = \frac{n1 + n4}{n1 + n2 + n3 + n4} \tag{7}$$

Other methods commonly used are calculating the **Kappa coefficient** and the **Modified kappa** coefficient. These values are correlation coefficients, so positive values closer to 1.00 than 0.00 are indications of good reliability. The Kappa and Modified kappa coefficients are discussed in measurement books such as Safrit and Wood (1989). Because the possible scores for dichotomously scored tests are one and zero rather than many different values, the reliability coefficient may not be high. The minimum score required to classify a person as passing influences the magnitude of the reliability coefficient. If the majority of the people receive the same classification, probably the reliability coefficient will be higher than the coefficient when about one-half the group receive each classification. Again, characteristics of the test and the group tested influence the magnitude of the reliability coefficient.

Reliability (Absolute)

The reliability techniques discussed so far have involved the use of a correlation coefficient or a percentage to indicate the degree of agreement between multiple-trial or multiple-day test scores of a group. If people who score high on one trial or on one

TABLE 14.7 Dichotomously Scored Test Data Arrangement for Reliability

		SECOND ADMINISTRATION	
		1	0
FIRST ADMINISTRATION	1	n1	n2
	0	n3	n4

n1 = the number of people classified as a 1 for both administrations
n2 = the number of people classified as a 1 for the first administration but 0 on the second administration

day score high on all trials or days and people who score low on one trial or day consistently score low, the degree of agreement will be high. Sometimes it is desirable to express reliability in actual test score units, indicating how much the test score of a person might change from trial to trial or day to day due to measurement error.

If each person is administered multiple trials of a test within a day or tested on multiple days, a standard deviation for the multiple measures could be calculated for each person and this standard deviation is the measurement error to expect for the person. However, if each person is administered only one trial or tested on only one day, the mean amount of measurement error in the data is estimated for the entire group by calculating the **standard error of measurement**

$$SEM = s\sqrt{1 - R} \, , \tag{8}$$

where SEM = standard error of measurement,
s = standard deviation of the data, and
R = reliability coefficient for the data.

For example, if s = 10 and R = .84, SEM = $10(\sqrt{1 - .84})$ = (10)(.4) = 4.0. The standard error of measurement is an estimate of how much one should expect a test score to vary due to measurement error, lack of reliability.

If, from a practical standpoint, the SEM is small enough to be tolerated because it does not change the interpretation of the data, then the data are sufficiently reliable. Many books, like Ferguson and Takane (1989) and Nunnally and Berstein (1994), contain a lengthy discussion of measurement theory and the SEM. Note that the SEM is based on the data of a group, and all members of the group may not follow the scoring pattern of the group. Darracot (1995) found the standard error of measurement tends to be an overestimate of the standard deviation of the repeated measures for an individual.

Validity

If acceptable objectivity and reliability are determined for the data, the validity of the data is determined. There are several basic approaches to estimating validity. Thus, each approach is just an estimate or indication of the data validity. In the past these approaches have been organized by types of validity. Presently, the use of validity types is losing popularity. The basic and commonly used approaches will be discussed so, as a researcher, you have a good understanding of what approaches are available to you and, as a consumer of research, you understand approaches used in a research article. All approaches can't be discussed and approaches can't be discussed in great detail. Thus, you may want to consult other sources, such as Baumgartner and Jackson (1999), Safrit and Wood (1989), or other measurement books. A very comprehensive source is *Standards for Educational and Psychological Testing* (American Educational Research Association 1999).

Logical Approach. Physical educators and exercise scientists use a logical approach, often called **(logical validity)**, when they state that a test provides valid data because based on all they know about the physical attribute to be measured and physical performance, the test measures that physical attribute. Note that this is usually a statement that the test yields valid data with no reference to the degree of validity (high, medium, or low). Also, note that the person using the logical approach may be wrong and/or all people will not agree with her/him. The logical approach is acceptable if there is no other approach possible. Many measurement experts believe that several indications of validity should be provided for the data, and so using the logical approach and some other approach would be acceptable. The term *content validity* probably originated with knowledge tests. The researcher claims the knowledge test yields valid data because the test is a comprehensive coverage of the content of the course, unit, program, and such. Since the opinions of several people are usually better than the opinion of one person, it is quite common for a researcher to use a jury of experts to estimate the validity of the data from a knowledge test, questionnaire, or any type of paper-and-pencil test. Basically the *jury of experts* examine the test and evaluate it as to whether it is a comprehensive coverage of the content to be tested, whether the test items are well constructed and understandable, whether the format of the test is conducive to obtaining valid data, and so on. The jury of experts may suggest improvements in the test or questionnaire and request to see the improved test before giving it their approval. When a jury of experts is used, the number of people in the jury, and their qualifications, must be determined. A jury of experts composed of two available graduate students, faculty, or peers hardly seems sufficient. Depending on a number of factors, a jury of experts is composed of three to twelve persons knowledgeable about some if not all aspects of the test and the attribute to be tested. A jury with some test construction experts and some content experts is fine. The jury of experts doesn't have to be the authorities in the profession but they should have qualifications which the average person in the profession does not possess. A jury composed entirely of peers, colleagues, or members of the same academic department or unit seldom would be considered a strong jury of experts.

Criterion Approach. This approach, often called **concurrent validity,** is quite traditional. It involves determining the correlation between scores on a test and scores on a criterion measure or standard which is known or accepted as being valid. Thus, each person in a group has a score on both the test and the criterion. If the correlation coefficient (r) is high enough, the test yields valid data, since people who have good scores on the test have good scores on the criterion and people who have poor scores on the test have poor scores on the criterion. In other words, the test is providing the same information as the criterion. The correlation coefficient obtained is often called the *validity coefficient.* The criterion is supposed to be the *gold standard,* the standard that is recognized by all people as being the best. For example, some laboratory measures of aerobic capacity and body composition are recognized as the gold standard.

Many times there is no gold standard, so one of the several good standards is used as the criterion. Thus, the magnitude of the validity coefficient obtained is influenced by the criterion selected. Sometimes there is disagreement among knowledgeable professionals as to which criterion to use. The criterion is a laboratory measure or some measure which is difficult, time consuming, and/or expensive to obtain. The test being validated is a field-based test which is easier, quicker, and/or less expensive to administer than the criterion measure. For example, in physical education and exercise science, the mile run test as a measure of aerobic capacity is validated using laboratory measures of oxygen consumption; the skinfold test as a measure of body composition is validated using underwater weighing measures from the laboratory. Another example is a field-based test of anxiety which practitioners could use is validated using measures of anxiety which only a trained psychologist can obtain. There are situations where scores on a test are correlated with a criterion which is the sum of judges' ratings to estimate test score validity. In this case several well-qualified judges independently rated each person in a group. Finding and assembling the judges is difficult and it is time consuming for them to do the ratings. The test can be administered by a practitioner with limited expertise in a short period of time. If the test yields valid data, it will be used in preference to judges' ratings.

There are numerous other criteria which could be used to determine the validity of data. The researcher must consider what possible criteria are available and how appropriate they are. In general, a criteria is anything the researcher and others who read and evaluate the research think is appropriate. Sometimes no acceptable criteria exists, so the concurrent approach to estimating the validity of the scores of a test is not used.

The magnitude of the validity coefficient is influenced by the test, the sex, age, and experience of the people tested, and the criterion used. The minimum acceptable value of the validity coefficient is dependent on how much validity is necessary and what other researchers have obtained for the same or similar groups and/or tests. Seldom is a validity coefficient less than .70 considered acceptable in a research setting. In some nonresearch settings where great accuracy in the data and the classification of people based on the data are not required, validity coefficients less than .70 are acceptable.

Construct Approach.   A **construct** is something which is known to exist although it may not be precisely defined and/or measured. A judge in a pornography trial said, "Pornography, I can't define it but I know it when I see it." Pornography is a construct. Feelings, attitudes, team work, total ability in a sport or job, and so on, are all potential constructs. The validity of the data from a test designed to measure a construct may be determined using a variety of different approaches. Any of the approaches already discussed may be used. For this reason some measurement experts maintain that all approaches to estimating the validity of the data are construct approaches.

Forming groups which are known to differ in terms of the construct to be measured and comparing them in regard to test scores is an accepted construct validity approach. If the best group has the highest mean score on the test, and the second best group has the second highest mean score on the test, and so on, this is evidence that the test yields data with at least some degree of validity. Groups which are known to differ might be formed based on sex, age, or any attribute which seems appropriate. However, comparing groups with extreme differences (for example, 6-year-old compared to 18-year-old individuals, professional athletes compared to nonathletes) may not make sense as an indicator of validity. Remember, the researcher is trying to determine if a test yields valid data for a defined classification of people, so each person in the groups used to determine validity basically must be a member of the defined classification of people (population). So, in the earlier example, if the researcher is trying to determine if a test yields valid data for 18-year-old individuals, comparing the data of 6-year-old and 18-year-old individuals makes no sense. In this example, if, by using appropriate techniques, the test is found to yield valid data, this indicates that the test has the ability to identify different levels of ability—that is, the better the test score, the more ability a person has.

Comparing an untrained group to a trained group or an uninstructed group to an instructed group in terms of mean test score is a common construct validity approach. If the trained or instructed group has a better mean test score than the other group, this is evidence of data validity. Comparing the data of a group before and after training or instruction and finding that the group had a better mean test score after training or instruction is evidence of data validity.

Other Approaches. Characteristics of dichotomously scored tests were discussed earlier in the reliability section of this chapter. Any of the techniques discussed up to this point could be used with dichotomously scored tests. However, two criterion approaches to estimating validity commonly used by researchers and, thus, commonly found in research articles are discussed here. In this case the validity question is whether the data from a test will classify people the same way as a criterion. For example, if the test score of a person is good enough to classify the person as proficient, is the performance of the person on the criterion sufficient to classify the person as proficient? Thus, the data format is as presented in table 14.8. The percent agreement coefficient, discussed in the reliability section, could be used here. A correlation coefficient called **phi** is often used as the validity coefficient in this situation. The phi coefficient is presented in most introductory statistics books and measurement books, like Ferguson and Takane (1989) and Baumgartner and Jackson (1999), and provided in many packages of statistical computer programs, like SPSS.

Reporting Validity. No matter what approach has been used to estimate validity of the data, the approach needs to be well described in the research report. The type of participant, number of participants, and validity evidence must be presented no matter whether the researcher or another person conducted the validity estimation work.

TABLE 14.8 Dichotomously Scored Test Data Arranged for Validity Estimation

		CRITERION	
		PROFICIENT	NONPROFICIENT
TEST	**PROFICIENT**	n1	n2
	NONPROFICIENT	n3	n4

where n1 = the number of people classified as proficient both on the test and on the criterion

n2 = the number of people classified as proficient with the test but nonproficient based on the criterion

Other Measurement Considerations

It should be noted that a desirable but not essential characteristic of a test is that it is economical. An economical test is inexpensive to purchase, and if it requires equipment, the equipment is not expensive to purchase. Also, the test is quick to administer. Further, administration of the test requires neither a large number of people nor people with great expertise. Finally, the time it takes to score the test and the cost of scoring the test is minimal.

There are some things which the researcher should do when preparing to test participants and actually collecting data on participants. These things will increase the chances of having acceptable objectivity, reliability, and validity for the data. Measurement books tend to have a chapter devoted to these topics. Experienced researchers tend to do these things and to describe them in the procedures section of the journal article.

Recognize that physical performance tests and paper-and-pencil tests may not be similar in terms of how participants are prepared to take the tests, how the tests are administered, and how participants perform the tests. Paper-and-pencil tests which include true-false items and/or multiple choice items, and questionnaires with the possible responses provided (see closed-ended items in chapter 8), are administered and taken in basically the same way, no matter what the content area of the test. Preparation for taking the test, test-taking strategy, and actual taking of the test, are similar for all true-false or multiple choice tests. However, each physical performance test has a unique set of directions and is administered in a unique manner. For example, a mile run test is different from a sit-up test. Having taken a mile run test does not prepare a person to take a sit-up test and certainly does not prepare a person to take a paper-and-pencil test.

There are some common elements with paper-and-pencil testing and physical performance testing. Participants need to be prepared to take the test. They need to know what the test is and to have had experience with the subject matter and, in physical performance, with the performance being tested. Participants need to know why they are being tested and what a test score indicates. There must be directions concerning test administration and scoring directions, which are presented to the participants in writing and/or verbally the day of the test. Sufficient time must be allowed for participants to take the test without feeling rushed. All participants must be encouraged to score at their highest level. Age often influences test performance, so one test or one set of procedures may not be appropriate for all people. Failure to address these things will likely decrease reliability and validity of the data.

There are some unique elements with paper-and-pencil testing and physical performance testing. Generally, with paper-and-pencil testing, many participants can be tested at the same time, whereas with physical performance testing, often only one participant can be tested at a time. So, testing time may be more of a concern and longer with physical performance tests than with paper-and-pencil tests. The reading level of participants is a concern with paper-and-pencil tests but not with physical performance tests. However, with physical performance tests, gender, height, and weight often influence the data but seldom influence paper-and-pencil data. As mentioned earlier, each physical performance test is unique and participants must have had prior experience with the test, where this is not a major problem with paper-and-pencil tests. Participants copying answers from the knowledge test paper of another person or not completing a questionnaire accurately or honestly are concerns with paper-and-pencil tests, but honesty is not a concern with a physical performance test if well-trained scorers are used (participants testing each other could be a problem). Again, failure to address these things will likely decrease reliability and validity of the data.

If the researcher has found in a pilot study, or other researchers have found for the type of participant in the study, that the test yields reliable and valid data, the researcher still must be careful to administer the test in a manner which will yield reliable and valid data. With paper-and-pencil tests this may not be too difficult because both the tester and participants have had experience with the test. The tester knows how to administer and score the test. The participants know how to perform the test. This may not be true with physical performance tests.

Planning and experience are the key to having acceptable objectivity, reliability, and validity for the data. Planning all aspects of the data collection is essential. When testing will occur, how long testing will take, what to do if measurement equipment malfunctions and/or participants don't take the test correctly, and preparing participants to be tested are just a few of the things which must be planned. No matter what the measurement and the characteristics of the participants, directions dealing with why the test is being administered, and how the test is administered, are essential. If people know why they are being tested and how to take the test, they are more likely to give their best effort, perform the test correctly, and receive a score approaching their best possible score. For example, physical performance tests each have different administrative procedures; people must have had experience with the test prior to being tested. Giving participants experience with the physical performance test in advance of the day they are tested is probably important for acceptable reliability and validity for the data. For maximum exertion physical performance tests, participants have to be prepared physiologically and psychologically to give their maximum effort.

For the data to be valid, the test administrator must have experience with the test used and the people tested. It is not enough to read the directions for a new test once. This is particularly true with physical performance tests, but generally true with all tests. Testing techniques appropriate for first-grade students, college students, and elderly individuals differ considerably. Lack of experience with the test and the people tested may jeopardize good data validity.

Summary

In this chapter we have discussed the three essential characteristics of data. Each of these characteristics has been defined, the importance of the characteristic discussed, and techniques for determining the characteristic identified. No matter whether you are a researcher or the consumer of research, you need to have a good understanding of these three essential characteristics of data. The goodness of the research is definitely influenced by the goodness of the data collected, which is influenced by the goodness of the test used to collect the data.

A concern is that some researchers make a mistake by using tests and techniques for which objectivity, reliability, and validity of the data have never been established or not established for the type of participants used in the research study. Further, it is not uncommon for researchers to use the wrong procedure or formula to determine objectivity, reliability, and/or validity of the data. It is hoped that, as a result of studying this chapter, you will not make these mistakes and will recognize these mistakes if they are made by other researchers.

Formative Evaluation of Objectives

Objective 1   Discuss objectivity in terms of what it is, why it is important, and how it is estimated.

1. What is objectivity in your own words, and why is it important?

2. What techniques are commonly used to estimate objectivity?

Objective 2   Discuss reliability in terms of what it is, why it is important, and how it is estimated.

1. What is reliability in your own words, and why is it important?

2. What are the two types of reliability, and why is each of them important?

3. What techniques are commonly used to estimate reliability?

Objective 3   Discuss validity in terms of what it is, why it is important, and how it is estimated.

1. What is validity in your own words, and why is it important?
2. What are techniques commonly used to estimate validity?

Objective 4   Identify things to consider when preparing to test participants in a research study and when actually testing them in the study.

1. What are similarities and differences between physical performance tests and paper-and-pencil tests?
2. What are three things which should be done to prepare participants for testing?
3. What are several things which should be done when testing participants?

Part Four

15

Writing the Research Report

OBJECTIVES

The function of a research report is to communicate a set of ideas and facts to those who are interested in the problem area in which the research was undertaken. Reports will differ in how they are treated, but, in general, the writers of the reports tend to follow similar style formats. Students completing research are usually required to follow a style of reporting selected by the faculty of the students' department. The style for published research will follow a format required by the journal to which the report is submitted for publication.

After reading chapter 15, you should be able to

1. Determine the characteristics of a good research report.
2. Understand the format for a report and the kinds of information required in each division of the report.
3. Differentiate between the style of writing a research report for a thesis or dissertation as opposed to a research report for publication in a journal.

The culmination of the research process is the disclosure of the findings to other professionals or interested persons. The researcher may present her/his findings through a journal article, a report to a sponsoring agency, a thesis or dissertation, an on-line publication, or presentation at a professional conference. Traditionally, a written research report of some type has been the option of choice.

The purpose of the written research report, whether it is in the form of a master's thesis, doctoral dissertation, or journal article, is to convey ideas and facts generated by the research to those who will read the report. To be effective, the information must be communicated in a manner that is clear and easily understood. *Clarity* is fundamental.

The Research Report

It is important to note that research is a shared enterprise among members of a professional group. The reports generated through research are perhaps the most common medium for researchers to communicate their findings to each other. Journal articles, master's degree theses, and doctoral dissertations all have the same objective—to disseminate ideas and information. The research procedure and results of an investigation become a record for posterity. The role of the report in the research process is important in that the preparation of a good, detailed report is a mechanism by which researchers can refine their thinking about the research problems they have investigated. In a way, the researcher evaluates the completed work through the research report.

Part IV of this book contains one detailed chapter titled "Writing the Research Report." Covered in this chapter are (1) examples of the elements typically included in a graduate student thesis or dissertation, and (2) how to prepare an article for publication.

The reader should not be required to guess how the research was performed or have to make any assumptions about what was found. The reader should hold no doubts or questions about the meaning of any statement included in the report.

Besides clarity, other important characteristics of the report include (1) *organization,* or the logic underlying the order in which the various parts of the report appear and the degree to which the transition between parts is clear and smooth; (2) *good and correct presentation,* which includes adherence to proper spelling, grammar, diction, punctuation, and the mechanics of a systematic format for presentation of the research material; (3) *completeness,* meaning that the total body of facts should be presented to enhance clarity; and (4) *conciseness,* an elimination of any material if it merely adds unnecessary length to the report rather than adding to its completeness and clarity.

Format of the Report

Published reports must conform to the style and format specified by the selected journal. The researcher is expected to check the format required and carefully follow the prescribed guidelines. The most frequently used style manuals include the *Publication Manual of the American Psychological Association*, 4th ed. (1994), *MLA Handbook for Writers of Research Papers*, 5th ed. (Gibaldi 1999), *The Chicago Manual of Style*, 14th ed. (1993), *Form and Style: Research Papers, Reports, Theses*, 9th ed. (Salde, Campbell, and Ballou 1994), and *A Manual for Writers of Term Papers, Theses, and Dissertations*, 6th ed. (Turabian 1996). Graduate students completing a thesis or dissertation are often required by their respective colleges or universities to follow a particular **thesis format** for organizing and presenting the report. If the institution has no established requirement, then the college, school, division, or department of HHP probably will. Various published and standardized formats are used, although special modifications are frequently made by the institution or department. Before commencing the written report, students are expected to become familiar with the prescribed style and format required at their institution.

Divisions of a Thesis or Dissertation

Usually, a research report, such as a thesis or dissertation, is arranged in three major parts: preliminary items, the text or body of the report, and supplementary items.

Preliminary Items

The **preliminary items** usually included are the title page, acceptance page, **acknowledgments page,** table of contents, list of tables, list of figures, and abstract. Example 15.1 provides samples of these items completed by former students of the authors of this textbook.

EXAMPLE 15.1A
Title Page
From J. K. Clark, *Two curricular settings of a HIV education unit related to secondary school students' HIV knowledge and attitude.* Doctoral dissertation, 1991. Reprinted by permission of Jeff K. Clark.

TWO CURRICULAR SETTINGS OF A HIV EDUCATION UNIT RELATED TO SECONDARY SCHOOL STUDENTS' HIV KNOWLEDGE AND ATTITUDE

by
Jeffrey K. Clark

Submitted in partial fulfillment of the requirements
for the Doctor of Health and Safety Degree
in the School of Health, Physical
Education, and Recreation
Indiana University

July 1991

(Clark 1991)

Accepted by the faculty of the School of Health, Physical Education, and Recreation, Indiana University, in partial fulfillment of the requirements for the Doctor of Physical Education degree.

_____
Director of Thesis

_____
Doctoral Committee: Chairperson

_____

_____

_____

(Clark 1991)

EXAMPLE 15.1B
Acceptance Page
From J. K. Clark, _Two curricular settings of a HIV education unit related to secondary school students' HIV knowledge and attitude._ Doctoral dissertation, 1991. Reprinted by permission of Jeff K. Clark.

EXAMPLE 15.1C
Acknowledgements Page

Acknowledgments

     The author wishes to express his gratitude to Dr. _____ , Dr. _____ , and Dr. _____ for their assistance and guidance in this investigation. The author is especially indebted to Dr. _____ whose help and encouragement was invaluable to the completion of this study.

     Special thanks is offered to the author's new young friends and their teachers who provided their time and energy so generously during the data-collection process.

B. J.

TABLE OF CONTENTS

EXAMPLE 15.1D
Table of Contents

From M. J. Major. *Effects of Special Olympics participation on self-esteem of adults with mental retardation.* Master's degree thesis, 1998. Reprinted by permission of M. J. Major.

EXAMPLE 15.1D
Concluded

(Major 1998)

EXAMPLE 15.1E
List of Tables

From R. J. Ogletree, *Selected
factors related to help-seeking
behavior in college women
victims of sexual coercion.*
Doctoral dissertation, 1991.
Reprinted by permission of
Roberta J. Ogletree.

List of Tables

(Ogletree 1991)

List of Figures

Abo-Abdo (1981)

EXAMPLE 15.1F
List of Figures
From H. E. Abo-Abdo, *Kinematic and kinetic analysis of the soccer instep kick.* Doctoral dissertation, 1981. Reprinted by permission of H. E. Abo-Abdo.

EXAMPLE 15.1G
Abstract

From W. Bian, *Physical activity patterns among physical education major students in selected institutions of China and the United States.* Master's degree thesis, 1999. Reprinted by permission of W. Bian.

Abstract

The benefits associated with regular physical activity have been well documented in recent years. Numerous studies have investigated physical activity patterns among children, adolescents, and adults, yet little work to date has examined the patterns of habitual physical activity participation among pre-service physical education (PE) majors. Furthermore, inasmuch as physical activity affords health benefits irrespective of one's nationality or culture, comparisons among the peoples of nations around the world becomes of greater interest.

This study was designed to examine the leisure-time physical activity patterns of physical education major students in selected institutions from the People's Republic of China (PRC) and the United States (U.S.). Data were collected from 184 PE major students enrolled in Beijing University of Physical Education ($n=98$) and the University of Northern Iowa ($n=86$) during April 1998 using a self-report questionnaire. The questionnaire was an adaptation of the Modifiable Activity Questionnaire designed to assess physical activity participation patterns and behaviors. With the exception of a few questions that were modified to reflect cultural differences, the questionnaires were indentical.

Results indicated that physical education major students in both the United States and China are more active than the general adult population. Approximately 62% of PRC students and 80% of U.S. students reported participation in leisure-time physical activities three or more of the previous seven days. U.S. students are generally more active than PRC students during their leisure-time, but less active during physical education activity classes. Students' preference of leisure-time physical activities as well as exercise behaviors often reflects cultural and ethnic differences between the two countries. Jogging and basketball were identified as the two most frequently participated in leisure-time physical activities for both PRC and U.S. students. For PRC students, the next most prevalent activities were swimming, soccer, ping-pong, and volleyball; while U.S. students reported weight training, bicycling, softball/baseball, and dancing. Results from the past-year physical activity participation of both groups indicated a notable seasonal variation in participation rates among the most common activities.

There is consideraable variance in the reasons for physical activity participation among physical education major students in the United States and China. For U.S. students, reasons related to self-feelings of physical activity participation were rated the most important. For PRC students, to improve fitness and develop sport skills were ranked higher than the reasons related to individual feelings. Although there were a few notable differences between the PRC and U.S. students, for the most part, the relative importance of the reasons given for discontinuing their physical activity participation was similar.

(Bian 1999)

The Text

The **text,** or body, of the thesis for most descriptive and experimental studies usually consists of five chapters. The first three chapters (**introduction, review of related literature,** and procedures or methods) are discussed in detail in chapter 2 of this book under the topic, "Developing the Research Proposal." The inclusions in these first three chapters are summarized.

Chapter 4, covering the results and discussion, and chapter 5, which includes the summary, conclusions, implementations, and **recommendations,** make up the remainder of the body of the thesis or dissertation. These chapters are discussed in some detail, and several examples for illustrating their content are included at the end of this chapter.

Summary of Chapters 1–5

Chapter 1 Introduction

Statement of the Problem: A clear and definitive statement of what was studied.

Purpose of the Study: A brief statement of why the study was done; a reason for the research or the potential uses for or contribution to be made by the results.

Need for the Study (Significance of the Study, Justification for the Study): An elaboration of the purpose, validating and establishing the importance of the problem.

Delimitations: The scope of the study as identified by including information on what subjects and variables were studied and what instrumentation was used; the methods and techniques incorporated; and the time and duration of the study.

Limitations: An indication of the inherent weaknesses in the study; factors that could not be controlled adequately and could have affected the results.

Assumptions: The particular facts taken for granted about the behaviors, conditions, methods, measures, and relationships inherent in the study.

Hypotheses: Predictions of the eventual outcome of the study.

Definition of Terms: A list of the terminology essential to consistent interpretation of the various concepts surrounding the problem being studied.

Chapter 2 Review of Related Literature.   This is a report of previous investigations related to the problem being studied. Theoretical formulations from other studies, the major issues of methodology, instrumentation, interpretation, and background information are presented. It is a well-organized chapter that shows how the present study may differ from previous ones, and at the same time add to their contributions. Knowledge gaps in the problem area are noted. Through a review of the literature, a theoretical basis and justification for the present study is formed.

Chapter 3 Procedures or Methods. This is a systematic and careful plan for attacking the problem. The procedures, methods, and techniques are detailed in a step-by-step set of instructions for conducting the study. The topics frequently included are selection of research participants, instrumentation, design of the study, administrative procedures for collecting the data, and treatment of the data.

Chapter 4 Results and Discussion. This is the reporting chapter of the thesis or dissertation in which the researcher (1) presents the data and (2) discusses and interprets those data. This chapter may also be called "Analysis of Data" or "Analysis and Discussion". This chapter should begin with an opening paragraph that restates the problem and tells how the chapter is organized (example 15.2). Following that paragraph will be several sections in which the data analysis and/or findings will be reported. Typical items that need to be included are the following indices: (1) What is in the chapter (example 15.2)? (2) How were the raw data scored or into what values were they converted for the analysis (example 15.3)? (3) Demographic information concerning research participants. (4) How were the data analyzed and what were the results of the analysis (examples 15.4 and 15.5)?

Note that the emphasis in the first section of chapter 4 is usually on *reporting only,* with no editorializing, discussion, or interpretation included. The standard procedure is to introduce a table containing data, present the table, and point out the significant findings in the table. The report of all of the data and findings should be followed by a detailed discussion and interpretation of the findings. This final section of the chapter may be labeled "Discussion of Findings." Here are some questions and thoughts concerning this section:

a. Are there any explanations for any of the findings? If so, these thoughts should be shared with the reader.

EXAMPLE 15.2

An Opening Paragraph

From T. L. Visker, *Self-consciousness and physical self-efficacy in relationship to exercise adherence.* Doctoral dissertation, 1986. Reprinted by permission of Tom L. Visker.

The problem of the study was to determine if the psychological factors of self-consciousness and physical self-efficacy discriminate between female adults who adhere to exercise programs and female adults who do not adhere to exercise programs. Included in the study was an attempt to identify the reasons exercise adherers give for continuing an exercise program and the reasons exercise non-adherers give for discontinuing exercise programs. The analysis of the data is presented in this chapter according to the following topics: (1) data-gathering instrument distribution, (2) demographic data, (3) chi-square analysis, (4) discriminant analysis data, (5) multiple regression data, (6) reasons for continuing or discontinuing an exercise program, and (7) discussion of findings.

(Visker 1986)

EXAMPLE 15.3
Data Reporting Table for
Response Rate Data
From T. L. Visker,
*Self-consciousness and
physical self-efficacy in
relationship to exercise
adherence.* Doctoral
dissertation, 1986.
Reprinted by permission of
Tom L. Visker.

Data-Gathering Instrument Distribution

The population of prospective subjects for the study consisted of 337 females who were enrolled in physical fitness classes at the Monroe County, Indiana, YMCA during the spring of 1985. Each of the 337 females was sent a letter in which they were asked to participate in the study. Each person was asked to return a postcard to the investigator regarding her intention to participate or not participate in the study. The results of this mailing are presented in Table 1.

TABLE 1 Letter Response Rate

	FIRST MAILING	SECOND MAILING	TOTAL
Letters Sent	350	196	546
Postcards Returned	141	139	280
Percent	40	71	83*
Postcards Not Returned	196	57	70
Percent	56	29	21*
Number Agreed to Participate	116	82	198
Percent	82	59	71**
Number Declined to Participate	25	57	82
Percent	18	41	29**
Invalid Addresses	13	0	13
Percent	4	0	4*

*of the 337 valid addresses
**of the 280 postcards returned

The initial mailing yielded a return of 141 postcards (40 percent). Of those subjects who returned the postcard, 116 (82 percent) agreed to participate in the study and 25 (18 percent) declined to participate in the study. There were 13 subjects (4 percent) for whom no valid address could be found. The number of prospective subjects who did not return a postcard was 196 (56 percent).

A second mailing of 196 letters yielded a return of 139 postcards (71 percent). Of those who returned the postcard after this mailing, 82 (59 percent) agreed to participate and 57 (41 percent) declined to participate in the study. Fifty-seven (29 percent) of those to whom a second letter was sent failed to return the postcard.

(Visker 1986)

EXAMPLE 15.4
Data Reporting Table for
Analysis: Chi-Square
Analysis

From T. L. Visker,
*Self-consciousness and
physical self-efficacy in
relationship to exercise
adherence.* Doctoral
dissertation, 1986.
Reprinted by permission of
Tom L. Visker.

Chi-Square Analysis

The chi-square test of association was used to test the hypothesis that there is no difference between exercise adherers and exercise non-adherers in terms of the type of fitness class attended, the highest educational degree earned, or the marital status of the subjects. This test was used since none of the parameters was known; the results of its application are presented in Tables 5 through 7.

TABLE 5 Chi-Square Test of Association for Fitness Class Attended of Exercise Adherers and Non-Adherers

CLASS	CLASSIFICATION		TOTAL
	Adherer	Non-Adherer	
Aerobics Plus	31	8	39
Percent	27	16	23
Aquaerobics	7	9	16
Percent	6	18	10
Fitness Fantasia	47	22	69
Percent	40	43	41
Fit-for-Life	29	11	40
Percent	25	22	24
General Aerobics	3	1	4
Percent	3	2	2
Group Total	117	51	168
Percent	70	30	

Chi-square value = 7.146
Chi-square required at .05 level of significance = 9.45

The chi-square value for the fitness classes was determined to be 7.146. A value of 9.45 was required for statistical significance at the .05 level with four degrees of freedom. Since the chi-square value for fitness classes was non-significant, the null hypothesis that there is no significant difference between exercise adherers and non-adherers in fitness class attended was accepted.

(Visker 1986)

EXAMPLE 15.5
Data Reporting Table for
Analysis: *F* Test

From T. D. Sells, *Selected
movement and anthropometric
variables of football defensive
tackles.* Doctoral dissertation,
1977. Reprinted by permission
of Thomas D. Sells.

The F-tests from the one-way analysis of variance of the difference between means of the first, second, and third team defensive tackles are presented in Table 2.

TABLE 2 One-Way Analysis of Variance of the Difference Between Means and the Level of Significance of Difference of the Means of the First Team, Second Team, and Third Team Defensive Tackles

VARIABLE	F-TEST	SIGNIFICANCE LEVEL*
Reaction	.2474	.7821
Movement time	1.8428	.1723
Five-yard sprint	1.7168	.1933
40-yard sprint	1.3740	.2654
Height	2.0586	.1416
Weight	.5299	.5929
Percent body fat	.0743	.9285

*Degrees of freedom = 2 and 38.

The significance of the separate F-tests based on the one-way analysis of variance of difference in group means did not reach the .05 level in the initial phase of the data analysis. At that point in the analysis, the null hypotheses stating an equality of group means across the three success groups could not be rejected for any of the variables.

(Sells 1977)

b. Do some findings defy explanation? Are some really surprising? If so, what are they? Speculate why these particular results may have come about in this way.

c. In answering the questions posed in a and b above, the element of hindsight in the procedure sometimes enters the discussion. The hindsight may be clear to the researcher, but not to the reader; so share that hindsight with the reader.

d. Are the findings consistent with findings in similar studies? Do the findings differ?

This part of the research report is often difficult to accomplish, but a feeling of satisfaction accompanies its completion. For an excellent example illustrating how some researchers have incorporated the information included in the comments made above, see example 15.6.

Chapter 5 Summary, Findings, Conclusions, Implementations, and Recommendations.

This is the final and, typically, the shortest chapter in a thesis or dissertation. A summary of the study and the general conclusions and recommendations resulting from the research should be placed in this chapter. Only material mentioned earlier in the report may be included in the summary.

In the summary, the problem should be restated, a general overview of the sources of data and the methods used should be provided, and the *more important* findings should be listed. For this reporting of the findings, brief statements will suffice rather than repeating the details already discussed.

General conclusions drawn from the findings should be presented in the same order as the findings on which they are based. In sampling studies, **conclusions** are population statements as are the hypotheses stated at the beginning of the research. The conclusions should be definitive and bring the study to an end. Conclusions should not be repetitions or summaries of findings but should answer this question: The data (findings) say this, so what does this tell me as to the conclusion that is warranted? Conclusions beyond the data obtained (i.e., the findings) should not be made. In stating the conclusions, avoid the use of "hedging" words such as "It seems as though . . ." or "It appears that . . ." The data tell the researcher what is or is not, and the conclusion statements should reflect such definitiveness. The distinction between a finding and the conclusion should be made abundantly clear.

The implementations section should indicate how the researcher envisions the findings being applied. How can the findings be used in a practical situation, or in what ways would the findings make a contribution? Could the findings also apply to a research setting? If so, how could they be implemented?

The recommendation section should appear last in the chapter, and the recommendations may be of more than one type. The researcher may recommend that certain specified action be taken in light of the findings; that further study be made of the problem using either the same data or a different sample; or that a study be made of a related problem or of the same problem in greater detail or after a certain length of time has elapsed. A typical chapter 5 of a thesis or dissertation is illustrated in example 15.7.

It is important to note that chapters 2, 3, and 4 always begin with an opening paragraph identifying what part of the problem is discussed in the chapter and indicating how the chapter is organized. Only in chapter 2 is a summary mandated. Each chapter is to start on a new page.

Discussion of Findings

The consistency in determining the significant contribution of perceived physical ability in the study was similar to the findings of other studies using perceived physical ability as a variable. Snyder and Spreitzer (1984), Spreitzer and Snyder (1983), and Snyder and Spreitzer (1981) found significant correlations between perceived athletic ability and involvement in vigorous physical activities. The finding of the present study reiterates the position that the higher an individual perceives her physical abilities to be, the more likely she will be to stay with an exercise program.

The findings of the study also supported Sonstroem's Physical Activity Model (1978, 1976, 1974). Sonstroem theorized that as one's estimation of physical ability increases, so will one's attraction to physical activity, which will result in an increase in physical activity. In the present study, the subjects who scored higher in perceived physical ability also were engaged in more minutes per week of vigorous physical activity than subjects who scored lower in perceived physical ability.

Since the data of the study were analyzed using multivariate correlational techniques, it would be inappropriate to suggest that a woman's perception of her physical abilities caused her to adhere to or discontinue an exercise program. All that can be inferred from this finding is that a significant positive relationship does exist between a woman's perceived physical ability and the likelihood that she will continue with an exercise program.

The lack of scientific inquiry into reasons for adhering to a program of exercise makes it difficult to draw parallels to other investigations. However, several of the reasons given for adhering to an exercise program have been investigated in other studies. Many of the reasons address the situational factors in which the exercise program is carried out. This alone provides credence to Dishman's (1984) conceptual model for exercise adherence which posits that whether a person stays with an exercise program or not is determined by an interaction between the exerciser and his or her environment. Specifically, the social reason of exercising with others has been found to be significant in other studies. Heinzelman and Bagley (1970) found that 90 percent of the subjects in their investigation preferred to exercise with others. Massie and Shepard (1971) found that exercise adherence was higher for subjects who exercised as a group than for subjects who exercised alone.

Exercise and mental health have been the subject of many research investigations (Sach, 1984; Folkins and Sime, 1981; and Morgan, 1981). It has consistently been shown that regular vigorous physical activity will enhance

EXAMPLE 15.6
Discussion of Findings
From T. L. Visker,
*Self-consciousness and
physical self-efficacy in
relationship to exercise
adherence.* Doctoral
dissertation, 1986.
Reprinted by permission
of Tom L. Visker.

EXAMPLE 15.6
Concluded

one's mental health. The frequency of the response of enhancing mental health found in this investigation is consistent with that found in other studies.

The exercise environment was also cited as a reason for adhering to an exercise program. One factor in the exercise environment which was specifically mentioned was the use of music. The use of music in an exercise setting is a dissociative technique which focuses the exerciser's attention away from the discomfort of exercise, resulting in more enjoyable exercise bouts. Martin, et al. (1984) found dissociative intervention strategy to be effective in increasing exercise adherence.

Several studies have investigated the reasons individuals give for discontinuing exercise programs (Lee and Owen, 1985; Andrew, et al. 1981; Boothby, Tungatt and Townsend, 1981). Two of the reasons exercise non-adherers cited in the present study are consistent with earlier findings. Perhaps the most frequent reason given for discontinuing an exercise program is lack of time. The frequency of this reason in the present study is parallel to studies by Boothby, Tungatt and Townsend (1981); Gettman, Pollock and Ward, (1983); and Lee and Owen (1985).

The distance traveled to the exercise setting was also cited as a reason for dropping out of an exercise program. While the frequency of this response is not as high as the response of lack of time, this response is consistent with other studies (Lee and Owen, 1985; Andrew and Parker, 1979; and Morgan, 1977).

Because the present investigation was composed entirely of women, some of the reasons given for adhering to or discontinuing an exercise program were unique to this investigation. Many of these reasons deal with traditional female roles. For example, some of the reasons given for adhering to an exercise program are the availability of babysitting services, reversing the effects of childbirth, and a child's nap schedule. The reasons given for discontinuing an exercise program are even more to the point. The demands of children and pregnancy-childbirth were two of the more frequent responses given. However, the fact that the response of demands of employment was one of the most frequent responses given for discontinuing an exercise program is, perhaps, an indication of the changing nature of women's roles in society.

(Visker 1986)

Summary

The problem of the study was to determine if the psychological factors of self-consciousness and physical self-efficacy discriminate between female adults who adhere to exercise programs and female adults who do not adhere to exercise programs. Included in the study was an attempt to identify the reasons exercise adherers give for continuing an exercise program and the reasons exercise non-adherers give for discontinuing an exercise program.

The subjects of the study were 168 females who had enrolled in physical fitness classes at the Monroe County YMCA, Bloomington, Indiana, during the spring of 1985. All subjects completed a survey instrument consisting of the self-consciousness scale, the physical self-efficacy scale, and questions designed to determine demographic data and exercise habits. The data for the study were collected during the months of May and June, 1986.

The data were analyzed using four statistical techniques. Chi-square test of association was used to test the differences in fitness class attended, education level, and marital status between exercise adherers and non-adherers. Discriminant analysis was used to determine if the independent variables of private self-consciousness, public self-consciousness, social anxiety, self-consciousness, perceived physical ability, physical self-presentation confidence, physical self-efficacy, age, and income could significantly predict the dependent variables of group membership (exercise adherer or non-adherer). Multiple regression analysis was used to determine if the independent variables of the study could significantly predict the number of minutes per week spent in vigorous physical activity. Finally, a frequency distribution of the reasons exercise adherers gave for continuing an exercise program and the reasons exercise non-adherers gave for discontinuing an exercise program was done. The Statistical Package for the Social Sciences (SPSS) was used for all statistical analysis except the frequency distributions.

Findings

The analysis of the data revealed the following significant findings:

1. The independent variables of private self-consciousness, public self-consciousness, social anxiety, self-consciousness, perceived physical ability, physical self-presentation confidence, physical self-efficacy, age, and income significantly predicted group membership as an exercise adherer or non-adherer.

EXAMPLE 15.7
Sample of a Chapter 5
From T. L. Visker,
*Self-consciousness and
physical self-efficacy in
relationship to exercise
adherence.* Doctoral
dissertation, 1986.
Reprinted by permission
of Tom L. Visker.

EXAMPLE 15.7
Continued

2. The independent variables of perceived physical ability and physical self-efficacy accounted for most of the function which discriminated between exercise adherers and non-adherers.

3. The optimal linear combination of the independent variables of private self-consciousness, public self-consciousness, social anxiety, self-consciousness, perceived physical ability, physical self-presentation confidence, physical self-efficacy, age, education level, marital status, and income, taken altogether, significantly predicted the number of minutes per week spent in vigorous physical activity.

4. By itself, only perceived physical ability significantly predicted the number of minutes per week spent in vigorous physical activity.

5. The most frequent reasons given by exercise adherers for continuing an exercise program were to maintain health, social, enhance mental health, relieve stress, and appearance.

6. The most frequent reasons given by exercise non-adherers for discontinuing an exercise program were lack of time, demands of employment, schedule conflicts, demands of children, and illness or injury.

Conclusions

Within the limitations of the study the following conclusions are warranted:

1. Significant psychological differences exist between female exercise adherers and non-adherers.

2. Females who adhere to a program of exercise perceive their physical abilities at a higher level than do females who discontinue a program of physical exercise.

3. Self-consciousness is not an important factor in the psychological differences between female exercise adherers and non-adherers.

4. Females who have a higher perception of their physical abilities exercise more than do females who have a lower perception of their physical abilities.

EXAMPLE 15.7
Continued

Implementations

The findings of the study may be implemented into either a professional practice situation or a research setting in the following ways:

1. The significance of perceived physical ability to discriminate between female exercise adherers and non-adherers should be considered in developing psychological profiles of exercise adherers and non-adherers. The use of these profiles may help to predict those who will continue an exercise program and those who will be inclined to drop out.

2. Adherence to an exercise program could be enhanced by the use of intervention strategies designed to increase the participants' perception of their physical ability. Programs involving the use of progression in skills and intensity of training could increase one's self-perception of physical ability and thereby increase the likelihood of an individual continuing in those exercise programs.

3. If exercise adherence is one of the major goals in physical activity programs, the enhancement of one's self-perceived physical abilities should be a major concern in elementary and secondary physical education programs. Exposure to a variety of skills will increase the likelihood of finding an activity in which the skills can be mastered, thus increasing the chance for regular life-long participation in that activity.

Recommendations for Further Study

The following recommendations are made for further research in the area of exercise adherence:

1. The present study should be replicated using both male and female participants.

2. The relationship of self-consciousness and physical self-efficacy to exercise adherence should be examined in an experimental type of study. This would permit more control in the variable of exercise adherence since it would not rely on the subjects' truthfulness regarding their exercise habits.

3. A study should be conducted to determine the cause and effect relationship between perceived physical ability and exercise adherence.

EXAMPLE 15.7
Concluded

4. Additional studies identifying other psychological variables which could be related to exercise adherence are needed.

5. The present investigation should be replicated in other communities to gain a large cross-section of the adult population from which data can be obtained.

6. The psychological variables of self-consciousness and physical self-efficacy related to exercise adherence should be investigated in a non-structured exercise program setting.

7. Additional studies identifying reasons exercise adherers give for continuing an exercise program are needed to corroborate the findings of the present study.

(Visker 1986)

References

The body of the text is always followed by an alphabetized list of **references.** It should be presented in accordance with whatever style format is required by the student's college or university or academic unit. With a relatively short list of sources to be referenced, different types of literary pieces may be incorporated. However, if the list of sources is quite long, they may be grouped according to type, such as books, documents, manuscripts, newspapers, pamphlets, and periodicals. The usual convention is to include only those sources that were referenced in the text. Occasionally, it may be necessary to include a source that was not cited, but the usual caution is not to pad the list of references. See example 15.8 for an illustration of a refernece list.

Supplementary Items

The appendices serve as the repository for **supplementary items** that are unnecessary for inclusion in the body of the text, but can be used by the reader to clarify various aspects of the thesis or research report. They provide additional specific information if the reader desires it. Typically, appendices will include the following types of items:

1. Copies of the verbal instruments (e.g., questionnaires, interview guides)
2. Instructions to subjects on how to engage in physical performance tests (e.g., fitness, skill tests)
3. Letters and similar documents
4. Human subject consent forms
5. Raw data from both a pilot study and the actual study
6. Diagrams of testing settings
7. Tables from related research
8. Supplementary reference lists
9. Credentials of the members of a jury of experts or committee of authorities
10. Interview and other data collection schedules
11. Legal codes

All such materials should be clearly labeled and lettered for quick and easy reference. Each appendix should bear a descriptive title of what is included.

Abstract

Example 15.1G is a sample of an **abstract** for a master's thesis (Bian, 1999). Most institutions require an abstract varying in length from 250 to 350 words. The abstract is one of the preliminary items of the thesis or dissertation. Most research journals

EXAMPLE 15.8
References

References

Cetron, M. J., & Rocha, W. (1987). Travel tomorrow: The hospitable future. *Futurist, 21*(4), (INFOTRAC 87–23310), 29–34.

Coates, J. F. (1989). Looking ahead: Travel marketing challenges of the next 25 years. *Travel and Tourism Executive Report, 1/2, 1.*

Cornish, E. (1986). Future free time: How will people use it? *Parks and Recreation, 5,* 57–59.

Davidson, T. L. (1984). Marketing travel in an emerging economy. *Journal of Travel Research, 22*(4), (INFOTRAC 84–15674), 38–39.

Dillman, D. A. (1978). *Mail and telephone surveys: The total design method.* New York: John Wiley & Sons, 44.

Fesenmaier, D. R. (1987). *Development of a market assistance program for tourist businesses along the Texas gulf coast.* Proposal for Texas A&M University Sea Grant College Program. College Station, Texas: Department of Recreation and Parks, Texas A&M University.

Fesenmaier, D. R. (1988). *A framework for tourism evaluation in Fredericksburg, Texas.* Unpublished report to the city of Fredericksburg, Texas.

Fesenmaier, D. R. (1989). *An assessment of information needs: Indiana convention and visitors bureaus.* Indiana University report. Bloomington, IN: Tourism Resource Center.

Gartrell, R. B. (1988). *Destination marketing for convention and visitors bureaus.* Dubuque, IA: Kendall/Hunt, 6–11.

Gee, C. Y. & Makens, J. C. (1985). The tourism board: Doing it right. *Cornell H.R.A. Quarterly, 11,* 25–33.

Glass, G. V., & Hopkins, K. D. (1984). *Statistical methods in education and psychology.* Englewood Cliffs, NJ: Prentice-Hall, 2.

Gunn, G. V. (1983). U.S. tourism policy development. *Journal of Physical Education, Recreation, and Dance, 4,* 10, 33.

Honomichi, J. (1984). Tourism industry big on research. *Advertising Age, 55,*(79), 24, 28.

(Pena 1990)

also require an abstract when researchers submit an article for publication. Though the length requirement varies among the journals, 150 to 200 words is typical. The researcher should use all of whatever abstract length is allowed, because the more that can be reported to the reader, the greater is the chance for good understanding of the research. Often abstracts are written as a single paragraph, but sometimes may include separate paragraphs for each section.

An abstract must be concise but should include enough detail to enable the reader to determine whether or not the entire research report, article, thesis, or dissertation needs to be read. The abstract should be brief and contain the overall essence of the information included in the larger work. The reader should be able to glean from the abstract all of the main ideas of the original research investigation.

An appropriate abstract will usually include comments concerning each of the following elements:

1. The *problem* that was investigated, including the rationale from which the problem was developed.

2. The *methods* by which the data for the problem were collected. Included here will be an identification of the variables studied, the procedure used in carrying out the research and collecting the data, and a discussion of how the data were analyzed.

3. A brief report of the *findings* resulting from the study. These results are usually not given in tables, figures, and graphs due to the limitations placed on the length of an abstract.

4. The *conclusions* made by the researcher based upon the findings. If room in the abstract exists, it could also include the researcher's interpretation of the possible implementation of the results or recommendations for further research in the problem area.

Thesis Format versus Published Article Format

On the foregoing pages, the format for a thesis or dissertation was described in some detail. The major difference between a thesis or dissertation and a research report is the length of the document. Researchers who publish articles are limited by the established publishing criteria of particular journals in the amount of detail they can submit. A six- to eight-page article, as prescribed by a specific publication, cannot possibly include all of the information contained in a 150-page thesis or dissertation. Although the precise format may vary depending upon the nature of the research, a published research report typically includes the following elements:

1. Preliminary Information
   a. Title

    b. Author and organizational affiliation

    c. Acknowledgements (if any)

    d. Abstract

2. Introduction

    a. Background information and literature review

    b. Rationale for study

    c. Problem statement

    d. Hypotheses or research questions

3. Methods

    a. Participants

    b. Instrumentation

    c. Procedures

    d. Statistical analysis

4. Results

    a. Presentation of data

5. Discussion

    a. Conclusions

    b. Recommendations

6. References

7. Appendix (if appropriate)

The style in which the published article is written will also be determined by whatever style manual is followed by the journal. Quite frequently, the style will be different from that found in a thesis or dissertation. Capitalization may differ, as will punctuation, the spelling of numbers, and abbreviations.

Theses or dissertations written by graduate students are considered "final" manuscripts. They usually have a long life span and will be read and referred to over a long time. A journal manuscript tends to be a "copy" manuscript that, in turn, becomes a typeset article. Copy manuscripts have a relatively short life. They are read by reviewers, editors, and typeset experts. The original content can sometimes be changed dramatically as a result of the publication process.

Students who complete a thesis or dissertation are encouraged to publish one or more articles derived from the document. Preparation of an article entails transposing selected thesis content to journal material according to the publishing restrictions of the journal in which the article will appear. This is not a particularly difficult task, although some people find it to be a laborious chore. Some confuse transposition with creating a whole new document. Students who write a thesis under one format are sometimes confused in following the guidelines imposed by the journal format requirements.

In recent years, some institutions, the University of Georgia among them, have adopted regulations that enable students to write their theses and dissertations in the form required by those journals in which the students hope to publish articles based upon their research. This would result in documents of twenty to thirty pages in length and containing only the essential information from the literature, procedures, and results sections. The more detailed information from the other thesis sections would become part of appendixes. The underlying idea is to make it quicker and easier for the student to create a journal article for publication from a document written to fulfill a degree requirement. Whether or not the movement away from the traditional thesis format will become large scale is yet to be seen.

Preparing a Manuscript for Publication

Before Writing

Prior to starting to prepare a manuscript for publication, the researcher should do several things. One, the researcher needs to select the journal to which the manuscript will be submitted. Two, the researcher needs to examine articles published in that journal to get a general idea of the format used, and needs to read the guidelines for submitting manuscripts to the journal. Guidelines are published in the journal. Select the journal primarily on its orientation and type of reader. Some journals are geared primarily toward researchers; others are more for practitioners. Some journals are highly specialized, while others are for a general audience. There is no use in submitting a manuscript to a journal that does not publish the type of research described in the manuscript. Also, the researcher should try to determine the manuscript acceptance rate of the journal. Acceptance rates vary from 10 percent for very prestigious and specialized research journals to as high as 70 percent for practical, general-audience state association journals.

By looking at articles in the selected journal, the researcher may discover a useful model to follow. Certainly the researcher will be able to determine whether an abstract is required as part of the manuscript, what organization and major headings are required in the manuscript, and the typical length of a manuscript based on the length of articles in the journal.

During Writing

Any manuscript starts with the title of the research study. The title needs to be short yet represent the research well and stimulate a person to read the entire article. If an abstract is required, that element appears next in the manuscript; it should be one to three paragraphs long. The abstract will contain the statement of purpose for the study, description of subjects, major procedures, major results, and conclusions.

The manuscript for most published articles begins with an introduction and brief review of the most important related literature. Somewhere, wherever appropriate, there should be a statement of the purpose of the study. This part of the manuscript is typically three to six paragraphs.

Next in a manuscript is a procedures or methods section. Typically included in this section are descriptions of research participants, how the research was conducted, data collection techniques, and data analysis procedures. The content and length of this section is dependent on the type of research conducted and the complexity of describing how the research was conducted. Tables and figures in this section are commonly used to clearly and economically present information. Not every small point concerning the conduct of the research can be presented, or the manuscript could not be kept to a reasonable length.

A results section follows the procedures section. This section usually makes up a relatively large portion of the manuscript because it includes all of the major data analysis and findings of the research study. Much of this information is presented in text form; however, the use of tables and figures is also common. The recommended organization when using tables and figures is to introduce a table or figure, present it, and then discuss it. This is not always possible, but the recommendation is a good rule of thumb. The discussion following the table or figure may be just a short sentence or two with the extensive discussion in a later section, or it may be quite extensive. The decision to present major discussion in this section or in a later section is left to the researcher. The majority of researchers probably place the extensive discussion in the next section.

The discussion and conclusions section are where the results previously reported are discussed at length and conclusions based on the results are stated. This part of the manuscript is usually of considerable length, also. The discussion may include comments on each finding followed by a discussion of all the findings as a whole. However, if each finding was discussed at length when introduced in the results section, then the discussion is reserved for the findings as a whole. Often included in the discussion of findings is a comparison of how the findings agree with those in the literature cited at the beginning of the manuscript. Usually, in the discussion are statements concerning the importance and application of the findings. No matter how the discussion is structured, the conclusions follow it. Anytime the research involves a population from which one or more samples were drawn, conclusions consist of statements concerning what the researcher thinks is true at the population level based on the findings from the samples used in the study.

The last section in a manuscript is a list of references. Included in the list are all sources cited in the manuscript. The length of this section is dependent on the number of sources cited. Normally, it is not a lengthy section and will contain from three to fifteen listings.

After Writing

After writing the first draft of the manuscript, one must spend considerable time proofing it. Attention to correctness of manuscript form, correctness of content, economy and clarity of presentation, and correctness of spelling and grammar are important. The more prestigious the journal where the manuscript will be submitted, the more important becomes the proofreading.

The spell check and grammar check options on most word processing computer programs are often quite helpful in revising the manuscript. However, they do not catch all problems and the final responsibility for correctness rests with the writer. Spell check will not catch words left out, the wrong word, confusing sentences, or misspelled words which are the correct spelling of another word.

When the manuscript is ready to be submitted to a journal, send the required number of copies and the necessary cover sheet containing author name(s) and contact information. If there are multiple authors, names are listed in order from major contribution to minor contribution to the research and manuscript. Major contributions would include such items as developing the problem, formulating hypotheses, setting up the design, selecting the data analysis procedures, interpreting the findings, and writing the majority of the report.

All manuscripts submitted to a journal are typically evaluated by two to four reviewers or associate editors for the journal. This evaluation takes one to three months. After the manuscript has been evaluated, the journal editor sends copies of the reviews to the author indicating whether the manuscript is accepted, needs revision, or is rejected. Authors should expect that the manuscript will not be acceptable in the form submitted. Thus, when the reviews are returned, revise the manuscript and return it to the original journal, or send it to another journal.

Guides to Preparation of the Research Report

Frequently Asked Questions about APA Style – http://www.apa.org/journals/faq.html

A Guide for Writing Research Papers – http://webster.commnet.edu/apa/apa_intro.htm

Cone, J. D. and Foster, S. L. (1993). *Dissertations and Theses from Start to Finish*. Washington, DC: American Psychological Association.

Alward, E. C. (1996). *Research Paper, Step-by-Step*. Westhampton, MA: Pine Island Press.

Day, R. A. (1998). *How to Write and Publish a Scientific Paper*. Philadelphia: ISI Press.

Dees, R. (1997). *Writing the Research Paper*. Boston: Allyn and Bacon.

Locke, L., Spirduso, W., and Silverman, S. (1999). *Proposals that Work: A Guide for Planning Dissertations and Grant Proposals*. Newbury Park, CA: Sage Publications.

Summary

The function of the written research report is to convey the results of the research effort. Clarity is a fundamental requirement of the report; the reader of the report should not have to make any assumptions as to what was done in the research and what was found. A typical format for the report has been presented, but this may be modified according to the particular requirements of the student's college, school, division, or department. Information regarding the difference between a thesis format and a published-article format has been presented. General guidelines for preparing an article for publication are detailed. As in the previous chapters, examples are presented to assist the student in understanding the research concepts inherent in a written report.

Formative Evaluation of Objectives

Objective 1   Determine the characteristics of a good research report.

1. Identify the characteristics of a good research report.
2. Why is effective writing so important in research reporting?

Objective 2   Understand the format for a report and the kinds of information required in each division of the report.

1. Identify the divisions of a typical research report.
2. Select a completed study and determine whether the content of each division of the report is appropriate.

Objective 3   Differentiate between the style of writing a research report for a thesis or dissertation as opposed to a research report for publication in a journal.

1. Select some completed research and analyze the style of writing in terms of desirable writing standards.

Appendix A

SPSS 10.0 for Windows Basics

Click with the left button of the mouse unless otherwise indicated.

1. Getting in to SPSS

   A. You should save your data on floppy disk. So, insert a floppy disk in the disk drive now.
   B. Click on **Start** in the lower left hand corner of the screen and then click on **Program** in the drop down menu.
   C. Click on **SPSS 10.0 for Windows** in the next menu.
   D. In the SPSS menu:

      (1) Click on **Tutorial** and then **OK** if you want information on using SPSS.
      (2) Click on **Type in Data** and then **OK** if you want to enter data.
      (3) Click on **Open an Existing File** and then **OK** if the data is already saved on disk.

2. Entering the data (see SPSS Base 10.0 Brief Guide in Reference section)

   A. Click on the **SPSS Data Editor** window title bar to make it the active window if it is not already highlighted. At the bottom of the window are two tabs: (1) Data View—to enter the data, edit the data, and see the data; and (2) Variable View—to name variables, and define variables. When you click on a tab it is displayed in dark letters. Define all variable names before entering the data.
   B. To define all variable names, click on the **Variable View** tab. Or to define one variable name, double click on the dimmed title *var* at the top of the column you want to name. This displays the headings (Name, Type, etc.) under which information can be entered.
   C. Enter a name for each variable under **Name**. [NOTE: The following rules apply to valid variable names and file names: 1) one word, 2) maximum 8 characters, 3) no special characters(!,*,?, -, etc).] You may backspace to correct typos. The other

information for each variable (Type, Width, etc.) are optional and may be left at the default (pre-set) values. Then click on the **Data View** tab and the entered names appear at the top of the columns. [NOTE: The first column you have not named is labeled **var00001**.]

D. After defining all variable names, put the cursor on the first empty cell (square) in the first column and click once. Type a score which is displayed in the space below the **SPSS Data Editor** menu. Each time you press **Enter**, the value appears with two decimal places in the cell, and the cursor will move down. If you press **Tab** rather than **Enter** the cursor will move to the right.

E. If a person has no score for a variable (score is missing), enter it as a blank (enter no score and press **Enter** or **Tab**). The missing score is represented by a period(.).

F. After entering all the data for a column or row, select the first cell in the next column (the next defined variable) or row (next person) by using the mouse to click on the cell or using the arrow keys on the keyboard or using the arrow keys on the right and bottom margin of the **SPSS Data Editor** to move to the cell.

G. Do step D and E until all data are entered.

H. Additional information: in the SPSS Data Editor window, note the buttons at the top of the window:

(1) 10th button from the left is Insert Case
(2) 11th button from the left is Insert Variable
(3) 12th button from the left is Split File
(4) 13th button from the left is Weight Cases
(5) 14th button from the left is Select Cases
(6) 15th button from the left is Value Labels

I. Additional information: when naming a variable, in addition to a title for the variable, labels for each level of the variable, changing the position of the decimal point, etc. are possible.

J. Example: variable is sex with 1 = female and 2 = male.

(1) In the Data Editor window click on the **Variable View** tab or click twice on **var** to name a column.
(2) The headings (Name, Type, etc.) are displayed
(3) Click on **Name** and type in the name of the variable: Sex
(4) Click on **Label** and type in the title of the variable: Sex of Person
(5) Click on **Values**, then the button for Values, and then type in the following:

Value: 1

Value Label: Female

click on **Add**

Value: 2

Value Label: Male

click on **Add**

click on **OK**

(6) This information will be shown in the output of any analysis (Frequencies used).

Sex of Person

Frequency

Female   35

Male   45

K.   Additional information: to remove a variable (column) in a data file, first highlight the column, then click on **Edit** on the menu bar, then click on **Cut.**

3. Saving the data

A.   To save the entered data in a file, Save does not have to be after the last score is entered. Click on **File** in the **SPSS Data Editor** menu and then click on **Save.** This opens the **Save Data As** dialog box. Enter a name for the data file (see rules in 2-C) in the **File name:** text box. Select the **a:** drive in the **Save in:** dialog box.

B.   At the **Save as type:** make sure the file is **SPSS(*.sav).** Click on **Save.**

C.   [NOTE: The untitled window will be changed to the drive and file name which you entered in 3-A.] The **SPSS Data Editor** window is still displayed. If this does not happen, save the data again.

D.   After a file is named, more data can be saved in it by clicking on **Save File** in the **SPSS Data Editor** menu.

4. Editing the data

A.   You can change data values which are incorrect, so the data entered should be still displayed on the screen.

B.   Where there are mistakes, click on the cell with the incorrect score or use the arrow keys to move to the incorrect score. Type in the correct value and press the **Enter** key. After editing, save the data again by clicking on **File** in the **SPSS Data Editor** menu and then clicking on **Save.** Make sure the **SPSS Data Editor**, and not an **Output** or **Syntax** window, is active because **Save** will save the active window. The light on the disk drive comes on while the data is being saved. Save again if the data is not save to the disk. The **SPSS Data Editor** window is still displayed.

C.   If you type in a score twice you may want to delete it rather than change it. If you leave out a score you may want to insert it. This may require deleting or inserting a row of data. To delete a row, click on the row to be deleted. The entire row will be highlighted. From the **SPSS Data Editor** menu click on **Edit** and then **Clear.** To insert a row (case) click on the row where you want to insert a row. Click on **Data** in the **SPSS Data Editor** menu. Click on **Insert Case,** the row you clicked on and all rows below it will be moved down, then enter the data. [NOTE: See the SPSS manuals for more details.]

5. Analyzing the data

A.   After doing steps 2-4 to enter the data, or the existing data file has been identified, click the analysis you want and then click on what options you want in the drop down menus. For data analysis, click **Analyze.** For graphs of the data, click **Graph.** For transformation of the data, click **Transform.**

B.   Since usually data analysis (Analyze) is desired, the options for Analyze are as follows: Report, Descriptive Statistics, Compare Means (3 t-tests, 1-Way ANOVA, Means), General Linear Model (other ANOVAs), Correlation, Regression, Loglinear,

Classify, Data Reduction, Scale, Nonparametric Tests, Survival, and Multiple Response. [NOTE: Put the cursor (no need to click) on any of these options and the screen will display a drop down menu of available options.]

C.   For specific information on using the options, see the SPSS 10.0 for Windows Statistical Procedures later in this document.

D.   The results of the analysis are displayed on the screen. After this you can print the output if desired or do another analysis on the same data. You can also enter another set of scores and analyze it or retrieve another set of scores on disk and analyze it.

6.   Printing output of the analysis

A.   To print the contents of the output of the analysis, make sure the **SPSS Output Navigator** is the active window at the top left of the screen. If it is not the active window, click on **Window** in the menu bar and then **SPSS Output Navigator**. The content of the active window is displayed on the right hand side of the screen (content pane) and the output objects on the left hand side of the screen (outline pane). Use the arrow keys to move around the screen.

B.   Before printing, indicate whether the entire contents (**All Visible Output**) (the default) or just part of the contents (**Selection**) of **Output Navigator** are to be printed. SPSS tends to produce many partially full pages of printout. To decrease the number of printed pages, select just the output desired.

(1)   In the left pane of Output Navigator highlight what contents of Output Navigator are to be printed.

(2)   From the Output Navigator click on **File** and then click on **Print**.

C.   The name of the file is shown in the dialog box. The printer name is also displayed. Click on the print option desired. By default, one copy is printed. If you want multiple copies, enter the number of copies you want to print. If there are too many columns (>7-8) to get on one vertical page (Portrait), or a line for the output can't be seen in full on the screen, select **Landscape** to print a horizontal page. To select Landscape print, click on **Properties**, click on **Landscape**, and then click on **Continue**. To print the contents, click on **OK**.

D.   Example:

(1)   Suppose the Descriptives and Frequencies programs have been run on scores for each person called jump, pullups, and run. The output from both programs is in Output Navigator.

(2)   The left pane of Output Navigator will look like this:

SPSS Output
     Descriptives
          Title
          Notes
          Descriptive Statistics
     Frequencies
          Title
          Notes
          Statistics
          Jump
          Pullups
          Run

(3) If SPSS Output in B. is clicked on, everything in B. will be highlighted and the entire output will be printed.

(4) If Descriptives in B. is clicked on, the Descriptives title and the three things under it will be highlighted and only that content will be printed.

(5) If Run which is under Frequencies in B. is clicked on, it will be highlighted and that content will be printed.

E. Situations for the Example in D

(1) If Descriptives is run, the Descriptives output is printed, and then Frequencies is run, all that needs to be printed is the Frequencies output by highlighting Frequencies in the left pane of Output Navigator.

(2) If Descriptives is run, and Frequencies is run, all of the output needs to be printed by highlighting **SPSS Output** in the left pane of Output Navigator.

F. Useful Information and Hints on Printing

(1) What is highlighted in the left pane is enclosed with a dark line box in the right pane of Output Navigator. If only part of the contents of Output Navigator is selected to be printed in the print menu, make sure Selection is highlighted as the print range.

(2) If both the Data Editor and Output Navigator are on the screen, be sure to click **File** or **Print** under Output Navigator to print the output.

(3) At the bottom of the screen both of the windows, Data Editor and Output, are shown. Click on one of them to make it the active window displayed on the screen.

(4) The content of the Output Navigator window can be eliminated by clicking on **File** for the Output Navigator window, then **Close**, and finally **No** (don't save content). This is useful when there is a lot of content no longer needed. The same thing can be accomplished by clicking on the **X** box in the upper right hand corner of the Output Navigator window.

G. If you want to print the contents of the **SPSS Data Editor** window, do steps B and C after activating the **SPSS Data Editor** window (see A and F-3).

7. Getting out of SPSS

A. To end an SPSS session, click of **File** under the **SPSS Data Editor** or **Output Navigator** and then, click on **Exit SPSS** in the drop down menu.

B. [NOTE: SPSS will ask whether you want to save the contents of the **Output Navigator** and **SPSS Data Editor** windows. If you want to save them, click on **Yes**. If not, click on **No**. Only if you want to keep the output on disk and/or you have not previously saved the data do you need to click on **Yes**.]

8. Retrieving data saved on disk (Data entered using **SPSS for Windows**)

A. If just getting into SPSS, see 1-D-(3).

B. If opening a saved data file, from the **SPSS Data Editor** menu click on **File** and then on **Open.**

C. Click on the drive **a:** or the drive to use from the **Look in:** dialog box and then click on **SPSS(*.sav)** in the **Files of type** list. You can click on a file from the list to use it or you can type in a filename. Then click on **Open.**

D. The retrieved data file is displayed on the screen.

9. Importing and exporting data

    A.   Importing data is using data not entered in SPSS (e.g. a word processing program).

    B.   Exporting data is using data entered in SPSS in some other program (e.g. Excel).

    C.   A file format must be selected when importing or exporting data. The file format can be either fixed field or free field. With fixed field the scores must be kept in specified columns and decimal points do not have to be entered whereas with free field the scores only have to be separated by one blank space and decimal points must be entered.

    D.   [NOTE: For more detailed procedures on importing and exporting data, see the SPSS Base 10.0 Brief Guide in Reference below.]

Reference

SPSS (1999). *SPSS Base 10.0 Applications Guide.* Chicago: SPSS Inc.

SPSS (2000). *SPSS 10.0 Brief Guide.* Chicago: SPSS Inc.

Norusis, M. J. (2000). *SPSS 10.0 Guide to Data Analysis.* Upper Saddle River, N.J.: Prentice-Hall.

Acknowledgment

Instructions for using SPSS were developed for earlier versions of SPSS by Suhak Oh and Ted Baumgartner. This document is an edited version of these instructions for SPSS 10.0 by Ted Baumgartner

SPSS 10.0 for Windows Statistical Procedures

Table of Contents for the SPSS 10.0 Programs Described in this Document

14. Percentile Ranks

15. Standard Scores (z-scores)

16. Transformation

17. Histograms

18. Line Chart (similar to frequency polygon)

19. Scatterplot

NOTE, click on **Analyze** or **Graphs** or **Transform** under the **SPSS Data Editor** menu and all of the sub-headings for it will be displayed. Click on one of the sub-headings and all of procedures under the sub-heading will be displayed.

SPSS has a **Help** feature which can be clicked on from the **SPSS for Windows** menu or any procedure menu. **Help** is excellent for learning about a statistical procedure or what to do in a procedure. To quit **Help,** click on **Cancel.**

1. Frequencies

    A. Click on **Analyze** under the **SPSS Data Editor** menu. Click on **Descriptive Statistics.** Click on **Frequencies** which opens the **Frequencies** dialog box.

    B. Click on one or more variables from the left variable box. The variable(s) is highlighted. Click on the arrow button and the variable(s) will show in the Variables box. By default, frequency tables are displayed with the data listed in ascending order (small to large). If small score is a good score, the data should be displayed in descending order. Click on **Format,** then on **Descending** (value), and finally click on **Continue** when through.

    C. To get optional descriptive and summary statistics, click on **Statistics** in the **Frequencies** dialog box. Click on the statistics desired. The **median** statistic is not provided by the Descriptives program, but is provided here. Many people use the Frequencies program to get descriptive statistics. When using Frequencies to get descriptive statistics, if you don't want frequencies for each variable, turn off the **Display Frequencies Tables** option before analyzing the data. Click on **Continue** when through.

    D. To get optional bar charts or histograms, click on **Charts** in the dialog box. Click on the charts or histograms desired in the dialog box. Click on **Continue** when through.

    E. Click on **OK** when ready to analyze the data.

2. Descriptives

    A. To get descriptive statistics, click on **Analyze** under the **SPSS Data Editor** menu. Click on **Descriptive Statistics.** Click on **Descriptives.** This opens the **Descriptives** dialog box.

    B. Click on one or more variables from the left variable box. The variable(s) is highlighted. Click on the arrow button and the variable(s) will show in the Variables box. By default, mean, standard deviation, minimum score, and maximum score will be displayed.

    C. If you want to get additional statistics, click on **Options** under the Descriptive dialog box. This opens the **Descriptives:Options** dialog box.

D. Click on one or more options from the box. [NOTE: the **median** statistic is not an option, but it can be obtained under optional statistics in the Frequencies program (see directions for Frequencies).] Click on **Continue** when through.

E. Click on **OK** when ready to analyze the data.

3. One-Sample T Test

A. Click on **Analyze** under the **SPSS Data Editor** menu. Click on **Compare Means.** Then click on **One-Samples T Test.**

B. Click on one or more variables from the left variable box to use in the analysis. The variable(s) is highlighted. Click on the arrow button to put the variables in the **Test Variable(s)** box. Click on the value in **Test Value** and enter a number which is the value of the mean against which the variable is tested (the hypothesized population mean).

C. By default, the confidence interval is 95%. If you want to change this value, click on **Options** in the dialog box then type the numeric value for the confidence interval. Click on **Continue** when through.

D. Click on **OK** when ready to analyze the data.

E. The mean is provided automatically in the analysis output.

4. Independent-Samples T Test (2 independent groups)

A. Click on **Analyze** under the **SPSS Data Editor** menu. Click on **Compare Means.** Click on **Independent-Samples T Test.**

B. Click on one or more variables from the left variable box to use in the analysis. The variable(s) is highlighted. Click on the arrow button to put the variable(s) in the **Test Variable(s)** box.

C. Click on a variable to form the two groups and then click on the arrow button for **Grouping Variable.**

D. You must define a value of the grouping variable for each groups. To define groups, click on **Define Groups.** Enter a value of the **Grouping Variable** which identified (is the code for) **Group 1.** Click on **Group 2** and enter a value for the grouping variable. Click on **Continue** when through.

E. By default, the confidence interval is 95% (alpha = .05). Click on **Options** to change it (see 3-C).

F. Click on **OK** when ready to analyze the data. Landscape print is suggested.

G. The means for the groups are provided automatically in the analysis output.

5. Paired-Samples T Test (dependent groups and repeated measures)

A. Click on **Analyze** under the **SPSS Data Editor** menu. Click on **Compare Means.** Click on **Paired-Samples T Test**.

B. Click on (highlight) one of the variables from the left variable box and click on the arrow button. It appears as **Variable 1** under **Current Selections.** Click on another variable from the left variable box and click on the arrow button to move the pair to the **Paired Variables:** dialog box. Other pairs can be entered.

C. To change the confidence interval, click on **Options** (see 3-C).

D. Click on **OK** when ready to analyze the data. Landscape print is suggested.

E. The means for the repeated measures are provided automatically in the analysis output.

6. One-Way ANOVA

   A. Click on **Analyze** under the **SPSS Data Editor** menu. Click on **Compare Means.** Click on **One-Way ANOVA.**

   B. Click on (highlight) one or more variables from the left variable box to test (analyze). Click on the arrow button to put the variable(s) in the **Dependent List:** box.

   C. Click on a variable for forming groups and click on the arrow button to put it in the **Factor** box.

   D. Click on **Options, Descriptive,** and any other options desired. You *must* select descriptive statistics like the mean and standard deviation for each group. When through click on **Continue.**

   E. If you want post hoc tests, click on **Post Hoc** and click on one of the 18 tests. When through, click on **Continue**.

   F. Click on **OK** when ready to analyze the data.

7. Two-Way Factorial ANOVA (and other ANOVAs)

   A. Click on **Analyze** under the **SPSS Data Editor** menu. Click on **General Linear Model.** Click on **Univariate**.

   B. On the left side, the variables available in the data set are listed in a box.

   C. On the right side are: Dependent Variable, Fixed Factors, Random Factors, and Covariance boxes.

   D. Put the variable to be the data analyzed in the Dependent Variable box.

   E. Put the variables for the rows and columns in the Fixed Factors box.

   F. Example: If the variables in the data set are named Row, Column, and Score, put Score in the Dependent Variable box, and Row and Column in the Fixed Factors box.

   G. Click on **Options** to get the means for rows, columns, and cells.

       (1) On the left side, in the Factors box, are listed Overall, the name of the row variable, the name of the column variable, and the name of the row x column interaction.

       (2) On the right side is the Display Means box.

       (3) Put everything from the Factors box into the Display Means box.

       (4) Click on **Continue** to return to the GLM-General Factorial Menu.

   H. Also, post hoc tests, effect size, observed power, etc. are available in Options. If post hoc tests are selected, it must be identified whether the post hoc tests are for rows, columns, or both.

   I. Click on **OK** to analyze the data.

8. One-Way Chi-Square

   A. Click on **Analyze** under the **SPSS Data Editor** menu. Click on **Nonparametric Tests.** Click on **Chi-Square.** This opens the **Chi-Square Test** dialog box.

   B. Click on (highlight) a variable from the left variable box and then click on the arrow button to put it in the **Test Variable List.** Do this for each variable to be analyzed.

   C. Under **Expected Range** the **Get from Data** should already be selected (marked; the default). If it is not selected, click on it.

   D. Under **Expected Values, All Categories Equal** will be marked (the default). If you do not want all categories equal, click on **Values** and enter an expected value for each category by typing in a value and then clicking on **Add.** The expected values are used with all the variables in the **Test Variable List.**

E. Click on **Options** and then click on **Descriptives** in the dialog box. When through selecting values you want, click on **Continue.**

F. Click on **OK** when ready to analyze the data. If the output is more than five columns, landscape print is suggested.

9. Two-Way Chi-Square

A. Click on **Analyze** under the **SPSS Data Editor** menus. Click on **Descriptive Statistics.** Click on **Crosstabs.** This opens the Crosstabs dialog box.

B. Click on (highlight) the variables in the left variable box you want to use as the row and column variables. Click on a variable to highlight it and then click on the arrow button for **Row(s)** or for **Column(s).**

C. Click on **Statistics** in the **Crosstabs** dialog box. Click on Chi-square, Contingency coefficient, Correlation, and anything else you want. When through, click on **Continue.**

D. Click on **Cell** in the **Crosstabs** dialog box. Click on **Observed, Expected,** and all three options under **Percentages**. When through, click on **Continue.**

E. Click on **OK** when ready to analyze the data.

10. Correlation

A. Click on **Analyze** under the **SPSS Data Editor** menu. Click on **Correlate.** Click on **Bivariate.**

B. Click on (highlight) two or more variables from the left variable box in the **Bivariate Correlations** dialog box. Click on the arrow button and the variable(s) will show in the **Variables** box.

C. Click on one or more of the correlation coefficients in the box (usually Pearson).

D. If you want a significance test, click on the type of significance test: **One-tailed** or **Two-tailed** (usually two-tailed).

E. Click on **OK** when ready to analyze the data.

11. Linear Regression

A. Click on **Analyze** under the **SPSS Data Editor** menu. Click on **Regression.** Click on **Linear.**

B. Click on (highlight) a variable from the left variable box for the dependent score (the Y-score). Click on the arrow button to put the variable in the **Dependent** box. Click on (highlight) a variable(s) from the left variable box for the independent variable (the X-score(s)). Click on the arrow button to put the variable(s) in the **Independent** box.

C. Click on one of the regression models (usually **Enter**).

D. Click on **OK** when ready to analyze the data.

12. Reliability Analysis

A. This analysis is in the SPSS standard version but not in the SPSS student version. See SPSS Base 10.0 Applications Guide, chapter 17.

B. Click on **Analyze** under the **SPSS Data Editor** menu. Click on **Scale**. Click on **Reliability Analysis.**

C. Click on (highlight) a variable from the left variable box and then click on the arrow button to put it in the **Items:** box. Do this for at least two variables. These are the repeated measure like trials or days.

D. The **Model:** box should have **Alpha** in it. If it does not, click on the down arrow in **Model:** and click on **Alpha**.

E. Click on **Statistics** in the **Reliability Analysis** dialog box. Click on **Item** under **Descriptives** to get item means and **F Test** under **ANOVA Table** to get the ANOVA summary table.

F. Also, in **Statistics,** click on **Intraclass Correlation Coefficient.** Set Model to One-Way or Two-Way Mixed depending on which ANOVA model is desired. **Confidence Interval** and **Test Value** can be changed but usually the default values are used. Click on **Continue** when through.

G. Click on **OK** when ready to analyze the data.

13. Percentiles

A. Analyze the data using the Frequencies procedure (see number 1 in this document). Click on **Analyze.** Click on **Descriptive Statistics.** Click on **Frequencies**.

B. After getting into **Frequencies,** making sure that the scores are listed from worst to best (ascending order if large score is good). If frequency tables are not desired, click on **Display Frequency Tables** to eliminate that option.

C. Click on **Statistics** and then on **Percentile(s):.**

D. The percentiles desired must be indicated by typing a number between 0 and 100 into the percentile box and then clicking on **Add.** Do this for each percentile desired. After indicating the percentiles desired, click on **Continue** to get out of **Statistics.**

Example: if the percentiles 5th, 10th , 15th, …, 100th are desired

Percentile Box	Add
5	click
10	click
•	•
•	•

E. The default for **Cut Points,** which is an alternative to typing in percentiles, is 10 equal groups yielding the 10th , 20th, etc. percentiles.

F. Click on **OK** when ready to analyze the data.

14. Percentile Ranks

A. Analyze the data using the **Frequencies** procedure (see number 1 in this document). Click on **Analyze**. Click on **Descriptive Statistics.** Click on **Frequencies**.

B. After getting into **Frequencies**, make sure that the scores are listed from worst to best (ascending order if large score is good).

C.   The output from the analysis will look like this example.

Value	Frequency	Percent	Valid Percent	Cum. Percent
15	4	20	20	20
16	6	30	30	50
17	8	40	40	90
19	2	10	10	100
	20	100	100	

D.   Calculate percentile ranks for a score (Value) by the formula:

$$PR = (\text{Cum. Percent above the score}) + (.5) (\text{Percent for the score})$$

$$PR \text{ for score} = 15: PR = 0 + (.5) (20) = 10$$

$$PR \text{ for score} = 16: PR = 20 + (.5) (30) = 35$$

15. Standard Scores (z-scores)

A.   See the SPSS 10.0 manuals for more information.

B.   A z-score for each variable analyzed is calculated assuming a large score is good whether or not the data is listed in ascending or descending order. If a small score is good, the sign of the z-score is reversed (e.g. –2.0 should be 2.0).

C.   Analyze the data using the **Descriptives** procedure (see number 2 in this document) by clicking on **Analyze**, then **Descriptive Statistics,** and finally **Descriptives**.

D.   Click on **Save standardized values as variables** in the **Descriptives** dialog box. Highlight the variables you want z-scores for in the left hand box. Click the arrow to move the variables into the right hand box. Click on **OK** when ready to analyze the data. The z-scores are calculated, and added to the file containing the original data. A message does appear in the output that this occurred. The names of the z-scores will be the names of the original data with a z in front of them (e.g. for the original variable CAT the z-score is ZCAT). Z-score can be seen by displaying the data file on the screen and printing it if desired. The data file must be saved again for the z-scores to be saved with the data. In most cases, saving the z-scores is not necessary. If saving the z-scores, it might be good to save them as a new file so the original data file is retained as one file, and the original data with z-scores are another file. When saving the z-scores use **Save As.**

E.   Sum of the z-scores can be obtained by using the Transformation procedure (presented in this document) and writing the formula for obtaining the sum of the z-scores allowing for the fact that some z-scores have the wrong sign (z-scores for scores when small score is good will have the wrong sign.) For example, if the original data were X1, X2, and X3 the z-scores are ZX1, ZX2, and ZX3, and if ZSUM is the name used for the sum of the z-scores:

$$ZSUM = ZX1 + ZX2 - ZX3 \text{ (for X3, small score is good)}$$

16. Transformation

A.   See the SPSS Base 10.0 Brief Guide, chapter 12 for more information.

B. Many things can be done with transformations such as changing the values of variables, grouping variables, creating new variables, etc. First, creating a new variable is presented. Then other examples are presented.

C. Click on **Transform** and then **Compute.** In the **Compute Variable** dialog box the name of the variable to be computed is typed in the **Target Variable:** box and the numeric expression or equation for calculating the target variable is typed in the **Numeric Expression:** box. Click on **OK** when ready to do the analysis. The computed variable is displayed on the screen and saved with the original data.

D. Example 1, creating a new variable: There are 3 scores named X1, X2 and X3 on each person and for all three scores a large score is good.

    (1) The sum (to be named SUMX) of the 3 scores is desired.
        Target Variable: SUMX
        Numerical Expression: X1 + X2 + X3

    (2) The data have already been analyzed calculating z-scores for each score (see Standard Score in this document). These z-scores are named ZX1, ZX2, and ZX3. The sum of the z-scores (to be named ZSUM) is desired.
        Target Variable: ZSUM
        Numerical Expression: ZX1 + ZX2 + ZX3
        [NOTE: The target variable is added to the file containing the original data (and z-scores in the case of ZSUM). The data file must be saved again for the target variable to be saved with the rest of the file (see 15-D for save procedures).]

E. Example 2, creating new variables by computing and by recoding: Each person has an X, Y, and ZZ score. X score values are from 1 to 10; Y score values are from 0 to 3; and ZZ score values are from 10 to 29.

    (1) Analysis 1: Calculate a new score for each person (Ratio) where Ratio = X/Y.
        (a) Click on **Transform** and then on **Compute**
        (b) Fill the Boxes:
            1. Target Variable Box: type in Ratio (name of new score)
            2. Numeric Expression Box: click on the box and type in X/Y or highlight X, click on the right arrow to put it in the box, click on /, highlight Y, and click on the right arrow to put it in the box.
            3. Click on **OK**
        (c) The new score (Ratio) is added to the data file as the last score for each person so now each person has an X, Y, ZZ, and Ratio score.
        (d) [NOTE: (1) When Y is zero, Ratio = X/Y will be set to missing value (period)(.) since division by zero is undefined; (2) The Ratio score is not saved on the data disk at this time. If Ratio should be saved, save the file (File, Save) or save the file with a new name (File, Save As) to preserve the original data file. If multiple transformations are to be done, saving could be done after doing all the transformations.]

    (2) Analysis 2: Calculate a new score for each person (Newz) using the ZZ scores and the Recode option as follows: (1) if ZZ = 10-14, Newz = 1; (2) if ZZ = 15-19, Newz = 2; (3) if ZZ = 20-24, Newz = 3, and if ZZ = 25-29, Newz = 4.
        (a) Click on **Transform** and then on **Recode.**
        (b) Click on **Into Different Variable.**

(c) Fill the Boxes:
    1. Numeric Variable Box: click on ZZ (the variable recoded), and click on the right arrow to put it in the box.
    2. Output Variable Box: click on it, and type in Newz (the name of the new variable)

(d) Click on **Old** and **New Values**
    1. Under Old Value, click on **Range**, enter 10, tab or click to the **Through Box,** and enter 14
    2. Under New Value, click on **Value** and enter 1
    3. Click on **Add**
    4. Do this for each variable change

ZZ	Newz
15-19	2
20-24	3
25-29	4

    5. Click on **Continue**
    6. Click on **Change**
    7. Click on **OK**

(e) The new score (Newz) is added to the data file as the last score for each person.

(f) [NOTE: The Newz score is not saved on the data disk at this time. Save it if necessary.]

17. Histogram

  A. See the Help feature for more information.
  B. Click on **Graphs**, and then on **Histogram.**
  C. In the **Histogram** dialog box, click on (highlight) a variable from the left variable box and then click on the arrow button so the variable is listed under the **Variable:** box. Note a variable can be removed from the **Variable:** box by clicking on it and then on the arrow button.
  D. If the default format for histogram is acceptable, click on **OK** to obtain the graph. The histogram is displayed in the **SPSS Viewer.** If you want to display the normal curve with the histogram, click on **Display normal curve** before clicking on **OK.** A normal curve will be superimposed over the histogram.
  E. [NOTE: Double click on a graph in the **SPSS Viewer** to bring it in the **SPSS Chart Editor.** Double clicking on a graph created from interactive graphics activates the chart manager. The **SPSS Chart Editor** on the chart manager can be used to edit the chart.]
  F. By default the histogram has bars showing the data divided into about 10 evenly spaced intervals. Usually 10-20 intervals are used with continuous data putting 2-5 different scores in an interval (e.g. 15-17 is interval size = 3). The base intervals of the histogram in the **SPSS Chart Editor** can be changed.

18. Line Chart (similar to frequency polygon)

  A. See the Help feature for more information.
  B. Click on **Graphs** and then on **Line.**

C.   In the Line Charts dialog box click on **Simple** line chart and **Summaries for Groups of Cases.** Then click on **Define**, click on (highlight) the variable from the left variable box to use, click on the arrow button to put the highlighted variable in the **Category Axis:** box, and click on **N of cases.** Click on **OK** when ready to obtain the graph. The line chart is displayed in the **SPSS Viewer** (see Histogram for details on the editing chart).

D.   By default the line chart has the data divided into about 15 intervals for the X-axis. Usually 10-20 labels (intervals) are used with continuous data putting 2-5 different score values in an interval (e.g., 15-17 is interval size = 3). The labels (intervals) for the X-axis can be altered.

19. Scatterplot

A.   See the Help feature for more information.

B.   Click on **Graphs**, then **Scatter,** and then **Simple** in the **Scatterplot** dialog box.

C.   Now click on **Define.** Click on (highlight) a variable from the left variable box and then click on the arrow button to put it in the **X Axis:** box. Do the same thing for a second variable to put it in the **Y Axis:** box.

D.   Click on **OK** when ready to obtain the graph.

E.   The scatterplot is displayed in the **SPSS Viewer** (see Histogram for details on the editing charts).

Acknowledgment

Instructions for using SPSS were developed for earlier versions of SPSS by Suhak Oh and Ted Baumgartner. This document is an edited version of these instructions for SPSS 10.0 by Ted Baumgartner.

Appendix B

	LEVEL OF SIGNIFICANCE FOR ONE-TAILED TEST					
	.10	.05	.025	.01	.005	.0005
	LEVEL OF SIGNIFICANCE FOR TWO-TAILED TEST					
df	.20	.10	.05	.02	.01	.001
1	3.078	6.314	12.706	31.821	63.657	636.619
2	1.886	2.920	4.303	6.965	9.925	31.598
3	1.638	2.353	3.182	4.541	5.841	12.941
4	1.533	2.132	2.776	3.747	4.604	8.610
5	1.476	2.015	2.571	3.365	4.032	6.859
6	1.440	1.943	2.447	3.143	3.707	5.959
7	1.415	1.895	2.365	2.998	3.499	5.405
8	1.397	1.860	2.306	2.896	3.355	5.041
9	1.383	1.833	2.262	2.821	3.250	4.781
10	1.372	1.812	2.228	2.764	3.169	4.587
11	1.363	1.796	2.201	2.718	3.106	4.437
12	1.356	1.782	2.179	2.681	3.055	4.318
13	1.350	1.771	2.160	2.650	3.012	4.221
14	1.345	1.761	2.145	2.624	2.977	4.140
15	1.341	1.753	2.131	2.602	2.947	4.073
16	1.337	1.746	2.120	2.583	2.921	4.015
17	1.333	1.740	2.110	2.567	2.898	3.965
18	1.330	1.734	2.101	2.552	2.878	3.922
19	1.328	1.729	2.093	2.539	2.861	3.883
20	1.325	1.725	2.086	2.528	2.845	3.850
21	1.323	1.721	2.080	2.518	2.831	3.819
22	1.321	1.717	2.074	2.508	2.819	3.792
23	1.319	1.714	2.069	2.500	2.807	3.767
24	1.318	1.711	2.064	2.492	2.797	3.745
25	1.316	1.708	2.060	2.485	2.787	3.725

Critical Values of *t*—Concluded

	LEVEL OF SIGNIFICANCE FOR ONE-TAILED TEST					
	.10	.05	.025	.01	.005	.0005
	LEVEL OF SIGNIFICANCE FOR TWO-TAILED TEST					
DF	.20	.10	.05	.02	.01	.001
26	1.315	1.706	2.056	2.479	2.779	3.707
27	1.314	1.703	2.052	2.473	2.771	3.690
28	1.313	1.701	2.048	2.467	2.763	3.674
29	1.311	1.699	2.045	2.462	2.756	3.659
30	1.310	1.697	2.042	2.457	2.750	3.646
40	1.303	1.684	2.021	2.423	2.704	3.551
60	1.296	1.671	2.000	2.390	2.660	3.460
120	1.289	1.658	1.980	2.358	2.617	3.373
∞	1.282	1.645	1.960	2.326	2.576	3.291

Appendix A is taken from Table III of Fisher & Yates; STATISTICAL TABLES FOR BIOLOGICAL, AGRICULTURAL AND MEDICAL RESEARCH Published by Longman Group UK Ltd., 1974. Reprinted by permission of Addison Wesley Longman Ltd.

Appendix C

DEGREES OF FREEDOM FOR DENOMINATOR	DEGREES OF FREEDOM FOR NUMERATOR											
	1	2	3	4	5	6	7	8	9	10	11	12
1	161	200	216	225	230	234	237	239	241	242	243	244
	4052	**4999**	**5403**	**5625**	**5764**	**5859**	**5928**	**5981**	**6022**	**6056**	**6082**	**6106**
2	18.51	19.00	19.16	19.25	19.30	19.33	19.36	19.37	19.38	19.39	19.40	19.41
	98.49	**99.01**	**99.17**	**99.25**	**99.30**	**99.33**	**99.34**	**99.36**	**99.38**	**99.40**	**99.41**	**99.42**
3	10.13	9.55	9.28	9.12	9.01	8.94	8.88	8.84	8.81	8.78	8.76	8.74
	34.12	**30.81**	**29.46**	**28.71**	**28.24**	**27.91**	**27.67**	**27.49**	**27.34**	**27.23**	**27.13**	**27.05**
4	7.71	6.94	6.59	6.39	6.26	6.16	6.09	6.04	6.00	5.96	5.93	5.91
	21.20	**18.00**	**16.69**	**15.98**	**15.52**	**15.21**	**14.98**	**14.80**	**14.66**	**14.54**	**14.45**	**14.37**
5	6.61	5.79	5.41	5.19	5.05	4.95	4.88	4.82	4.78	4.74	4.70	4.68
	16.26	**13.27**	**12.06**	**11.39**	**10.97**	**10.67**	**10.45**	**10.27**	**10.15**	**10.05**	**9.96**	**9.89**
6	5.99	5.14	4.76	4.53	4.39	4.28	4.21	4.15	4.10	4.06	4.03	4.00
	13.74	**10.92**	**9.78**	**9.15**	**8.75**	**8.47**	**8.26**	**8.10**	**7.98**	**7.87**	**7.79**	**7.72**
7	5.59	4.74	4.35	4.12	3.97	3.87	3.79	3.73	3.68	3.63	3.60	3.57
	12.25	**9.55**	**8.45**	**7.85**	**7.46**	**7.19**	**7.00**	**6.84**	**6.71**	**6.62**	**6.54**	**6.47**
8	5.32	4.46	4.07	3.84	3.69	3.58	3.50	3.44	3.39	3.34	3.31	3.28
	11.26	**8.65**	**7.59**	**7.01**	**6.63**	**6.37**	**6.19**	**6.03**	**5.91**	**5.82**	**5.74**	**5.67**
9	5.12	4.26	3.86	3.63	3.48	3.37	3.29	3.23	3.18	3.13	3.10	3.07
	10.56	**8.02**	**6.99**	**6.42**	**6.06**	**5.80**	**5.62**	**5.47**	**5.35**	**5.26**	**5.18**	**5.11**
10	4.96	4.10	3.71	3.48	3.33	3.22	3.14	3.07	3.02	2.97	2.94	2.91
	10.04	**7.56**	**6.55**	**5.99**	**5.64**	**5.39**	**5.21**	**5.06**	**4.95**	**4.85**	**4.78**	**4.71**
11	4.84	3.98	3.59	3.36	3.20	3.09	3.01	2.95	2.90	2.86	2.82	2.79
	9.65	**7.20**	**6.22**	**5.67**	**5.32**	**5.07**	**4.88**	**4.74**	**4.63**	**4.54**	**4.46**	**4.40**
12	4.75	3.88	3.49	3.26	3.11	3.00	2.92	2.85	2.80	2.76	2.72	2.69
	9.33	**6.93**	**5.95**	**5.41**	**5.06**	**4.82**	**4.65**	**4.50**	**4.39**	**4.30**	**4.22**	**4.16**
13	4.67	3.80	3.41	3.18	3.02	2.92	2.84	2.77	2.72	2.67	2.63	2.60
	9.07	**6.70**	**5.74**	**5.20**	**4.86**	**4.62**	**4.44**	**4.30**	**4.19**	**4.10**	**4.02**	**3.96**
14	4.60	3.74	3.34	3.11	2.96	2.85	2.77	2.70	2.65	2.60	2.56	2.53
	8.86	**6.51**	**5.56**	**5.03**	**4.69**	**4.46**	**4.28**	**4.14**	**4.03**	**3.94**	**3.86**	**3.80**

From G. W. Snedecor and W. G. Cochran, *Statistical Methods,* 7th edition, Table of Critical Values of *F,* 1980. Copyright © 1980 Iowa State University Press, Ames, Iowa. Reprinted by permission.

14	16	20	24	30	40	50	75	100	200	500	∞
245	246	248	249	250	251	252	253	253	254	254	254
6142	**6169**	**6208**	**6234**	**6258**	**6286**	**6302**	**6323**	**6334**	**6352**	**6361**	**6366**
19.42	19.43	19.44	19.45	19.46	19.47	19.47	19.48	19.49	19.49	19.50	19.50
99.43	**99.44**	**99.45**	**99.46**	**99.47**	**99.48**	**99.48**	**99.49**	**99.49**	**99.49**	**99.50**	**99.50**
8.71	8.69	8.66	8.64	8.62	8.60	8.58	8.57	8.56	8.54	8.54	8.53
26.92	**26.83**	**26.69**	**26.60**	**26.50**	**26.41**	**26.35**	**26.27**	**26.23**	**26.18**	**26.14**	**26.12**
5.87	5.84	5.80	5.77	5.74	5.71	5.70	5.68	5.66	5.65	5.64	5.63
14.24	**14.15**	**14.02**	**13.93**	**13.83**	**13.74**	**13.69**	**13.61**	**13.57**	**13.52**	**13.48**	**13.46**
4.64	4.60	4.56	4.53	4.50	4.46	4.44	4.42	4.40	4.38	4.37	4.36
9.77	**9.68**	**9.55**	**9.47**	**9.38**	**9.29**	**9.24**	**9.17**	**9.13**	**9.07**	**9.04**	**9.02**
3.96	3.92	3.87	3.84	3.81	3.77	3.75	3.72	3.71	3.69	3.68	3.67
7.60	**7.52**	**7.39**	**7.31**	**7.23**	**7.14**	**7.09**	**7.02**	**6.99**	**6.94**	**6.90**	**6.88**
3.52	3.49	3.44	3.41	3.38	3.34	3.32	3.29	3.28	3.25	3.24	3.23
6.35	**6.27**	**6.15**	**6.07**	**5.98**	**5.90**	**5.85**	**5.78**	**5.75**	**5.70**	**5.67**	**5.65**
3.23	3.20	3.15	3.12	3.08	3.05	3.03	3.00	2.98	2.96	2.94	2.93
5.56	**5.48**	**5.36**	**5.28**	**5.20**	**5.11**	**5.06**	**5.00**	**4.96**	**4.91**	**4.88**	**4.88**
3.02	2.98	2.93	2.90	2.86	2.82	2.80	2.77	2.76	2.73	2.72	2.71
5.00	**4.92**	**4.80**	**4.73**	**4.64**	**4.56**	**4.51**	**4.45**	**4.41**	**4.36**	**4.33**	**4.31**
2.86	2.82	2.77	2.74	2.70	2.67	2.64	2.61	2.59	2.56	2.55	2.54
4.60	**4.52**	**4.41**	**4.33**	**4.25**	**4.17**	**4.12**	**4.05**	**4.01**	**3.96**	**3.93**	**3.91**
2.74	2.70	2.65	2.61	2.57	2.53	2.50	2.47	2.45	2.42	2.41	2.40
4.29	**4.21**	**4.10**	**4.02**	**3.94**	**3.86**	**3.80**	**3.74**	**3.70**	**3.66**	**3.62**	**3.60**
2.64	2.60	2.54	2.50	2.46	2.42	2.40	2.36	2.35	2.32	2.31	2.30
4.05	**3.98**	**3.86**	**3.78**	**3.70**	**3.61**	**3.56**	**3.49**	**3.46**	**3.41**	**3.38**	**3.36**
2.55	2.51	2.46	2.42	2.38	2.34	2.32	2.28	2.26	2.24	2.22	2.21
3.85	**3.78**	**3.67**	**3.59**	**3.51**	**3.42**	**3.37**	**3.30**	**3.27**	**3.21**	**3.18**	**3.16**
2.48	2.44	2.39	2.35	2.31	2.27	2.24	2.21	2.19	2.16	2.14	2.13
3.70	**3.62**	**3.51**	**3.43**	**3.34**	**3.26**	**3.21**	**3.14**	**3.11**	**3.06**	**3.02**	**3.00**

Critical Values of *F*—*Continued*

DEGREES OF FREEDOM FOR DENOMINATOR					DEGREES OF FREEDOM FOR NUMERATOR							
	1	2	3	4	5	6	7	8	9	10	11	12
15	4.54	3.68	3.29	3.06	2.90	2.79	2.70	2.64	2.59	2.55	2.51	2.48
	8.68	6.36	5.42	4.89	4.56	4.32	4.14	4.00	3.89	3.80	3.73	3.67
16	4.49	3.63	3.24	3.01	2.85	2.74	2.66	2.59	2.54	2.49	2.45	2.42
	8.53	6.23	5.29	4.77	4.44	4.20	4.03	3.89	3.78	3.69	3.61	3.55
17	4.45	3.59	3.20	2.96	2.81	2.70	2.62	2.55	2.50	2.45	2.41	2.38
	8.40	6.11	5.18	4.67	4.34	4.10	3.93	3.79	3.68	3.59	3.52	3.45
18	4.41	3.55	3.16	2.93	2.77	2.66	2.58	2.51	2.46	2.41	2.37	2.34
	8.28	6.01	5.09	4.58	4.25	4.01	3.88	3.71	3.60	3.51	3.44	3.37
19	4.38	3.52	3.13	2.90	2.74	2.63	2.55	2.48	2.43	2.38	2.34	2.31
	8.18	5.93	5.01	4.50	4.17	3.94	3.77	3.63	3.52	3.43	3.36	3.30
20	4.35	3.49	3.10	2.87	2.71	2.60	2.52	2.45	2.40	2.35	2.31	2.28
	8.10	5.85	4.94	4.43	4.10	3.87	3.71	3.56	3.45	3.37	3.30	3.23
21	4.32	3.47	3.07	2.84	2.68	2.57	2.49	2.42	2.37	2.32	2.28	2.25
	8.02	5.78	4.87	4.37	4.04	3.81	3.65	3.51	3.40	3.31	3.24	3.17
22	4.30	3.44	3.05	2.82	2.66	2.55	2.47	2.40	2.35	2.30	2.26	2.23
	7.94	5.72	4.82	4.31	3.99	3.76	3.59	3.45	3.35	3.26	3.18	3.12
23	4.28	3.42	3.03	2.80	2.64	2.53	2.45	2.38	2.32	2.28	2.24	2.20
	7.88	5.66	4.76	4.26	3.94	3.71	3.54	3.41	3.30	3.21	3.14	3.07
24	4.26	3.40	3.01	2.78	2.62	2.51	2.43	2.36	2.30	2.26	2.22	2.18
	7.82	5.61	4.72	4.22	3.90	3.67	3.50	3.36	3.25	3.17	3.09	3.03
25	4.24	3.38	2.99	2.76	2.60	2.49	2.41	2.34	2.28	2.24	2.20	2.16
	7.77	5.57	4.68	4.18	3.86	3.63	3.46	3.32	3.21	3.13	3.05	2.99
26	4.22	3.37	2.98	2.74	2.59	2.47	2.39	2.32	2.27	2.22	2.18	2.15
	7.72	5.53	4.64	4.14	3.82	3.59	3.42	3.29	3.17	3.09	3.02	2.96
27	4.21	3.35	2.96	2.73	2.57	2.46	2.37	2.30	2.25	2.20	2.16	2.13
	7.68	5.49	4.60	4.11	3.79	3.56	3.39	3.26	3.14	3.06	2.98	2.93
28	4.20	3.34	2.95	2.71	2.56	2.44	2.36	2.29	2.24	2.19	2.15	2.12
	7.64	5.45	4.57	4.07	3.76	3.53	3.36	3.23	3.11	3.03	2.95	2.90
29	4.18	3.33	2.93	2.70	2.54	2.43	2.35	2.28	2.22	2.18	2.14	2.10
	7.60	5.42	4.54	4.04	3.73	3.50	3.33	3.20	3.08	3.00	2.92	2.87
30	4.17	3.32	2.92	2.69	2.53	2.42	2.34	2.27	2.21	2.16	2.12	2.09
	7.56	5.39	4.51	4.02	3.70	3.47	3.30	3.17	3.06	2.98	2.90	2.84
32	4.15	3.30	2.90	2.67	2.51	2.40	2.32	2.25	2.19	2.14	2.10	2.07
	7.50	5.34	4.46	3.97	3.66	3.42	3.25	3.12	3.01	2.94	2.86	2.80
34	4.13	3.28	2.88	2.65	2.49	2.38	2.30	2.23	2.17	2.12	2.08	2.05
	7.44	5.29	4.42	3.93	3.61	3.38	3.21	3.08	2.97	2.89	2.82	2.76
36	4.11	3.26	2.86	2.63	2.48	2.36	2.28	2.21	2.15	2.10	2.06	2.03
	7.39	5.25	4.38	3.89	3.58	3.35	3.18	3.04	2.94	2.86	2.78	2.72

14	16	20	24	30	40	50	75	100	200	500	∞
2.43	2.39	2.33	2.29	2.25	2.21	2.18	2.15	2.12	2.10	2.08	2.07
3.56	**3.48**	**3.36**	**3.29**	**3.20**	**3.12**	**3.07**	**3.00**	**2.97**	**2.92**	**2.89**	**2.87**
2.37	2.33	2.28	2.24	2.20	2.16	2.13	2.09	2.07	2.04	2.02	2.01
3.45	**3.37**	**3.25**	**3.18**	**3.10**	**3.01**	**2.96**	**2.89**	**2.86**	**2.80**	**2.77**	**3.75**
2.33	2.29	2.23	2.19	2.15	2.11	2.08	2.04	2.02	1.99	1.97	1.96
3.35	**3.27**	**3.16**	**3.08**	**3.00**	**2.92**	**2.86**	**2.79**	**2.76**	**2.70**	**2.67**	**2.65**
2.29	2.25	2.19	2.15	2.11	2.07	2.04	2.00	1.98	1.95	1.93	1.92
3.27	**3.19**	**3.07**	**3.00**	**2.91**	**2.83**	**2.78**	**2.71**	**2.68**	**2.62**	**2.59**	**2.57**
2.26	2.21	2.15	2.11	2.07	2.02	2.00	1.96	1.94	1.91	1.90	1.88
3.19	**3.12**	**3.00**	**2.92**	**2.84**	**2.76**	**2.70**	**2.63**	**2.60**	**2.54**	**2.51**	**2.49**
2.23	2.18	2.12	2.08	2.04	1.99	1.96	1.92	1.90	1.87	1.85	1.84
3.13	**3.05**	**2.94**	**2.86**	**2.77**	**2.69**	**2.63**	**2.56**	**2.53**	**2.47**	**2.44**	**2.42**
2.20	2.15	2.09	2.05	2.00	1.96	1.93	1.89	1.87	1.84	1.82	1.81
3.07	**2.99**	**2.88**	**2.80**	**2.72**	**2.63**	**2.58**	**2.51**	**2.47**	**2.42**	**2.38**	**2.36**
2.18	2.13	2.07	2.03	1.98	1.93	1.91	1.87	1.84	1.81	1.80	1.78
3.02	**2.94**	**2.83**	**2.75**	**2.67**	**2.58**	**2.53**	**2.46**	**2.42**	**2.37**	**2.33**	**2.31**
2.14	2.10	2.04	2.00	1.96	1.91	1.88	1.84	1.82	1.79	1.77	1.76
2.97	**2.89**	**2.78**	**2.70**	**2.62**	**2.53**	**2.48**	**2.41**	**2.37**	**2.32**	**2.28**	**2.26**
2.13	2.09	2.02	1.98	1.94	1.89	1.86	1.82	1.80	1.76	1.74	1.73
2.93	**2.85**	**2.74**	**2.66**	**2.58**	**2.49**	**2.44**	**2.36**	**2.33**	**2.27**	**2.23**	**2.21**
2.11	2.06	2.00	1.96	1.92	1.87	1.84	1.80	1.77	1.74	1.72	1.71
2.89	**2.81**	**2.70**	**2.62**	**2.54**	**2.45**	**2.40**	**2.32**	**2.29**	**2.23**	**2.19**	**2.17**
2.10	2.05	1.99	1.95	1.90	1.85	1.82	1.78	1.76	1.72	1.70	1.69
2.86	**2.77**	**2.66**	**2.58**	**2.50**	**2.41**	**2.36**	**2.28**	**2.25**	**2.19**	**2.15**	**2.13**
2.08	2.03	1.97	1.93	1.88	1.84	1.80	1.76	1.74	1.71	1.68	1.67
2.83	**2.74**	**2.63**	**2.55**	**2.47**	**2.38**	**2.33**	**2.25**	**2.21**	**2.16**	**2.12**	**2.10**
2.06	2.02	1.96	1.91	1.87	1.81	1.78	1.75	1.72	1.69	1.67	1.65
2.80	**2.71**	**2.60**	**2.52**	**2.44**	**2.35**	**2.30**	**2.22**	**2.18**	**2.13**	**2.09**	**2.06**
2.05	2.00	1.94	1.90	1.85	1.80	1.77	1.73	1.71	1.68	1.65	1.64
2.77	**2.68**	**2.57**	**2.49**	**2.41**	**2.32**	**2.27**	**2.19**	**2.15**	**2.10**	**2.06**	**2.03**
2.04	1.99	1.93	1.89	1.84	1.79	1.76	1.72	1.69	1.66	1.64	1.62
2.74	**2.66**	**2.55**	**2.47**	**2.38**	**2.29**	**2.24**	**2.16**	**2.13**	**2.07**	**2.03**	**2.01**
2.02	1.97	1.91	1.86	1.82	1.76	1.74	1.69	1.67	1.64	1.61	1.59
2.70	**2.62**	**2.51**	**2.42**	**2.34**	**2.25**	**2.20**	**2.12**	**2.08**	**2.02**	**1.98**	**1.96**
2.00	1.95	1.89	1.84	1.80	1.74	1.71	1.67	1.64	1.61	1.59	1.57
2.66	**2.58**	**2.47**	**2.38**	**2.30**	**2.21**	**2.15**	**2.03**	**2.04**	**1.98**	**1.94**	**1.91**
1.98	1.93	1.87	1.82	1.78	1.72	1.69	1.65	1.62	1.59	1.56	1.55
2.62	**2.54**	**2.43**	**2.35**	**2.26**	**2.17**	**2.12**	**2.04**	**2.00**	**1.94**	**1.90**	**1.87**

Critical Values of F—Concluded

DEGREES OF FREEDOM FOR DENOMINATOR	DEGREES OF FREEDOM FOR NUMERATOR											
	1	2	3	4	5	6	7	8	9	10	11	12
38	4.10	3.25	2.85	2.62	2.46	2.35	2.26	2.19	2.14	2.09	2.05	2.02
	7.35	**5.21**	**4.34**	**3.86**	**3.54**	**3.32**	**3.15**	**3.02**	**2.91**	**2.82**	**2.75**	**2.69**
40	4.08	3.23	2.84	2.61	2.45	2.34	2.25	2.18	2.12	2.07	2.04	2.00
	7.31	**5.18**	**4.31**	**3.83**	**3.51**	**3.29**	**3.12**	**2.99**	**2.88**	**2.80**	**2.73**	**2.66**
42	4.07	3.22	2.83	2.59	2.44	2.32	2.24	2.17	2.11	2.06	2.02	1.99
	7.27	**5.15**	**4.29**	**3.80**	**3.49**	**3.26**	**3.10**	**2.96**	**2.86**	**2.77**	**2.70**	**2.64**
44	4.06	3.21	2.82	2.58	2.43	2.31	2.23	2.16	2.10	2.05	2.01	1.98
	7.24	**5.12**	**4.26**	**3.78**	**3.46**	**3.24**	**3.07**	**2.94**	**2.84**	**2.75**	**2.68**	**2.62**
46	4.05	3.20	2.81	2.57	2.42	2.30	2.22	2.14	2.09	2.04	2.00	1.97
	7.21	**5.10**	**4.24**	**3.76**	**3.44**	**3.22**	**3.05**	**2.92**	**2.82**	**2.73**	**2.66**	**2.60**
48	4.04	3.19	2.80	2.56	2.41	2.30	2.21	2.14	2.08	2.03	1.99	1.96
	7.19	**5.08**	**4.22**	**3.74**	**3.42**	**3.20**	**3.04**	**2.90**	**2.80**	**2.71**	**2.64**	**2.58**
50	4.03	3.18	2.79	2.56	2.40	2.29	2.20	2.13	2.07	2.02	1.98	1.95
	7.17	**5.06**	**4.20**	**3.72**	**3.41**	**3.18**	**3.02**	**2.88**	**2.78**	**2.70**	**2.62**	**2.56**
55	4.02	3.17	2.78	2.54	2.38	2.27	2.18	2.11	2.05	2.00	1.97	1.93
	7.12	**5.01**	**4.16**	**3.68**	**3.37**	**3.15**	**2.98**	**2.85**	**2.75**	**2.66**	**2.59**	**2.53**
60	4.00	3.15	2.76	2.52	2.37	2.25	2.17	2.10	2.04	1.99	1.95	1.92
	7.08	**4.98**	**4.13**	**3.65**	**3.34**	**3.12**	**2.95**	**2.82**	**2.72**	**2.63**	**2.56**	**2.50**
65	3.99	3.14	2.75	2.51	2.36	2.24	2.15	2.08	2.02	1.98	1.94	1.90
	7.04	**4.95**	**4.10**	**3.62**	**3.31**	**3.09**	**2.93**	**2.79**	**2.70**	**2.61**	**2.54**	**2.47**
70	3.98	3.13	2.74	2.50	2.35	2.23	2.14	2.07	2.01	1.97	1.93	1.89
	7.01	**4.92**	**4.08**	**3.60**	**3.29**	**3.07**	**2.91**	**2.77**	**2.67**	**2.59**	**2.51**	**2.45**
80	3.96	3.11	2.72	2.48	2.33	2.21	2.12	2.05	1.99	1.95	1.91	1.88
	6.96	**4.88**	**4.04**	**3.56**	**3.25**	**3.04**	**2.87**	**2.74**	**2.64**	**2.55**	**2.46**	**2.41**
100	3.94	3.09	2.70	2.46	2.30	2.19	2.10	2.03	1.97	1.92	1.88	1.85
	6.90	**4.82**	**3.98**	**3.51**	**3.20**	**2.99**	**2.82**	**2.69**	**2.59**	**2.51**	**2.43**	**2.36**
125	3.92	3.07	2.68	2.44	2.29	2.17	2.08	2.01	1.95	1.90	1.86	1.83
	6.84	**4.78**	**3.94**	**3.47**	**3.17**	**2.95**	**2.79**	**2.65**	**2.56**	**2.47**	**2.40**	**2.33**
150	3.91	3.06	2.67	2.43	2.27	2.16	2.07	2.00	1.94	1.89	1.85	1.82
	6.81	**4.75**	**3.91**	**3.44**	**3.14**	**2.92**	**2.76**	**2.62**	**2.53**	**2.44**	**2.37**	**2.30**
200	3.89	3.04	2.65	2.41	2.26	2.14	2.05	1.98	1.92	1.87	1.83	1.80
	6.76	**4.71**	**3.88**	**3.41**	**3.11**	**2.90**	**2.73**	**2.60**	**2.50**	**2.41**	**2.34**	**2.28**
400	3.86	3.02	2.62	2.39	2.23	2.12	2.03	1.96	1.90	1.85	1.81	1.78
	6.70	**4.66**	**3.83**	**3.36**	**3.06**	**2.85**	**2.69**	**2.55**	**2.46**	**2.37**	**2.29**	**2.23**
1000	3.85	3.00	2.61	2.38	2.22	2.10	2.02	1.95	1.89	1.84	1.80	1.76
	6.66	**4.62**	**3.80**	**3.34**	**3.04**	**2.82**	**2.66**	**2.53**	**2.43**	**2.34**	**2.26**	**2.20**
∞	3.84	2.99	2.60	2.37	2.21	2.09	2.01	1.94	1.88	1.83	1.79	1.75
	6.64	**4.60**	**3.78**	**3.32**	**3.02**	**2.80**	**2.64**	**2.51**	**2.41**	**2.32**	**2.24**	**2.18**

14	16	20	24	30	40	50	75	100	200	500	∞
1.96	1.92	1.85	1.80	1.76	1.71	1.67	1.63	1.60	1.57	1.54	1.53
2.59	**2.51**	**2.40**	**2.32**	**2.22**	**2.14**	**2.08**	**2.00**	**1.97**	**1.90**	**1.86**	**1.84**
1.95	1.90	1.84	1.79	1.74	1.69	1.66	1.61	1.59	1.55	1.53	1.51
2.56	**2.49**	**2.37**	**2.29**	**2.20**	**2.11**	**2.05**	**1.97**	**1.94**	**1.88**	**1.84**	**1.81**
1.94	1.89	1.82	1.78	1.73	1.68	1.64	1.60	1.57	1.54	1.51	1.49
2.54	**2.46**	**2.35**	**2.26**	**2.17**	**2.08**	**2.02**	**1.94**	**1.91**	**1.85**	**1.80**	**1.78**
1.92	1.88	1.81	1.76	1.72	1.66	1.63	1.58	1.56	1.52	1.50	1.48
2.52	**2.44**	**2.32**	**2.24**	**2.15**	**2.06**	**2.00**	**1.92**	**1.88**	**1.82**	**1.78**	**1.75**
1.91	1.87	1.80	1.75	1.71	1.65	1.62	1.57	1.54	1.51	1.48	1.46
2.50	**2.42**	**2.30**	**2.22**	**2.13**	**2.04**	**1.98**	**1.90**	**1.86**	**1.80**	**1.76**	**1.72**
1.90	1.86	1.79	1.74	1.70	1.64	1.61	1.56	1.53	1.50	1.47	1.45
2.48	**2.40**	**2.28**	**2.20**	**2.11**	**2.02**	**1.96**	**1.88**	**1.84**	**1.78**	**1.73**	**1.70**
1.90	1.85	1.78	1.74	1.69	1.63	1.60	1.55	1.52	1.48	1.46	1.44
2.46	**2.39**	**2.26**	**2.18**	**2.10**	**2.00**	**1.94**	**1.86**	**1.82**	**1.76**	**1.71**	**1.68**
1.88	1.83	1.76	1.72	1.67	1.61	1.58	1.52	1.50	1.46	1.43	1.41
2.43	**2.35**	**2.23**	**2.15**	**2.06**	**1.96**	**1.90**	**1.82**	**1.78**	**1.71**	**1.66**	**1.64**
1.86	1.81	1.75	1.70	1.65	1.59	1.56	1.50	1.48	1.44	1.41	1.39
2.40	**2.32**	**2.20**	**2.12**	**2.03**	**1.93**	**1.87**	**1.79**	**1.74**	**1.68**	**1.63**	**1.60**
1.85	1.80	1.73	1.68	1.63	1.57	1.54	1.49	1.46	1.42	1.39	1.37
2.37	**2.30**	**2.18**	**2.09**	**2.00**	**1.90**	**1.84**	**1.76**	**1.71**	**1.64**	**1.60**	**1.56**
1.84	1.79	1.72	1.67	1.62	1.56	1.53	1.47	1.45	1.40	1.37	1.35
2.35	**2.28**	**2.15**	**2.07**	**1.98**	**1.88**	**1.82**	**1.74**	**1.69**	**1.62**	**1.56**	**1.53**
1.82	1.77	1.70	1.65	1.60	1.54	1.51	1.45	1.42	1.38	1.35	1.32
2.32	**2.24**	**2.11**	**2.03**	**1.94**	**1.84**	**1.78**	**1.70**	**1.65**	**1.57**	**1.52**	**1.49**
1.79	1.75	1.68	1.63	1.57	1.51	1.48	1.42	1.39	1.34	1.30	1.28
2.26	**2.19**	**2.06**	**1.98**	**1.89**	**1.79**	**1.73**	**1.64**	**1.59**	**1.51**	**1.46**	**1.43**
1.77	1.72	1.65	1.60	1.55	1.49	1.45	1.39	1.36	1.31	1.27	1.25
2.23	**2.15**	**2.03**	**1.94**	**1.85**	**1.75**	**1.68**	**1.59**	**1.54**	**1.46**	**1.40**	**1.37**
1.76	1.71	1.64	1.59	1.54	1.47	1.44	1.37	1.34	1.29	1.25	1.22
2.20	**2.12**	**2.00**	**1.91**	**1.83**	**1.72**	**1.66**	**1.56**	**1.51**	**1.43**	**1.37**	**1.33**
1.74	1.69	1.62	1.57	1.52	1.45	1.42	1.35	1.32	1.26	1.22	1.19
2.17	**2.09**	**1.97**	**1.88**	**1.79**	**1.69**	**1.62**	**1.53**	**1.48**	**1.39**	**1.33**	**1.28**
1.72	1.67	1.60	1.54	1.49	1.42	1.38	1.32	1.28	1.22	1.16	1.13
2.12	**2.04**	**1.92**	**1.84**	**1.74**	**1.64**	**1.57**	**1.47**	**1.42**	**1.32**	**1.24**	**1.19**
1.70	1.65	1.58	1.53	1.47	1.41	1.36	1.30	1.26	1.19	1.13	1.08
2.09	**2.01**	**1.89**	**1.81**	**1.71**	**1.61**	**1.54**	**1.44**	**1.38**	**1.28**	**1.19**	**1.11**
1.69	1.64	1.57	1.52	1.46	1.40	1.35	1.28	1.24	1.17	1.11	1.00
2.07	**1.99**	**1.87**	**1.79**	**1.69**	**1.59**	**1.52**	**1.41**	**1.36**	**1.25**	**1.15**	**1.00**

Appendix D

Critical Values of Chi-Square

PROBABILITY UNDER H₀ THAT $X^2 \geq$ CHI-SQUARE

df	.99	.98	.95	.90	.80	.70	.50	.30	.20	.10	.05	.02	.01	.001
1	.00016	.00063	.0039	.016	.064	.15	.46	1.07	1.64	2.71	3.84	5.41	6.64	10.83
2	.02	.04	.10	.21	.45	.71	1.39	2.41	3.22	4.60	5.99	7.82	9.21	13.82
3	.12	.18	.35	.58	1.00	1.42	2.37	3.66	4.64	6.25	7.82	9.84	11.34	16.27
4	.30	.43	.71	1.06	1.65	2.20	3.36	4.88	5.99	7.78	9.49	11.67	13.28	18.46
5	.55	.75	1.14	1.61	2.34	3.00	4.35	6.06	7.29	9.24	11.07	13.39	15.09	20.52
6	.87	1.18	1.64	2.20	3.07	3.83	5.35	7.23	8.56	10.64	12.59	15.03	16.81	22.46
7	1.24	1.56	2.17	2.83	3.82	4.67	6.35	8.38	9.80	12.02	14.07	16.62	18.48	24.32
8	1.65	2.03	2.73	3.49	4.59	5.53	7.34	9.52	11.03	13.36	15.51	18.17	20.09	26.12
9	2.09	2.53	3.32	4.17	5.38	6.39	8.34	10.66	12.24	14.68	16.92	19.68	21.67	27.88
10	2.56	3.06	3.94	4.86	6.18	7.27	9.34	11.78	13.44	15.99	18.31	21.16	23.21	29.59
11	3.05	3.61	4.58	5.58	6.99	8.15	10.34	12.90	14.63	17.28	19.68	22.62	24.72	31.26
12	3.57	4.18	5.23	6.30	7.81	9.03	11.34	14.01	15.81	18.55	21.03	24.05	26.22	32.91
13	4.11	4.76	5.89	7.04	8.63	9.93	12.34	15.12	16.98	19.81	22.36	25.47	27.69	34.53
14	4.66	5.37	6.57	7.79	9.47	10.82	13.34	16.22	18.15	21.06	23.68	26.87	29.14	36.12
15	5.23	5.98	7.26	8.55	10.31	11.72	14.34	17.32	19.31	22.81	25.00	28.26	30.58	37.70
16	5.81	6.61	7.96	9.31	11.15	12.62	15.34	18.42	20.46	23.54	26.30	29.83	32.00	39.29
17	6.41	7.26	8.67	10.08	12.00	13.53	16.34	19.51	21.62	24.77	27.59	31.00	33.41	40.75
18	7.02	7.91	9.39	10.86	12.86	14.44	17.34	20.60	22.76	25.99	28.87	32.35	34.80	42.31
19	7.63	8.57	10.12	11.65	13.72	15.35	18.34	21.69	23.90	27.20	30.14	33.69	36.19	43.82
20	8.26	9.24	10.85	12.44	14.58	16.27	19.34	22.78	25.04	28.41	31.41	35.02	37.57	45.82
21	8.90	9.92	11.59	13.24	15.44	17.18	20.34	23.86	26.17	29.62	32.67	36.34	38.93	46.80
22	9.54	10.60	12.34	14.04	16.31	18.10	21.34	24.94	27.30	30.81	33.92	37.66	40.29	48.27
23	10.20	11.29	13.09	14.85	17.19	19.02	22.34	26.02	28.43	32.01	35.17	38.97	41.64	49.73
24	10.86	11.99	13.85	15.66	18.06	19.94	23.34	27.10	29.55	33.20	36.42	40.27	42.98	51.18
25	11.52	12.70	14.61	16.47	18.94	20.87	24.34	28.17	30.68	34.38	37.65	41.57	44.31	52.62
26	12.20	13.41	15.38	17.29	19.82	21.79	25.34	29.25	31.80	35.58	38.88	42.86	45.64	54.05
27	12.88	14.12	16.15	18.11	20.70	22.72	26.34	30.32	32.91	36.74	40.11	44.14	46.96	55.48
28	13.56	14.85	16.93	18.94	21.59	23.65	27.34	31.39	34.03	37.92	41.34	45.42	48.28	56.89
29	14.26	15.57	17.71	19.77	22.48	24.58	28.34	32.46	35.14	39.09	42.56	46.69	49.59	58.30
30	14.95	16.31	18.49	20.60	23.36	25.51	29.34	33.53	36.25	40.26	43.77	47.96	50.89	59.70

From Table IV of Fisher & Yates; STATISTICAL TABLES FOR BIOLOGICAL, AGRICULTURAL AND MEDICAL RESEARCH Published by Longman Group UK Ltd., 1974. Reprinted by permission of Addison Wesley Longman Ltd.

References

Books

Albreck, P. L. and Settle, R. B. (1995). *The survey research handbook* (2nd ed.). Chicago, IL: Irwin.

Alward, E. C. (1996). *Research paper, step-by-step.* Westhampton, MA: Pine Island Press.

American Educational Research Association. (1999). *Standards for educational and psychological testing.* Washington, DC: Author.

American Psychological Association. (1994). *Publication manual of the American Psychological Association* (4th ed.). Washington, DC: Author.

Ary, D., Jacobs, L. C., and Razaveih, A. (1996). *Introduction to research in education* (5th ed.). Orlando, FL: Harcourt Brace.

Babbie, E. (1990). *Survey research methods* (2d ed.). Belmont, CA: Wadsworth.

Babbie, E. (1992). *The practice of social research* (6th ed.). Belmont, CA: Wadsworth.

Barlow, D. H., and Hersen, M. (1984). *Single case experimental designs: Strategies for studying behavior change.* New York: Pergamon.

Baumgartner, T. A., and Jackson, A. S. (1999). *Measurement for evaluation in physical education and exercise science* (6th ed.). New York: McGraw-Hill.

Berryman, J. W. (1995). *Out of many, one: A history of the American College of Sports Medicine.* Champaign, IL: Human Kinetics.

Best, J. W. (1981). *Research in education* (4th ed.). Englewood Cliffs, NJ: Prentice-Hall.

Best, J. W., and Kahn, J. V. (1998). *Research in education* (8th ed.). Boston, MA: Allyn & Bacon.

Blommers, P. J., and Forsyth, R. A. (1983). *Elementary statistical methods.* Lanham, MD: University Press of America.

Blumer, H. (1969). *Symbolic interactionism: Perspective and method.* Englewood Cliffs, NJ: Prentice-Hall.

Bogdan, R., and Biklen, S. (1997). *Qualitative research for education* (3rd ed.). Boston: Allyn & Bacon.

Bookwalter, C. W., and Bookwalter, K. W. (1959). Library techniques. In M. G. Scott (Ed.), *Research methods in health, physical education, and recreation* (pp. 20-38). Washington, DC: American Association for Health, Physical Education, and Recreation.

Borg, W. R. (1987). *Applying educational research: A practical guide for teachers* (2d ed.). New York: Longman.

Campbell, D., and Stanley, J. (1963). *Experimental and quasi-experimental designs for research.* Chicago: Rand McNally.

Campbell, W. G., and Ballou, S. V. (1984). *Form and style: Theses, reports, term papers* (9th ed.). Boston: Houghton Mifflin.

Cohen, J. (1988). *Statistical power analysis for the behavioral sciences* (2d ed.). Hillsdale, NJ: Lawrence Erlbaum Associates, Publishers.

Cohen, J., and Cohen, P. (1975). *Applied multiple regression/correlation analysis for the behavioral sciences.* New York: Wiley.

Cook, T. D., and Campbell, D. T. (1979). *Quasi-experimentation: Design and analysis issues for field settings.* Boston: Houghton Mifflin.

Cook, T. D., and Reichardt, C. S. (Eds.). (1979). *Qualitative and quantitative methods in evaluation research.* Beverly Hills, CA: Sage.

Cone, J. D., and Foster, S. L. (1993). *Dissertations and theses from start to finish.* Washington, DC: American Psychological Association.

Crocker, L., and Algina, J. (1986). *Introduction to classical and modern test theory.* New York: Harcourt Brace Jovanovich.

Dattilo, A. M. (1992). Meta-analysis in nutrition and dietetics. In E. R. Monsen (Ed.), *Research: Successful approaches.* Chicago: The American Dietetic Association.

Day, R. A. (1998). *How to write and publish a scientific paper* (2d ed.). Philadelphia: ISI.

Dees, R. (1987). *Writing the research paper.* Boston: Allyn & Bacon.

Denzin, N. (1992). *Symbolic interactionism and cultural studies: The politics of interpretation.* Oxford: Blackwell.

Denzin, N. K., and Lincoln, Y. S. (1994). Entering the field of qualitative research. In N. K. Denzin and Y. S. Lincoln (Eds.), *Handbook of qualitative research.* (pp. 1-22). Thousand Oaks, CA: Sage Publications.

Dillman, D. A. (1978). *Mail and telephone surveys: The total design method.* New York: John Wiley and Sons.

Dishman, R. K., Heath, G., and Washburn, R. (in press). *Physical activity epidemiology.* Champaign, IL: Human Kinetics.

Dooley, D. (1990). *Social research methods* (2d ed.). Englewood Cliffs, NJ: Prentice-Hall.

Drew, C. J., Hardman, M. L., and Hart, A. W. (1996). *Designing and conducting research: inquiry into education and social science* (2d ed.). Needham Heights, MA: Allyn and Bacon.

Drowatzky, J. N. (1996). *Ethical decision making in physical activity research:* Champaign, IL: Human Kinetics.

Ferguson, G. A., and Takane, Y. (1989). *Statistical analysis in psychology and education* (6th ed.). New York: McGraw-Hill.

Fielding, N. G., and Lee, R. (1993). *Using computers in qualitative research.* London: Sage Publications.

Fox, D. J. (1969). *The research process in education.* New York: Holt, Rinehart and Winston.

Gay, L. R., and Airasian, P. (2000). *Educational research: competencies for analysis and application.* Upper Saddle River, NJ: Prentice-Hall.

Geertz, C. (1973). *The interpretation of cultures.* New York: Basic Books.

Gibaldi, J. (1988). *MLA handbook: For writers of research papers* (5th ed.). New York: Modern Language Association.

Glaser, B. (1978). *Theoretical sensitivity: Advances in the methodology of grounded theory.* Mill Valley, CA: Sociology Press.

Glaser, B., and Strauss, A. (1967). *The discovery of grounded theory: Strategies for qualitative research.* Chicago: Aldine.

Good, C. V. (1972). *Essentials of educational research.* New York: Appleton-Century-Crofts.

Gorden, R. (1975). *Interviewing: Strategy, techniques, and tactics.* Homewood, IL: Dorsey.

Green, L., and Lewis, F. M. (1986). *Measurement and evaluation in health education and health promotion.* Mountain View, CA: Mayfield.

Greenbaum, T. L. (1998). *The handbook of focus group research.* Thousand Oaks, CA: Sage Publications.

Griffin, P. (1983). Gymnastics is a girl's thing: Student participation and interaction patterns in a middle school gymnastic's unit. In T. J. Templin and J. K. Olson (Eds.), *Teaching in physical education* (pp. 71-85). Champaign, IL: Human Kinetics.

Guba, E., and Lincoln, Y. (1981). *Effective evaluation.* San Francisco: Jossey-Bass.

Harris, M. B. (1995). *Basic statistics for behavioral science research* (2d ed.). Needham Heights, MA: Allyn & Bacon.

Harris, R. J. (1985). *A primer of multivariate statistics.* Orlando, FL: Academic Press.

Henderson, K. A. (1991). *Dimensions of choice: A qualitative approach to recreation, parks, and leisure research.* State College, PA: Venture.

Hollander, M., and Wolfe, D. A. (1973). *Nonparametric statistical methods.* New York: Wiley.

Huck, S. W. (2000). *Reading statistics and research* (3rd ed.). New York: Addison Wesley Longman.

Huck, S. W., and Cormier, W. H. (1996). *Reading statistics and research* (2nd ed.). New York: Harper Collins.

Hult, J. S., and Trekell, M. (Eds.). (1991). *A century of women's basketball.* Reston, VA: American Alliance for Health, Physical Education, Recreation and Dance.

Hyllegard, R., Mood, D. P., and Morrow, J. R. (1996). *Interpreting research in sport and exercise science.* St. Louis, MO: Mosby.

Isaac, S., and Michael, W. B. (1982). *Handbook in research and evaluation.* San Diego: EdITS.

Isaac, S., and Michael, W. B. (1995). *Handbook in research and evaluation.* San Diego: EdITS.

Johnson, J. M., and Pennypacker, H. S. (1993). *Strategies and tactics of behavioral research* (2d ed.). Hillsdale, NJ: Lawrence Erlbaum Associates.

Kazdin, A. E. (1982). Single-case experimental designs in clinical research and practice. In A. E. Kazdin & A. H. Tuma (Eds.), *New directions for methodology of social and behavioral sciences: Single-case research designs,* 13, 33-47. San Francisco: Jossey-Bass.

Keppel, G. (1991). *Design and analysis: A researcher's handbook.* Englewood Cliffs, NJ: Prentice-Hall.

Kirk, J., and Miller, M. (1986). *Reliability and validity in qualitative research.* Beverly Hills, CA: Sage.

Kraemer, H. C., and Thiemann, S. (1987). *How many subjects?* Newbury Park, CA: Sage Publications.

Kratochwill, T. R., and Levin, J. R. (Eds.). (1992). *Single case research design and analysis: New directions for psychology and education.* Hillsdale, NJ: Lawrence Erlbaum Associates.

Kuzma, J. W. (1998). *Basic statistics for the health sciences* (3rd ed.). Mountain View, CA: Mayfield.

Larose, T. L., and Jin, C. (1998). *READY, SET, RUN! A student guide to SAS® software for Microsoft® Windows®.* Mountain View, CA: Mayfield.

Lecompte, M., Preissle, J., and Tesch, R. (1993). *Ethnography and qualitative design in educational research* (2d ed.). Orlando: Academic Press.

Leininger, M. (1985). Nature, rationale importance of qualitative research in nursing. In M. Leininger (Ed.), *Qualitative research methods in nursing.* Orlando, FL: Grune & Stratton.

Lincoln, Y., and Guba, E. (1985). *Naturalistic inquiry.* Beverly Hills, CA: Sage.

Lipsey, M. W. (1990). *Design Sensitivity: Statistical power for experimental research.* Newbury Park, CA: Sage.

Locke, L. F., Spirduso, W. W., and Silverman, S. J. (2000). *Proposals that work: A guide for planning dissertations and grant proposals.* Thousand Oaks, CA: Sage Publications.

Marascuilo, L. A., and McSweeney, M. (1977). *Nonparametric and distribution-free methods for the social sciences.* Monterey, CA: Brooks/Cole.

Marshall, C., and Rossman, G. (1999). *Designing Qualitative Research* (3rd ed.). Walnut Creek, CA: Altamira Press.

McCuen, G. E. (1998). *Human experimentation: When research is evil.* Hudson, WI: GEM Publications, Inc.

McMillan, J. H., and Schumacher, S. (2001). *Research in education* (5th ed.). New York: Addison Wesley Longman.

Merriam, S. B. (1997). *Qualitative research and case study applications in education.* San Francisco: Jossey-Bass.

Miles, M. B., and Huberman, A. M. (1994). *Qualitative data analysis: An expanded sourcebook* (2d ed.). Thousand Oaks, CA: Sage Publications.

Monette, D. R., Sullivan, T. J., & DeJong, C. R. (1990). *Applied social research: tool for human services* (2d ed.). Fort Worth, TX: Holt, Rinehart and Winston.

Neutens, J. J., and Rubinson, L. (1997). *Research techniques for the health sciences* (2d ed.). Boston: Allyn & Bacon.

Nevins, A. (1938). *The gateway to history.* New York: McGraw-Hill.

Nie, N. H., et al. (1975). *Statistical package for the social sciences* (2d ed.). New York: McGraw-Hill.

Norusis, M. J. (2000). *SPSS 10.0 Guide to Data Analysis.* Upper Saddle River, N.J.: Prentice Hall.

Nunnally, J. C., and Bernstein, I. H. (1994). *Psychometric Theory* (3rd ed.). New York: McGraw-Hill.

Patton, M. Q. (1990). *Qualitative evaluation and research methods* (2d ed.). Thousand Oaks, CA: Sage Publications.

Pavkov, T. W., and Pierce, K. A. (2001). *READY, SET, GO! A student guide to SPSS® 10.0 for Windows®.* Mountain View, CA: Mayfield.

Pedhazur, E. J. (1982). *Multiple regression in behavioral research: Explanation and prediction* (2d ed.). New York: Holt, Rinehart & Winston.

Pelegrino, D. A. (1979). *Research methods for recreation and leisure: A theoretical and practical guide.* Dubuque, IA: Wm. C. Brown.

Poling, A., and Fuqua', R. W. (Eds.). (1986). *Research methods in applied behavior analysis: Issues and advances.* New York: Plenum.

Pyrczak, F., and Bruce, R. R. (2000). *Writing empirical research reports: A basic guide for students of the social and behavioral sciences* (3rd ed.). Los Angeles: Psyczak.

Reason, P., and Rowan, J. (Eds.). (1981). *Human inquiry: A sourcebook of new paradigm research.* New York: John Wiley & Sons.

Rosenthal, R. (1991). *Meta-analytic procedures for social researchers* (Rev. ed.). Thousand Oaks, CA: Sage.

Rubin, H. J. (1983). *Applied social research.* Columbus, OH: Charles E. Merrill.

Rubin, H. J., and Rubin, I. S. (1995). *Qualitative interviewing: The art of hearing data.* Thousand Oaks, CA: Sage Publications.

Safrit, M. J., and Wood. T. M. (1989). *Measurement concepts in physical education and exercise science.* Champaign, IL: Human Kinetics.

Sarvela, P., and McDermott, R. J. (1993). *Health education evaluation and measurement: A practitioner's perspective.* Madison, WI: Brown & Benchmark.

Sax, G. (1979). *Foundations of educational research* (2d ed.). Englewood Cliffs, NJ: Prentice-Hall.

Siegel, S. (1956). *Nonparametric statistics for the behavioral sciences.* New York: McGraw-Hill.

Siegel, S., and Castellan, N. J. (1988). *Nonparametric statistics for the behavioral sciences* (2d ed.). New York: McGraw-Hill.

Spradley, J. P. (1997). *The ethnograhic interview* (textbook ed). Ft. Worth: Harcourt College Publishers.

Stevens, J. (1986). *Applied multivariate statistics for the social sciences.* Hillsdale, NJ: Erlbaum.

Stunkard, A. J., Sorenson, T., and Schulsinger, F. (1983). Use of the Danish adoption register for the study of obesity and thinness. In S. S. Kety, L. P. Rowland, R. L. Sidman and S. W. Matthysee (Eds.), *Genetics of neurological and psychiatric disorders.* New York: Raven.

Sudman, S., and Bradburn, N. M. (1988). *Asking questions: A practical guide to questionnaire design.* San Francisco: Jossey-Bass.

Tabachnick, B. G., and Fidell, L. S. (1989). *Using multivariate statistics.* New York: Harper & Row.

Tatsuoka, M. M. (1988). *Multivariate analysis: Techniques for educational and psychological research.* New York: Wiley.

Thomas, J. R., and Nelson, J. K. (1985). *Introduction to research in health, physical education, recreation, and dance.* Champaign, IL: Human Kinetics.

Thomas, J. R., and Nelson, J. K. (1996). *Research methods in physical activity* (3rd ed.). Champaign, IL: Human Kinetics.

Thorndike, R. M., Cunningham, G. K., Thorndike, R. L., and Hagen, E. P. (1991). *Measurement and evaluation in psychology and education.* New York: Macmillan.

Tuckman, B. W. (1999). *Conducting educational research* (5th ed.). Orlando, FL: Harcourt Brace.

Turabian, K. L. (1996). *A manual for writers of term papers, theses, and dissertations* (6th ed.). Chicago: University of Chicago Press.

Tutko, T. A., Lyon, L. P., and Ogilvie, B. C. (1969). *Athletic motivation inventory.* San Jose: Institute for the Study of Athletic Motivation, California State University.

University of Chicago (1993). *The Chicago manual of style* (14th ed.). Chicago: Author.

Van Dalen, D. B. (1959). The historical method. In M. G. Scott (Ed.), *Research methods in health, physical education, and recreation* (pp. 465-481). Washington, DC: American Association for Health, Physical Education, and Recreation.

Van Dalen, D. B. (1964). *Understanding educational research.* New York: McGraw-Hill.

Van Dalen, D. B. (1979). *Understanding educational research: An introduction* (4th ed.). New York: McGraw-Hill.

Vidich, A. J., and Lyman, S. M. (1994). Qualitative methods: Their history in sociology and anthropology. In N. K. Denzin & Y. S. Lincoln (Eds.), *Handbook of qualitative research.* (pp. 23-59). Thousand Oaks, CA: Sage Publications.

Weisberg, H. F., and Bowen, B. D. (1977). *An introduction to survey research and data analysis.* San Francisco: W. H. Freeman.

Wiersma, W. (1991). *Research methods in education* (5th ed.). Boston: Allyn & Bacon.

Winer, B. J., Brown, D. R., and Michels, K. N. (1991). *Statistical principles in experimental design* (3d ed.). New York: McGraw-Hill.

Wolcott, H. (1990). *Writing up qualitative research.* Newbury Park, CA: Sage.

Catalogs

Lawrence Erlbaum Associates. (2000). Publications Catalog. Lawrence Erlbaum Associates, Inc., 10 Industrial Ave., Mahwah, NJ 07430-2262.

Sage Publications. (1996). Publications Catalog. Sage Publications, Inc., P.O. Box 5084, Thousand Oaks, CA, 91359-9924.

Dissertations and Theses

Abo Abdo, H. E. (1981). *Kinematic and kinetic analysis of the soccer instep kick.* Doctoral dissertation, Indiana University, Bloomington.

Bian, W. (1999). *Physical activity patterns among physical education major students in selected institutions of China and the United States.* Master's thesis, University of Northern Iowa, Cedar Falls.

Baptista, R. C. (1962). *A history of intercollegiate soccer in the United States of America.* Doctoral dissertation, Indiana University, Bloomington.

Bishop, R. (1963). *The origin and development of adapted physical education in the United States.* Doctoral dissertation, Indiana University, Bloomington.

Clark, J. K. (1991). *Two curricular settings of a HIV education unit related to secondary school students' HIV knowledge and attitude.* Doctoral dissertation, Indiana University, Bloomington.

Collins, M. E. (1989). *Body figure perceptions and preferences among preadolescent children.* Doctoral dissertation, Indiana University, Bloomington.

Cotter, L. L. (1978). *Group cohesiveness and team success among women's intercollegiate basketball teams.* Doctoral dissertation, Indiana University, Bloomington.

Darracott, S. H. (1995). *Individual differences in variability and pattern of performance as a consideration in the selection of a representative score from multiple trial physical performance data.* Doctoral dissertation, University of Georgia, Athens, GA.

Fey, M. A. (1998). *Relationship between self-esteem, eating behaviors, and eating attitudes among female collegiate swimmers.* Master's thesis, University of Northern Iowa, Cedar Falls.

Fratzke, M. R. (1973). *Discriminant analysis of intramural basketball officials.* Doctoral dissertation, Indiana University, Bloomington.

Frye, P. A. (1977). *Selected coefficients for estimating the reliability of multiple trail motor performance tests.* Doctoral dissertation, Indiana University, Bloomington.

Gaunt, S. J. (1979). *Factor structure of basketball playing ability.* Doctoral dissertation, Indiana University, Bloomington.

Grosshans, I. R. (1975). *Delbert Oberteuffer: His professional activities and contributions to the fields of health and physical education.* Doctoral dissertation, Indiana University, Bloomington.

Hashim, T. J. (1988). *A health knowledge test for male college freshmen in Saudi Arabia.* Doctoral dissertation, Indiana University, Bloomington.

Hendrick, J. (1981). *Biomechanical analysis of selected parameters in the field hockey drive.* Master degree thesis, Indiana University, Bloomington.

Henry, G. M. (1974). *The shooting accuracy of third grade students who practiced shooting at goals less than ten feet high.* Doctoral dissertation, Indiana University, Bloomington.

Holland, J. C. (1970). *Heart rates of Indiana high school basketball officials as measured by electrocardiographic radio telemetry.* Doctoral dissertation, Indiana University, Bloomington.

Luedke, G. C. (1980). *Range of motion as the focus of teaching the overhand throwing pattern to children.* Doctoral dissertation, Indiana University, Bloomington.

Major, M. J. (1998). *Effects of Special Olympics participation on self-esteem of adults with mental retardation.* Master's thesis, University of Northern Iowa, Cedar Falls.

Mintah, J. K. (2000). *Teacher's perceptions about the impact of authentic assessment use on students' skill achievement, motivation, and self-concept.* Doctoral dissertation, University of Northern Iowa, Cedar Falls.

Ogletree, R. J. (1991). *Selected factors related to help-seeking behavior in college women victims of sexual coercion.* Doctoral dissertation, Indiana University, Bloomington.

Peña, C. (1990). *Needs assessment of Indiana convention and visitor bureaus.* Master's thesis, Indiana Univeristy, Bloomington.

Peters, G. J. (1999). *Characteristics of highly successful high school football programs in Iowa.* Master's thesis, University of Northern Iowa, Cedar Falls.

Piercy, I. (1978). *The extent of influence of Lloyd Bridges Sharp as identified in the lives and professional careers of selected educators and youth leaders.* Doctoral dissertation, University of Oregon, Eugene.

Sells, T. D. (1977). *Selected movement and anthropometric variables of football defensive tackles.* Doctoral dissertation, Indiana University, Bloomington.

Stoner, J. (1990). *George Warren Donaldson: His professional philosophy, influences and contributions to outdoor education.* Doctoral dissertation, Indiana University, Bloomington.

Umansky, W. (1976). *Prediction of preschool performance in selected areas from perinatal factors.* Doctoral dissertation, Indiana University, Bloomington.

Van Oteghen, S. L. (1973). *Two speeds of isokinetic exercise as related to the vertical jump performance of women.* Doctoral dissertation, Indiana University, Bloomington.

Visker, T. L. (1986). *Self-consciousness and physical self-efficacy in relationship to exercise adherence.* Doctoral dissertation, Indiana University, Bloomington.

Wasilak, J. M. (1988). *Training at various velocities on the biokinetic swim bench related to the three-dimensional pattern of the front crawl stroke.* Doctoral dissertation, Indiana University, Bloomington.

West, J. (1989). *Perceptions of self and physical activity in a culturally diverse physical education class.* Doctoral dissertation, University of Georgia, Athens.

Government Documents

45 C.F.R. 46 (1991). Protection of human subjects. Code of Federal Regulations, Vol 45, Part 46. Retrieved October 15, 2000, from the World Wide Web: http://ohrp.osophs.dhhs.gov/humansubjects/guidance/45cfr46.htm

Interagency Research Animal Committee (1985). U. S. government principles for utilization and care of vertebrate animals used in testing, research, and training. Federal Register, May 20, 1985.

National Commission for the Protection of Human Subjects on Biomedical and Behavioral Research (1979). The Belmont report: Ethical principles and guidelines for the protection of human subjects of research. Washington, DC: U. S. Government Printing Office. Retrieved October 5, 2000, from the World Wide Web: http://ohrp.osophs.dhhs.gov/humansubjects/guidance/belmont.htm

National Science Foundation (1991). Misconduct in science and engineering. Federal Register, May 14, 1991, 22286-22290.

Nuremberg Code (1949). Reprinted in trials of war criminals before the Nuremberg military tribunals under control council law No. 10, Vol. 2, Washington, DC: U. S. Government Printing Office.

Office of Research Integrity (1999). Case Summaries, ORI Newsletter, 7(2), March 1999. Retrieved October 17, 2000, from the World Wide Web: http://ori.dhhs.gov/html/publications/newsletters_vol7no2.asp

Public Health Service (1989). Responsibilities of awardee and applicant institutions for dealing with and reporting possible misconduct in science. Federal Register, August 8, 1989, 32446-32451.

Public Health Service (1996). Public health policy on humane care and use of laboratory animals. Washington, DC: U. S. Department of Health and Human Services.

U.S. Department of Health and Human Services (1996). Physical activity and health: A report of the Surgeon General. Washington, DC: Author.

Nonprint Media

Andrews, J., and Drake, A. (Hosts). (1991). *Hanya: Portrait of a pioneer: The story of dancer/choreographer Hanya Holm* (Cassette Recording No. 243-28682). Reston, VA: American Alliance for Health, Physical Education, Recreation and Dance.

The Ethnograph (software). (1998). Qualis Research Associates.

Johnson, B. J. (1993). *DSTAT 1.10 Software for the meta-analytic review of research literature.* Hillsdale, NJ: Lawrence Erlbaum Associates.

*NUD*IST* (software). (1998). QSR International.

NVivo (software). (1998). QST International.

SAS. (1998). StatView Software, Version 5. Cary, NC: SAS.

Schwarzer, R. (1991). *Meta: Programs for secondary data analysis, 5.3.* Berlin: Free University of Berlin.

SPSS. (1999). *SPSS 10.0.* Chicago, IL: SPSS.

SPSS. (2000). *SPSS 10.0 Student Version.* Chicago, IL: SPSS.

Periodicals

American College of Sports Medicine (1999). Policy statement regarding the use of human subjects and informed consent. *Medicine and Science in Sports and Exercise, 31*(7), vi.

American Educational Research Association (1992). Ethical standards of the American educational research association. *Educational Researcher, 21*(7), 23-26.

American Psychological Association (1992). Ethical principles of psychologists and code of conduct. *American Psychologist, 47,* 1597-1611.

Amorose, A, J., and Horn, T. S. (2000). Intrinsic motivation: Relationships with collegiate athletes' gender, scholarship status, and perceptions of their coaches' behavior. *Journal of Sport and Exercise Psychology, 22*(1), 63-84.

Bain, L., Wilson, T., and Chaikind, E. (1989). Participant perceptions of exercise programs for overweight women. *Research Quarterly for Exercise and Sport, 60*(2), 134-143.

Balog, L. F., and Scheidt, D. M. (2000). Assessing student learning outcomes and validation of the "self-assessment for health educators" in an undergraduate health education program. *Journal of Health Education, 31*(4), 219-224.

Bates, B. T. (1996). Single-subject methodology: An alternative approach. *Medicine and Science in Sports and* Exercise, *28,* 631-638.

Bates, B. T., Dufek, J. S., and Davis, H. P. (1992). The effect of trial size on statistical power. *Medicine and Science in Sports and Exercise, 24,* 1059-1068.

Baumgartner, T. A. (1969). Stability of physical performance scores. *Research Quarterly, 40,* 257-261.

Behlendorf, B., MacRae, P. G., and Vos Strache, C. (1999). Children's perceptions of physical activity for adults: competence and appropriateness. *Journal of Aging and Physical Activity, 7*(4), 354-373.

Blinde, E. M., and McCallister, S. G. (1999, September). Women, disability. and sport and physical fitness activity: The intersection of gender and disability dynamics. *Research Quarterly for Exercise and Sport, 70*(3), 303-312.

Bouffard, M. (1993). The perils of averaging data in adapted physical activity research. *Adapted Physical Activity Quarterly, 10,* 371-391.

Brody, E. B., Hatfield, B. D., Spalding, T. W., Frazer, M. B., and Cahery, F. J. (2000). The effect of psyching strategy on neuromuscular activation and force production in strength-trained men. *Research Quarterly for Exercise and Sport, 71*(2), 162-170.

Brown, W. J., Mishra, G., Lee, C., and Bauman, A. (2000). Leisure time physical activity in Australian women: Relationship with well being and symptoms. *Research Quarterly for Exercise and Sport, 71*(3), 206-216.

Bukowski, B. J., and Stinson, A. D. (2000). Physical Educators' Perceptions of Block Scheduling in Secondary School Physical Education. *Journal of Physical Education, Recreation and Dance, 71*(1), 53-57.

Cardinal, B. J. (2000). (Un)Informed consent in exercise and sport science research? A comparison of forms written for two reading levels. *Research Quarterly for Exercise and Sport, 71*(3), 295-301.

Cardinal, B. J., Martin, J. J., and Sachs, M. L. (1996). Readability of written informed consent forms used in exercise and sport psychology research. *Research Quarterly for Exercise and Sport, 67,* 360-362.

Caster, B. L., and Bates, B. T. (1995). The assessment of mechanical and neuromuscular response strategies during landing. *Medicine and Science in Sports and Exercise, 27,* 736-744.

Cheatham, C. C, Manon, A. D., Brown, J. D., and Bolster, D. R. (2000). Cardiovascular responses during prolonged exercise at ventilatory threshold. *Medicine and Science in Sports and Exercise, 32*(3), 1080-1087.

Chilcott, J. (1987). Where are you coming from and where are you going? The reporting of ethnographic research. *American Educational Research Journal, 24*(2), 199-218.

Cobb, L. E., Stone, W. J., Anonsen, L. J., and Klein, D. A. (2000). The influence of goal setting on exercise adherence. *Journal of Health Education, 31*(5), 277-281.

Cooper, J. M., and Andrews, E. W. (1975). Rhythm as a linguistic art: Signs, symbols, sounds and motions. *Quest, 23,* 68-74.

Damsgaard, R., Bencke, J., Matthiesen, G., Petersen, J. H., and Miller, J. (2000). Is prepubertal growth adversely affected by sport? *Medicine and Science in Sports and Exercise, 32*(10), 1698-1703.

Dempsey, K. (1990). Women's life and leisure in an Australian rural community. *Leisure Studies, 9,* 35-44.

DeLuca, R. V., and Holborn, S. W. (1992). Effects of a variable-ratio reinforcement schedule with changing criteria on exercise in obese and nonobese boys. *Journal of Applied Behavior Analysis, 25,* 671-679.

Dishman, R. K., and Buckworth, J. (1996). Increasing physical activity: A quantitative synthesis. *Medicine and Science in Sports and Exercise, 28,* 706-719.

Dixey, R. (1987). It's a great feeling when you win: Women and bingo. *Leisure Studies, 6,* 199-214.

Edginton, E. S. (1987). Randomized singel-subject experiments and statistical tests. *Journal of Counseling Psychology,* 34, 437–442.

Eisner, E. (1981). On the differences between scientific and artistic approaches to qualitative research. *Educational Researcher, 10*(4), 5-9.

Engels, H. J., Zhu, W., and Moffatt, R. J. (1998). An empirical evaluation of the prediction of maximal heart rate. *Research Quarterly for Exercise and Sport, 69*(1), 94-98.

Ennis, C., and Chepyator-Thomson, J. (1990). Learning characteristics of field-dependent children within an analytical concept-based curriculum. *Journal of Teaching in Physical Education, 10,* 170-187.

Ennis, C., Ross, J., and Chen, A. (1992). The role of value orientations in curricular decision-making: A rationale for teacher's goals and expectations. *Research Quarterly for Exercise and Sport, 35*(4), 38-47.

Ennis, C.D., Solmon, M. A., Satina, B., Loftus, S. J., Mensch, J., and McCauley, M. T. (1999, September). Creating a sense of family in urban schools using the "Sport for Peace" curriculum. *Research Quarterly for Exercise and Sport, 70*(3), 273-285.

Etnier, J. L., and Landers, D. M. (1998). Motor performance and motor learning as function of age and fitness. *Research Quarterly for Exercise and Sport, 69*(2), 139-146.

Everhart, C. B., and Chelladurai, P. (1998). Gender differences in preferences for coaching as an occupation: The role of self-efficacy, valence, and perceived barriers. *Research Quarterly for Exercise and Sport, 69*(2), 188-200.

Faucette, N., Sallis, J. F., McKenzie, T., Alcaraz, J., Kolody, B., and Nugent, P. (1995). Comparison of fourth grade students' out-of-school physical activity levels and choices by gender: Project SPARK. *Journal of Health Education, 26*(2), S82-S89.

Graham, C. (1991). The influence of teacher education on preservice development: Beyond a custodial orientation. *Quest, 43,*1-19.

Graham, A., and Reid, G. (2000). Physical fitness of adults with an intellectual disability: A 13-year follow-up study. *Research Quarterly for Exercise and Sport, 71*(2), 152-161.

Grant, B. C., Ballard, K. D., and Glynn, T. L. (1990). Teaching feedback intervention, motor on-task behavior and successful task performance. *Journal of Teaching in Physical Education, 9*(2), 123-139.

Gould, D., Guinan, D., Greenleaf, C., Medbery, R., and Peterson, K. (1999). Factors affecting olympic performance: Perceptions of athletes and coaches from more and less successful teams. *The Sport Psychologist 13*, 371-394.

Griffin, P. (1984). Girls participation pattern in a middle school team sport unit. *Journal of Teaching in Physical Education, 4,* 30-38.

Griffin, P. (1985). Boys participation styles in a middle school physical education sports unit. *Journal of Teaching in Physical Education, 4,* 100-110.

Hamdan, S. M., and Maratinex, R. (2000). An exploration of ethnic/cultural violence perceptions among urban middle and high school students. *Journal of Health Education, 31*(4), 238-246.

Hastie, P. A., and Buchannan, A. M. (2000, March). Teaching responsibility through sport education: Prospects of a coalition. *Research Quarterly for Exercise and Sport, 71*(1), 25-35.

Henderson, K. A., and Bedini, L. A. (1995, June). "I have a soul that dances like Tina Turner, but my body can't: Physical activity and women with mobility impairments. *Research Quarterly for Exercise and Sport, 66*(2), 151-161.

Houston-Wilson, C., Dunn, J. M., van der Mars, H., and McCubbin, J. (1997). The effect of untrained and trained peer tutors on the motor performance of students with developmental disabilities in integrated physical education classes. *Adapted Physical Activity Quarterly, 14,* 298-313.

Ingram, D., and Hutchinson, S. (2000, January). Double binds and the reproductive and mothering experiences of HIV-positive women. *Qualitative Health Research, 110*(1), 117-132.

Kann, L., Collins, J. L., Pateman, B. C., Small, M. L., Ross, J. G., and Kolbe, L.T. (1995). The school health policies and programs study (SHPPS): Rationale for a nationwide status report on school health programs. *Journal of School Health, 65*(8), 291-294.

Kandakai, T. L., and King, K. A. (1999). Perceived self-efficacy in performing lifesaving skills: An assessment of the American Red Cross's responding to emergencies course. *Journal of Health Education, 30*(4), 235-241.

Katz, D.L., Brunner, R.L., St. Jeor, S. T., Scott, B., Jekel, J. F., and Brownell, K. D. (1998). Dietary fat consumption in a cohort of American adults, 1985-1991: Covariates, secular trends, and compliance with guidelines. *American Journal of Health Promotion, 12*(6), 382-390.

Krejcie, R. V., and Margan, D. W. (1970). Determining sample size for research activities. *Educational and Psychological Measurements, 30,* 607-610.

Langley, D. J., and Knight, S. M. (1996, December). Exploring practical knowledge: A case study in an experienced senior tennis performer. *Research Quarterly for Exercise and Sport, 67*(4), 433-443.

Lewis, P. C., Harrell, J. S., Deng, S., and Bradley, C. (1999). Smokeless tobacco use in adolescents: The cardiovascular health in children study. *Journal of School Health, 69*(8), 320-325.

Lincoln, Y., and Guba, E. (1990). Judging the quality of case study reports. *Qualitative Studies in education, 3*(1), 53-59.

Locke, L. (1989). Qualitative research as a form of scientific inquiry in sport and physical education. *Research Quarterly for Exercise and Sport, 60*(1), 1-20.

LoVerde, M. E., Prochazka, A.V., and Byyny, R. L. (1989). Research consent forms: Continued unreadability and increasing length. *Journal of General Internal Medicine, 4,* 410-412.

Maatz-Majestic, E., and Tapp, M. (1992). College students' definitions of responsible alcohol use and perceived strategies for avoiding alcohol-related problems. *Research Quarterly for Exercise and Sport, 63*(1), A-40.

McKenzie, T. L., Marshall, S. J., Sallis, J. F., and Conway, T. L. (2000). Student activity levels, lesson context, and teacher behavior during middle school physical education. *Research Quarterly for Exercise and Sport, 71*(3), 249-259.

McLachlan, L., (1992). A Model of constraints to family leisure: A study of families who have a child with Down's syndrome. *Research Quarterly for Exercise and Sport Supplement, 63*(1), A-50.

McLaughlin, J., Owen, S., Fors, S., and Levinson, R. (1992). The school child as health educator: Diffusion of hypertension information from sixth grade children to their parents. *Qualitative Studies in Education, 5*(2), 135-156.

McLaughlin, J., and Sliepcevich, F. (1985). The self-care behavior inventory: A model for behavioral instrument development. *Patient Education and Counseling, 7,* 289-301.

McLaughlin, J., and Zeeberg, I. (1993). Self-care and multiple sclerosis: A view from two cultures. *Social Science and Medicine, 37*(3), 315-329.

Mobley, T. A. (1980). Practitioner/researcher: A team. *Parks & Recreation, 15*(4), 40-43.

Morgan, D., and Laing, D. (1991). The diagnosis of Alzheimer's disease: Spouse's perspectives. *Qualitative Health Journal, 1*(3), 370-387.

Mull, S. S. (1991). The role of the health educator in development of self-esteem. *Journal of Health Education, 22*(6), 349-351.

Ogloff, J. R. P., and Otto, R. K. (1991). Are research participants truly informed? Readability of informed consent forms used in research. *Ethics and Behaviour, 1,* 239-252.

O'Neill, D. E. T., Thayer, R. E., Taylor, A. W., Dzialoznski, T. M., and Noble, E. G. (2000). Effects of short-term resistance training on muscle strength and morphology in the elderly. *Journal of Aging and Physical Activity, 8*(4), 312-324.

Paffenbarger, R. S. Jr. (1988). Contributions of epidemiology to exercise science and cardiovascular health. *Medicine and Science in Sports and Exercise, 20,* 426-438.

Papaioannou, A. (1998). Students' perceptions of the physical education class environment for boys and girls and the perceived motivational climate. *Research Quarterly for Exercise and Sport, 69*(3), 267-275.

Payne, V. G., and Morrow, J. R. Jr. (1993). Exercise and VO2max in children: A meta-analysis. *Research Quarterly for Exercise and Sport, 64,* 305-313.

Payne, V. G., Morrow, J. R. Jr., Johnson, L., and Dalton, S. N. (1997). Resistance training in children and youth: A meta-analysis. *Research Quarterly for Exercise and Sport, 68,* 80-88.

Pesa, J. (1998). The association between smoking and unhealthy behaviors among a national sample of Mexican-American adolescents. *Journal of School Health, 68*(9), 376-379.

Poon, P. P. L., and Rodgers, W. M. (2000). Learning and remembering strategies of novice and advanced jazz dancers for skill level appropriate dance routines. *Research Quarterly for Exercise and Sport, 71*(2), 135-144.

Prohaska, T. R., Peters, K., and Warren, J. S. (2000). Sources of attrition in a church-based exercise program for older African-Americans. *American Journal of Health Promotion, 14*(6), 380-385.

Rushall, B. S., and Pettinger, J. (1969). An evaluation of the effects of various reinforcers used as motivators in swimming. *Research Quarterly, 40,* 540-545.

Sallis, J. F., Patterson, T. L., Buono, M. J., and Nader, P. R. (1988). Relation of cardiovascular fitness and physical activity to cardiovascular disease risk factors in children and adults. *American Journal of Epidemiology, 127*(5), 933-941.

Schutz, R. J., and Goodman, D. (1982). The interpretation of data from single-subject studies: Some cautions and concerns. *Journal of Teaching in Physical Education, 1*(3), 39-45.

Sharpe, T., and Lounsbery, M., and Bahls, V. (1997). Description and effects of sequential behavior practice in teacher education. *Research Quarterly for Exercise and Sport, 68,* 222-232.

Smith, M. (1987). Publishing qualitative research. *American Educational Research Journal, 24*(2), 178-183.

Spencer, L. (1999). College freshmen smokers versus nonsmokers: Academic, social and emotional expectations and attitudes toward college. *Journal of Health Education, 30*(5), 274-281.

Steckler, A., Eng, E., and Goodman, R. (1991). Integrating qualitative and quantitative evaluation methods. *Hygie, 10,* 16-20.

Steckler, A., McLeroy, K., Goodman, R., McCormick, L., and Bird, S. (Eds.). (1992). Integrating qualitative and quantitative methods [Special edition]. *Health Education Quarterly, 19*(1).

Telama, R., Yang, X., Laakso, L., and Viikari, J. (1997). Physical activity in childhood and adolescence as predictor of physical activity in young adulthood. *American Journal of Preventive Medicine, 13,* 317-323.

Thomas, D. Q., Bowdoin, B. A., Brown, D. D., and McCaw, S. T. (1998). Nasal strips and mouthpieces do not affect power output during anaerobic exercise. *Research Quarterly for Exercise and Sport, 69*(2), 201-204.

Thomas, J. R, and French, K. E. (1986). The use of meta-analysis in exercise and sport: A tutorial. *Research Quarterly for Exercise and Sport, 57,* 196-204.

Torabi, M. R., and Yarber, W. (1992). Alternate forms of HIV prevention attitude scales for teenagers. *Aids Education and Prevention, 4*(2), 172-182.

Tucker, L. A. (1986). The relationship of television viewing to physical fitness and obesity. *Adolescence, 21,* 797-806.

Weiss, M. R., McCullagh, P., Smith, A. L., and Berlant, A. R. (1998). Observational learning and the fearful child: Influence of peer models on swimming skill performance and psychological responses. *Research Quarterly for Exercise and Sport, 69*(4), 380-394.

Welschimer, K. J., and Harris, S. E. (1994). A Survey of Rural Parents' Attitudes Toward Sexuality Education. *Journal of School Health, 64*(9), 347-351.

Weston, A. R., Mbambo, Z., and Myburgh, K. H. (2000). Running economy of African and Caucasian distance runners. *Medicine and Science in Sports and Exercise, 32*(6), 1130-1134.

Wiggins, D. K. (1991). Prized performers, but frequently overlooked students: The involvement of black athletes in intercollegiate sports in predominantly white university campuses, 1890-1972. *Research Quarterly for Exercise and Sport, 62*(2), 164-177.

Williamson, K. (1990). The ivory tower: Myth or reality? *Journal of Teaching in Physical Education, 9,* 95-105.

Wilson, S. (1997). The use of ethnographic techniques in educational research. *Review of Educational Research, 47,* 245-265.

Presentations

Lincoln, Y. (1991, January). *Ethics and the new paradigm.* Presented at the Qualitative Methods in Education Conference, Athens, GA.

van der Mars, H. (1998, April). *Single subject research designs.* Workshop presented at the American Alliance for Health, Physical Education, Recreation and Dance National Convention, Reno, NV.

Published Proceedings

James, C. R., and Bates, B. T. (1997). Experimental and statistical design issues in human movement research. In T. M. Wood (Ed.), *Exploring the kaleidoscope: Proceedings of the 8th measurement and evaluation symposium* (pp. 68-81). Oregon State University.

Zhu, W. (1997). A leaf tells the story: A commentary on the James and Bates paper. In T. M. Wood (Ed.), *Exploring the kaleidoscope: Proceedings of the 8th measurement and evaluation symposium (*pp. 83-89). Oregon State University.

Reports

The University of Georgia. (1995). *Guidelines for appointment, promotion, and tenure.* Athens, GA: Author.

Unpublished Manuscripts

Miller, D. E. (1990). *Challenge education programs related to the development of selected personality characteristics in psychologically troubled adolescents.* Unpublished research proposal, Indiana University, Bloomington.

Padilla, S. (1986). *Five options related to the improvement of smoking-damaged air quality in the military workplace.* Unpublished research proposal, Indiana University, Bloomington.

Pate, D. J. (1987). *Sea kayak touring and self-concept of persons with low level spinal cord injury.* Unpublished research proposal, Indiana University, Bloomington.

Sun, D. C. (1988). *Fat loss in moderately obese women using two walking protocols.* Unpublished research proposal, Indiana University, Bloomington.

Welcher, C. L. (1991). *Shift rotation related to night nurse performance and frequency of medication errors in a hospital setting.* Unpublished research proposal, Indiana University, Bloomington.

Index